LIBRARY OF NEW TESTAMENT STUDIES

639

Formerly the Journal for the Study of the New Testament Supplement series

Editor
Chris Keith

Editorial Board
Dale C. Allison, Lynn H. Cohick, R. Alan Culpepper, Craig A. Evans,
Jennifer Eyl, Robert Fowler, Simon J. Gathercole, Juan Hernández Jr.,
John S. Kloppenborg, Michael Labahn, Matthew V. Novenson, Love L.
Sechrest, Robert Wall, Catrin H. Williams, Brittany E. Wilson

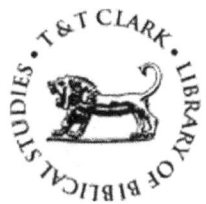

"This book offers an impressive survey of the different practices and practitioners that were deemed effective in healing sickness and injuries in the Roman Empire, in order to situate Paul's relative disinterest in such issues in a wider context. In so doing, it sheds much light on ancient understandings of health and illness, and on the 'magical,' 'religious,' and 'medical' healers who competed with each other in the world in which Paul preached, and to which he offered his own vision of a life in Christ."

Gideon Bohak, Tel-Aviv University, Israel

"This wide-ranging and informative book places the ideas and practices of healing in the New Testament firmly in the context of the many recent discoveries about healing in the Greco-Roman and Middle Eastern worlds."

Vivian Nutton, University College London, UK

"Christopher D. Stanley's new book, Paul and Asklepios: The Greco-Roman Quest for Healing and the Apostolic Mission, is broad, thoroughly researched, and engagingly written. It compares many different notions of disease and kinds of healing practices from ancient Greek, Roman, Jewish, and other sources, finally concentrating on what we can say, and what we cannot say, about disease and healing in early Christian communities. The study concentrates most on Paul and Pauline Christianity, seeking to explain why we hear so little from Paul and his own healing practices, or those among his churches. But the study also goes much further afield, including much of what we know from ancient Christian groups and writing otherwise. This study is excellent. It should become a classic of early Christian studies."

Dale B. Martin, Yale University, USA

"Christopher D. Stanley's Paul and Asklepios gives a thorough investigation of Greco-Roman and early Christian healing practices in their historical contexts and then applies concepts of medical anthropology to these, developing a unique picture of Paul's approaches to healing and its importance for the spread of Christianity. To reconcile the conflict between Paul's paucity of medical advice and Luke-Acts' imagery of Paul the healer, Stanley delves into eight useful scenarios, settling on one that captures the nuances of Paul's missionary activity in a mixed and changing society."

Laura Zucconi, Stockton University, USA

Paul and Asklepios

The Greco-Roman Quest for Healing and the Apostolic Mission

Christopher D. Stanley

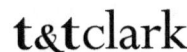

LONDON • NEW YORK • OXFORD • NEW DELHI • SYDNEY

T&T CLARK
Bloomsbury Publishing Plc
50 Bedford Square, London, WC1B 3DP, UK
1385 Broadway, New York, NY 10018, USA
29 Earlsfort Terrace, Dublin 2, Ireland

BLOOMSBURY, T&T CLARK and the T&T Clark logo are trademarks of
Bloomsbury Publishing Plc

First published in Great Britain 2023
Paperback edition published 2024

Copyright © Christopher D. Stanley, 2023, 2024

Christopher D. Stanley has asserted his right under the Copyright, Designs and
Patents Act, 1988, to be identified as Author of this work.

All rights reserved. No part of this publication may be reproduced or transmitted
in any form or by any means, electronic or mechanical, including photocopying,
recording, or any information storage or retrieval system, without prior
permission in writing from the publishers.

Bloomsbury Publishing Plc does not have any control over, or responsibility for, any
third-party websites referred to or in this book. All internet addresses given in this
book were correct at the time of going to press. The author and publisher regret any
inconvenience caused if addresses have changed or sites have ceased to exist,
but can accept no responsibility for any such changes.

A catalogue record for this book is available from the British Library.

Library of Congress Cataloging-in-Publication Data

Names: Stanley, Christopher D., author.
Title: Paul and Asklepios: the Greco-Roman quest for healing and the apostolic mission /
Christopher D. Stanley.
Description: London: New York: T&T CLARK, 2022. | Series: Library of New Testament
studies, 2513-8790; 639 | Includes bibliographical references and index. | Summary: "This
book explores the nature and extent of sickness and healing in the Greco-Roman world,
and assesses what the apostle Paul might have thought, said, and done regarding "pagan"
modes of medical treatment"– Provided by publisher.
Identifiers: LCCN 2022011291 (print) | LCCN 2022011292 (ebook) | ISBN 9780567696557
(hardback) | ISBN 9780567708151 (paperback) | ISBN 9780567696564 (pdf) |
ISBN 9780567696588 (epub)
Subjects: LCSH: Medicine, Greek and Roman. | Medicine in the Bible. |
Paul, the Apostle, Saint–Theology.
Classification: LCC R138.S73 2022 (print) | LCC R138 (ebook) |
DDC 610.938–dc23/eng/20220523
LC record available at https://lccn.loc.gov/2022011291
LC ebook record available at https://lccn.loc.gov/2022011292

ISBN: HB: 978-0-5676-9655-7
PB: 978-0-5677-0815-1
ePDF: 978-0-5676-9656-4
ePUB: 978-0-5676-9658-8

Series: Library of New Testament Studies, volume 639
ISSN 2513-8790

Typeset by Deanta Global Publishing Services, Chennai, India

To find out more about our authors and books visit www.bloomsbury.com and
sign up for our newsletters.

Contents

Introduction	1
Part I The Greco-Roman Health Care System	
1 Sickness and Disability in the Greco-Roman World	15
2 Home Remedies	26
3 "Magical" Treatments	52
4 Religious Healing	87
5 Medical Care	106
6 Overlapping Health Care Systems	125
Part II Judean and Christian Health Care Systems	
7 Judean Approaches to Health Care	135
8 Christian Approaches to Health Care	166
9 Paul and the Greco-Roman Health Care System	188
10 Sickness, Healing, and the Mission of Paul	213
Bibliography	237
Index of Ancient Authors	250
Subject Index	251

Introduction

A Healing Religion?

What role did physical healing (or the hope of receiving it) play in the missionary success of the early Christian movement? Interpreters are divided on this point.

Over a century ago, Adolf von Harnack in his magisterial work *Die Mission und Ausbreitung des Christentums in den ersten drei Jahrhunderten* described the early Christian movement as a "religion of healing" ("Religion der Heilung").[1] A careful perusal of his book, however, reveals that he was referring not to promises of bodily healing for the sick but to offers of spiritual healing for the soul from the effects of sin.[2] Only in the case of Jesus does he acknowledge that bodily healing played any notable role in the success of the Christian mission; after his time, it was the church's compassionate care for the sick that attracted new followers, not any miraculous power to remove sickness.[3]

Two decades later, Shirley Jackson Case used similar language but with a different sense when he asserted that "Christianity is from the start a healing religion."[4] According to Case, early Christians like Paul not only told stories about Jesus's healing miracles but also claimed similar powers to heal physical illness and cast out demons as part of their strategy for evangelizing their neighbors. Such claims were necessary to succeed in a religious marketplace where "the quest for health was one of the most urgent personal demands made upon the deities."[5] Without them, he implies, the Christ-movement might not have attracted enough followers to survive. By framing itself as a healing religion, "Christianity proved itself capable of ministering to one of the most insistent demands within the life of the contemporary Graeco-Roman world."[6]

After Harnack and Case, the question of whether physical healing played any notable role in the early success of the Christian movement received little attention until it was revived in the 1980s and 1990s by a number of historians and biblical scholars.[7] One of the central theses of Ramsay MacMullen's *Christianizing the Roman*

---

[1] (2nd edn; Leipzig: J. C. Hinrichs, 1906), 104; Eng. transl., *The Mission and Expansion of Christianity in the First Three Centuries*, trans. and ed. James Moffatt (Grand Rapids, MI: Christian Classics Ethereal Library, 2005), 81.
[2] Ibid., 69–80.
[3] Ibid., 70–1, 81–3, 105–6.
[4] "The Art of Healing in Early Christian Times," *JR* 3 (1923): 238–55.
[5] Shirley Jackson Case, *Experience with the Supernatural in Early Christian Times* (New York and London: The Century Co., 1929), 229.
[6] Ibid., 255.
[7] Other scholars besides those discussed herein wrote helpful studies of early Christian healing during this period, but they limited their attention to Jesus and the Gospels, saying little or nothing about

Empire (1984) is that claims of miraculous healing and exorcisms were vital to the winning of Christian converts during the first few centuries.

> Driving all competition from the field head-on was crucial. The world, after all, held many dozens and hundreds of gods. Choice was open to everybody. It could thus be only an exceptional force that would actually displace alternatives and compel allegiance; it could only be the most probative demonstrations that would work. We should therefore assign as much weight to this, the chief instrument of conversion, as the best, earliest reporters do.[8]

MacMullen was talking primarily about the patristic period, but he implicitly includes the New Testament era in his pronouncements. Medical historian Vivian Nutton offered a similar judgment: "The New Testament emphasizes the power of Christ and his apostles to cure diseases, and this was one of the features that secured for Christianity the primacy among competing religions."[9]

Writing in 1992, medical historian Gary Ferngren offered what he viewed as a corrective to the theses of Case, MacMullen, and Nutton.[10] According to his analysis, references to physical healing and exorcism are uncommon in Christian literature from the first two centuries (including the New Testament), and those that do appear are not often cited as evidence for the truth of Christian preaching.[11] Such stories become more common in the third century and ubiquitous in the fourth, a trend that Ferngren traces to "the credulity of the age, found in pagan and Christian alike, which lessened the appeal of rational medicine and encouraged frequent resort to exorcism and other forms of supernatural healing."[12] "It was not until the fourth century," he concludes, "that Christianity can be called, in the broadest sense, a religion of healing. . . . Specific cases of healing were increasingly used for apologetic purposes, and they proved successful in convincing a credulous age."[13]

---

the post-Jesus community. Examples (listed in chronological order) include Morton Smith, *Jesus the Magician* (New York: Harper & Row, 1978); Howard Clark Kee, *Medicine, Miracle and Magic in New Testament Times* (SNTSMS 55; Cambridge: Cambridge University Press, 1986); Harold Remus, *Jesus as Healer* (Cambridge: Cambridge University Press, 1997); John J. Pilch, *Healing in the New Testament: Insights from Medical and Mediterranean Anthropology* (Minneapolis: Fortress, 2000); and Elaine M. Wainwright, *Women Healing/Healing Women: The Genderization of Healing in Early Christianity* (London: Equinox: 2006).

[8] (New Haven: Yale University Press, 1984), 27. See the broader discussion in 22–9, 40–1.

[9] "From Galen to Alexander: Aspects of Medicine and Medical Practice in Late Antiquity," *Dumbarton Oaks Papers* 38 (1984): 5.

[10] "Early Christianity as a Religion of Healing," *Bulletin of the History of Medicine* 66 (1992): 1–15.

[11] Ibid., 4–6. In a later work, Ferngren offers his judgment regarding how the earliest Christians treated health problems: "The evidence, scattered and circumstantial as it is, suggests that first-century Christians relied on ordinary means of healing, such as conventional medicine or folk or traditional remedies. When those failed, they encouraged the sufferer to patiently endure." See *Medicine and Religion: A Historical Introduction* (Baltimore, MD: Johns Hopkins University Press, 2014), 78–9.

[12] "Early Christianity as a Religion of Healing," 10. According to Ferngren, "There are more instances of miraculous healing reported from the fourth century that from all three preceding centuries combined" (10).

[13] Ibid., 12–13. René Josef Rüttimann lays out the patristic evidence in much greater detail in his unpublished 1986 Harvard dissertation, *Asclepius and Jesus: The Form, Character and Status of the*

Ferngren's findings were largely affirmed by J. Keir Howard in his 2001 study of sickness and healing in the New Testament.[14] According to Howard, virtually all of the references to healing in the book of Acts, the letters of Paul, and other parts of the New Testament can be explained either as sudden releases from psychosomatic disorders or as the product of ordinary modes of healing intensified by the application of communal prayer and supportive care. "Healing thus becomes a sharpened and enhanced natural skill coupled with intuitive knowledge that is able to deal with the needs of the sick person within a context of prayer."[15] Paul himself says little about these activities due to his awareness that "'miracles' could be performed through trickery and deception like conjuring tricks before a gullible audience."[16] As a result, they say nothing about the genuineness of an apostle or the truth of the apostle's message. The mark of a genuine apostle, Paul insists, is a willingness to suffer humbly in the service of Christ.[17] Thus "the evidence of the Pauline writings would militate against the view that an emphasis on the healing of physical disease was a major aspect of early Christianity" until at least the second century CE when both church and society show a growing interest in the supernatural.[18]

Others have disputed these characterizations of the New Testament materials. Bernd Kollman (1996) finds in the Gospels evidence for bands of wandering charismatics in the post-Jesus era who used healings and exorcisms to validate their evangelistic message (Lk. 10:1-5 par, Mt. 7:15-23, Mk 9:38-40, 16:15-20, Mt. 11:1-6).[19] The fact that these wandering preachers offered healing and exorcism free of charge (Mt. 10:8) would have enhanced their appeal to the masses. According to Kollman, a band of them made their way to Corinth as the "super-apostles" whom Paul opposes in 2 Corinthians 10-12. Paul concedes that these intruders performed "signs, wonders, and miracles" as part of their missionary efforts, just as he did (2 Cor. 12:12; cf. Rom. 15:18-19), but he rejects their claim that such activities qualified one to be labeled as an apostle of Christ.[20] Similar references to "signs and wonders" are scattered throughout the New Testament, including several texts where they are cited to validate a speaker's claims (Acts 2:14-22, 2 Thess. 2:9-12, Heb. 2:2-4).[21] Taken together, these observations lead Kollman to the conclusion that

Asclepius Cult in the Second Century CE *and Its Influence on Early Christianity* (ThD dissertation, Harvard Divinity School, 1986). He argues that the growing emphasis on physical healing in the early centuries can be traced to a competitive need to overcome the challenge posed by Asklepios, the Greek god of healing, whose story in many ways resembled that of Jesus.

[14] *Disease and Healing in the New Testament: An Analysis and Interpretation* (Lanham, MD: University Press of America, 2001).
[15] Ibid., 232.
[16] Ibid., 235.
[17] Ibid., 236.
[18] Ibid., 238, 292–3. A similar view can be seen in Audrey Dawson, *Healing, Weakness and Power: Perspectives on Healing in the Writings of Mark, Luke and Paul* (Milton Keynes: Paternoster, 2008). Noting the paucity of references to physical healing in Paul's letters, she concludes that for Paul, "Converting the ill to physical health was not an important part of Gentile soteriology. Salvation was a spiritual result of God's grace, and Paul found that the important function of the Spirit, to transform lives, enabled even those sick and disabled (like himself) to live a life that was valuable to Christ" (201).
[19] *Jesus und die Christen als Wunderttäter: Studien zu Magie, Medizin und Schamanismus in Antike und Christentum* (Göttingen: Vandenhoeck & Ruprecht, 1996), 316–40, 358–61.
[20] Ibid., 318–33, 376.
[21] Ibid., 328.

"Dämonenaustreibungen und Krankenheilungen waren ein entscheidender Grund für die Ausbreitung und Etablierung des Christentums."[22]

Hector Avalos (1999) approaches the question from a different angle. Applying the methods and insights of medical anthropology, he analyzes the systems of health care[23] that were available to people in the Greco-Roman world (including Jewish communities) and compares them with the care offered by the early Christian community. Though he does not think it is possible to determine whether the healings and exorcisms performed by Christians were any more efficacious than what was available in other healing traditions, he does see a number of factors in the early Christian movement that could have made their system more attractive than some of their competitors. He points especially to their willingness to reach out to people who were regarded as "unclean" by other groups; the simplicity of their healing techniques (faith, prayer, laying on of hands, etc.); the fact that they charged no fees; and their practice of visiting the sick in their homes rather than requiring them to venture to a local temple or a distant healing shrine.[24] On the whole, he concludes, "The ideas of health care reflected in early Christianity constitute a system that was an important factor in attracting converts. As such, these ideas about health care constitute an important factor in the rise of Christianity itself."[25]

Stefan Schreiber (1996), writing specifically about Paul, is more ambivalent in his judgment. On the one hand, he finds a close link between the performance of miracles (including healing) and Christian preaching in the book of Acts, including its depiction of the apostle Paul.[26] In Paul's letters, on the other hand, the evidence is less clear. Paul affirms that miraculous deeds occurred in his churches, but he does not assign a single meaning to their presence. In some cases he cites them as evidence for the continuity of the church with biblical Israel, while in others he links them with the eschatological presence of God's Spirit working in the Christian assemblies.[27] In the few texts where he speaks about "signs and wonders" and works of "power" occurring in conjunction with his ministry, he links them closely to his evangelistic preaching as if that were the only time when they took place.[28] Even in these cases it is not clear that he views them as a legitimation of his message since elsewhere he questions their value

---

[22] Ibid., 378.
[23] Both "health care" (two words) and "healthcare" are common in the literature. "Health care" is preferred by the major news outlets (*New York Times, Washington Post, Wall Street Journal*, Associated Press) and medical journals (*New England Journal of Medicine, Journal of the American Medical Association, Annals of Internal Medicine*), so that is the form that will be used in this study except when quoting sources that use "healthcare." See the discussion by Michael L. Millenson, "'Healthcare' vs. 'Health Care': The Definitive Word(s)," *The Health Care Blog*, August 17, 2012, https://thehealthcareblog.com/blog/2012/08/17/%E2%80%9Chealthcare%E2%80%9D-vs-%E2%80%9Chealth-care%E2%80%9D-the-definitive-words/.
[24] *Health Care and the Rise of Christianity* (Peabody, MA: Hendrickson, 1999), 67–70, 81–4, 91–5, 102–6, 113–14.
[25] Ibid., 3.
[26] *Paulus also Wundertäter: Redakstionsgeschichtliche Untersuchungen zur Apostelgeschichte und den authentischen Paulusbriefen* (BZNW 79; Berlin and New York: de Gruyter, 1996), 53–76, 137, 147.
[27] Ibid., 175–6, 195–6, 201–2, 217–19, 272–3.
[28] Ibid., 205–7, 243–4, 272, 293–4. Like many authors, Schreiber simply assumes that the "signs and wonders" that Paul mentions included miraculous healings, though Paul never makes such an association and the phrase is never used in that sense in the Jewish Scriptures.

for validating his own or his opponents' apostolic authority.[29] For Paul, the miracles are largely incidental, whereas they take center stage in Luke's depiction of Paul in Acts.[30]

A different kind of ambiguity is evident in Graham Twelftree's 2013 analysis of what he terms "the miraculous" in the letters of Paul.[31] The driving concern of this study is "to solve the riddle of the profound difference between, on the one hand, the miraculous ethos of Jesus's ministry, the Gospels and Acts, and the Christianity reflected there and, on the other hand, the letters of Paul, in which miracles and the miraculous appear of much less or perhaps no interest."[32] As a Pharisaic Jew, says Twelftree, Paul would have been familiar with a variety of traditions that interpreted miracles as evidence of the presence and power of the Jewish god and as harbingers of the impending "end of the age." As a Christ-follower, he believed that the final days had now dawned. Yet he does not seem to have experienced miraculous healings in his own life, and he does not interpret the ability to perform "signs and wonders" as a sure marker of apostolic election.[33] Such observations are hard to square with Paul's repeated references to "signs and wonders" that accompanied his missionary preaching and his expectation that his audiences should view these acts as divine validations of his message.[34] Twelftree resolves this tension by positing that Paul's "signs and wonders" were spontaneous acts of healing and exorcism that occurred at the sole instigation of the Spirit, similar to the *charismata* of "healings" and "works of power" that the Spirit is said to distribute in 1 Corinthians 12.[35] Paul says little about them not because they were unimportant to him—according to Twelftree, "miracles are a high-profile, integral, and regular part of his thinking and ministry strategy"[36]—but because they were beyond his control. Both types of events served to reveal the presence and power of the God of Israel in the Christian community and thus implicitly affirmed the truth of the Christian gospel.

The most recent efforts to assess whether physical healing might have played a role in Paul's evangelistic mission come from Heidi Wendt (2016) and Jennifer Eyl (2019). Both authors view healing as part of a broader set of strategies that Paul deployed to authenticate his message and entice people to join the nascent community of Christ-followers. Wendt classes Paul as one of many "freelance religious experts" who "competed intensely and with great creativity for potential followers or students"

---

[29] Ibid., 195-6, 203-5, 226-34, 271-6, 277-81.
[30] Ibid., 292-302. Schreiber's analysis and conclusions mostly parallel the ideas presented in less detail a decade earlier by Helge Kjaer Nielsen, *Heilung und Verkündigung: Das Verständnis der Heilung und ihres Verhältnisses zur Verkündigung bei Jesus und in der Ältesten Kirche* (Leiden: Brill, 1987), 172-210. She in turn relies on an even shorter study by Karl Gatzweiler from the decades in the middle of the twentieth century when such issues received little attention—see "La Conception Paulinienne du Miracle," *ETL* 37 (1961): 813-46.
[31] *Paul and the Miraculous: A Historical Reconstruction* (Grand Rapids, MI: Baker, 2013).
[32] Ibid., ix.
[33] Ibid., 49-86, 142-62.
[34] Ibid., 180-224. Passages in which Twelftree sees likely reference to "miraculous" activity include Rom. 15:18-19, 1 Cor. 2:1-5, 1 Cor. 4:19-20, 2 Cor. 6:6-7, 2 Cor. 12:11-12, 1 Thess. 1:5, and Gal. 3:1-5.
[35] Ibid., 215-17, 224-5, 313-22. This idea that "signs and wonders" occurred spontaneously during Paul's preaching by the uncontrollable working of God's Spirit rather than through some "gifting" that Paul could exercise at will was anticipated by Jacob Jervell, *The Unknown Paul: Essays on Luke-Acts and Early Christian History* (Minneapolis, MN: Augsburg, 1984), 77-95.
[36] *Paul and the Miraculous*, 222.

during the era when Paul was seeking to win converts.[37] The term "freelance religious expert" in her usage refers to "any self-authorized purveyor of religious teachings and other practices who drew upon such abilities in pursuit of various social benefits and often more transparent forms of profit."[38] According to Wendt, Paul developed a unique strategy for attracting followers in this marketplace, "an ambitious religious program whose elements included exegesis of Judean writings, philosophical discourses, initiation into divine mysteries, and after-life rewards."[39] This combination proved attractive to some but not to others. Whether physical healing played any role in this program is unclear from Wendt's study. She mentions it several times as a strategy used by Paul's competitors and refers briefly to the performance of "signs and wonders" as an element of Paul's appeal,[40] but she never states clearly whether she views Paul himself as a healer. The closest she gets is when she refers to "health or healing" as one of several benefits ("gifts of the Spirit") that one might acquire by joining Paul's group.[41]

No such reticence can be seen in Jennifer Eyl's work. Near the beginning of her book she states without qualification that "Paul's performance of miracles, his interpretation of signs, and his engagement in practices of prophecy and speaking in tongues, constitute a significant and legitimating aspect of his teaching."[42] Healing and other "miraculous" activities are included in this list of legitimating acts: Paul "performs miracle healings with no medical training, and he refers to a host of unnamed signs, wonders, and 'mighty works.'"[43] In Eyl's analysis, these displays were part of a broader program of "divinatory practices" (along with tongues and prophecy, revelatory interpretations of sacred oracles, promises of miraculous transformation through baptism, and claims of heavenly visitations) that Paul used to portray himself as a mediator of divine power and presence, a wonder-worker who offered similar abilities to his followers under the label of *charismata pneumatika*.[44] Eyl does not explicitly address the question of how such claims and activities might have affected the success of Paul's missionary efforts, but it seems fairly clear that she regards them as divisive: some people would have been attracted to a leader who displayed such divine powers, while others would have classed him among the purported sorcerers and magicians whom they rejected as "quacks, phonies, and charlatans."[45]

---

[37] *At the Temple Gates: The Religion of Freelance Experts in the Roman Empire* (Oxford: Oxford University Press, 2016), 29.
[38] Ibid., 10.
[39] Ibid., 28.
[40] Ibid., 151.
[41] Ibid., 184.
[42] *Signs, Wonders, and Gifts: Divination in the Letters of Paul* (Oxford: Oxford University Press, 2019), 2.
[43] Ibid., 3.
[44] These claims are expounded at length in *Signs*, 87–114, but similar statements can be found throughout the book.
[45] The terms appear repeatedly in her book—see especially *Signs*, 3, 7, 116–19, and 219. Eyl is more interested in situating Paul in relation to his historical peers than in drawing sweeping analytical or theological conclusions, but she does insist in her conclusion that Pauline scholars have paid too little attention to this important aspect of Paul's belief and practice due to their own discomfort with such activities.

In short, there seems to be general agreement that offers of physical healing played an important role in causing people to be open to the Christian message during the third and fourth centuries CE, and perhaps as early as the second century. These offers included "miraculous" cures, the application of standard medical treatments, and the self-sacrificial nursing of the sick and wounded.[46] During this era, Christianity can rightly be described as a "religion of healing." But whether such a label is accurate for the early decades of the Christian movement remains a point of contention, especially as it relates to the apostle Paul.

Sickness and Healing in the Letters of Paul

Much of the scholarly uncertainty regarding the role of physical healing in the missionary strategy of Paul can be attributed to a paucity of evidence. For a man who endured so much bodily suffering during the course of his ministry (1 Cor. 4:11-13; 2 Cor. 4:7-12, 11:23-9, 12:7-10; Gal. 4:13-14; Phil. 4:11-13), Paul has very little to say about health, medical care, or healing in his letters. Forms of the Greek verb ἰάομαι appear only three times in the assuredly Pauline corpus, all in 1 Corinthians 12 where Paul speaks rather vaguely about "gifts of healings" (χαρίσματα ἰαμάτων) when listing the abilities that the Spirit has distributed to the Christ-followers in Corinth.[47] The verb θεραπεύω and its cognates are entirely absent from Paul's letters, while the twenty or so uses of the verb σώζω never refer to healing as in the Gospels.[48]

The same is true for words relating to sickness. The common Greek noun νόσος appears nowhere in Paul's letters, while the partial synonym ἀσθένεια and cognates, which are used some forty times, refer in most cases to (literal or metaphorical) "weakness" rather than "illness." The only clear exceptions are Gal. 4:13 (δι' ἀσθένειαν τῆς σαρκός), Phil. 2:26-27 (καὶ γὰρ ἠσθένησεν παραπλήσιον θανάτῳ), and 1 Cor. 11:30 (διὰ τοῦτο ἐν ὑμῖν πολλοὶ ἀσθενεῖς καὶ ἄρρωστοι καὶ κοιμῶνται ἱκανοί) in the assured letters, and 1 Tim. 5:23 (καὶ τὰς πυκνάς σου ἀσθενείας) and 2 Tim. 4:20 (Τρόφιμον δὲ ἀπέλιπον ἐν Μιλήτῳ ἀσθενοῦντα) in the Pastorals. Other verses where physical illness might conceivably be in view include Rom. 8:26, 1 Cor. 2:3, 1 Cor. 4:10, 2 Cor. 10:10, 2 Cor. 11:29, 2 Cor. 12:9-10, and 1 Thess. 5:14, though most interpreters have understood these texts to be referring to "weakness," not illness. Only once does Paul speak of a sick person being restored to health (Epaphroditus in Phil. 2:26-27), and he says nothing about how it transpired (i.e., by "natural" or "supernatural" means). The illness was apparently serious, since he refers to death as a real possibility.

Such observations are unremarkable to modern Western readers who are accustomed to viewing illness as a problem to be addressed by secular means (physicians, hospitals, medications, etc.) and not by religious leaders. Even among the devout, the role of

---

[46] More will be said on this point in Chapter 8.
[47] The only other use anywhere in the Pauline correspondence is Col. 4:14, where Luke is described as an ἰατρός.
[48] Similar observations can be made about the nine instances where the word appears in the disputed letters.

religion is generally limited to asking God to guide the hands of medical professionals and to comfort those who are suffering. Few see physical healing as a central concern of their religion, and even fewer (primarily Pentecostals and charismatics) have any real expectation that God might effect a miraculous cure in cases deemed hopeless by the medical profession. In short, most contemporary readers would not expect a religious figure like Paul to have anything to say about sickness or healing except perhaps to pray and endure.

In Paul's day, by contrast, religion and health care were intricately intertwined. Hippocratic physicians worshipped the Greek god Asklepios as their patron deity, encouraged their patients to pray for healing, and gave credit to the gods for their successes, while priests and doctors worked hand in hand at healing shrines across the Greco-Roman world. Folk healers, sorcerers, root-cutters, exorcists, and other quasi-medical practitioners straddled the boundaries between what Western traditions regard as "secular" and "religious" modes of treatment. Reports of miraculous cures were fairly common, while the number of people who discounted such stories and sought healing without reference to the gods was small. In a world where disease was pervasive, treatments were unsystematic, and outcomes were unpredictable, people at all levels of society used every means at their disposal to preserve or restore their health.

Deities who were thought to have healing powers were especially popular in the areas where Paul plied his ministry. Every city that Paul visited would have had its temple to Asklepios where residents could present prayers and offerings for the sick and even spend the night in hopes of receiving medical advice or a miraculous cure from the deity in a dream. Indigenous deities and foreign gods (especially those from Egypt) served the same purpose. Regional centers were available for those who lived outside the cities or who were dissatisfied with the results that they received from local physicians and religious personnel.[49] "Medical tourism" was popular among the urban elites, who visited hot springs like those at Hierapolis and Carura in western Asia Minor or submitted to more rigorous systems of religio-medical treatment at larger Asklepian sanctuaries such as Pergamon and Epidaurus. Gods and cults that made no provision for treating illness stood at a competitive disadvantage with those who offered such services unless they could promise other benefits that people valued as much or more.[50]

Given these realities, how do we explain the fact that Paul's letters say nothing about Jesus as a healing deity?[51] It is hard to see how he could have been unaware of this

---

[49] Cécile Nissen, in *Entre Asclépios et Hippocrate: Études des cultes guérisseurs et des médecins en Carie* (Liège, Belgium: Centre International d'Étude de la Religion Grecque Antique, 2009), identifies thirty healing centers devoted to nine different divine patrons in the region of Caria (southwestern Asia Minor) alone. More details on these and other religious facilities where people went for healing will be presented in Chapter 4.

[50] More will be said on this point in Chapter 10.

[51] A handful of scholars have remarked on this omission when analyzing Paul's views on sickness and healing, but few have tried to explain it. Exceptions include Twelftree, *Paul and the Miraculous*, who sees possible allusions to Jesus's miracle-working power in Rom. 15:18-19, 1 Cor. 1:22, 4:20, 13:2, Phil. 1:8, 1 Thess. 1:5, 2:12, and 5:14, and in passages where Paul speaks of Christ living and working through him (124–41); Dawson, *Healing, Weakness and Power*, who posits several possible reasons

important element of the Jesus-traditions in view of his contacts with Peter and others from the Jerusalem community (Gal. 1:18-19, 2:1-10; 1 Cor. 9:5-6; cf. Rom. 15:25, 15:31) and the evident link between the Christ-followers in Antioch and Jerusalem (Gal. 2:1-14; cf. Acts 11:19-30, 15:1-35). It is equally unlikely that Luke created from whole cloth the entire panoply of healings and other miraculous activities narrated in the book of Acts, where instantaneous cures "in the name of Jesus" are common. Luke's depiction of Paul as a healer (14:8-10, 19:11-12, 28:7-9), exorcist (16:16-18), and wonder-worker (20:7-12, 28:1-6) whose mighty acts cause him to be fêted as a god (14:11-13, 28:6) only compounds the problem.

What are we to make of these data? The easiest (and most common) solution is to reject Luke's picture of a wonder-working Paul in favor of the "theological" Paul of the letters. But we still have the problem of why Paul might have chosen to distance himself from the "miraculous" elements of both the Jesus-traditions and the earliest Christian narratives unless we take all of the miracle stories in both the Gospels and Acts as pious fictions that were unknown to Paul. An explanation is also required for Paul's references to "signs and wonders" (Rom. 15:18-19, 2 Cor. 12:12) and works of "power" (Gal. 3:5, 1 Cor. 2:4-5, 1 Thess. 1:5; cf. 1 Cor. 4:20, 2 Cor. 6:7) that accompanied his missionary preaching.[52] Whether these texts relate to miraculous healings or any of the other "wonders" that Paul performs in Acts is hard to assess, but his language clearly poses problems for attempts to frame a non-miraculous Paul.

Of course, none of these problems are new. But the specific question of what Paul thought about physical healing (whether natural or "miraculous") and what role it might have played in his missionary strategy (and the instruction that he gave to his followers) has never been addressed with any degree of thoroughness. If we focus specifically on these issues, we discover a host of unanswered questions. Did Paul perform acts that others viewed as miraculous as a means of attracting converts and advancing his mission, or is this a Lucan construct? Did he present Jesus as a healing god whom people could approach for cures, or did he downplay or ignore this aspect of the Jesus-traditions? Did the "gifts of healings" that are mentioned in 1 Corinthians 12 play any role in the evangelistic outreach of Paul and his congregations, or did they only serve members? Did these "gifts" involve extraordinary occurrences that might have served to authenticate the Christian message, or was Paul referring to the Spirit-guided use of human healing skills, like the gifts of wisdom and knowledge in the same chapter? In short, did Paul or the members of his congregations use the promise of physical healing as an evangelistic tool? If not, how did their failure to address this need affect their competitive position in a world where other gods did offer such services?

for the omission while also pointing to possible allusions in 2 Cor. 10:1 and Phil. 1:8 (180–5); and Nielsen, *Heilung und Verkündigung*, who infers that Paul did not attach much significance to Jesus's healings (188). By contrast, second century CE Christian authors often refer to Jesus as *Christus medicus*, though usually in relation to the healing of souls, not bodies (noted by Gary B. Ferngren and Darrel W. Amundsen, "Medicine and Christianity in the Roman Empire: Compatibilities and Tensions," *ANRW* II.37.3 [1996]: 2964).

[52] These and other verses that might refer to miraculous activity will be discussed more fully in Chapter 9.

Similar questions can be raised about Paul's attitudes toward the various types of health care that were available outside the community of Christ-followers. Most of Paul's converts were gentiles who were accustomed to using the normal healing practices of the Greco-Roman world, including consulting a local physician; presenting offerings and/or vows to a deity either at home or in a local temple; visiting a folk-healer, midwife, or "sorcerer" in search of an amulet, medication, or incantation that would avert the illness or the demon that was causing it; or traveling to a regional healing sanctuary in hopes of receiving a sacred dream, a miraculous cure, or a course of medical treatment through the intervention of a priest or physician. Similar means would have been used to prevent illness from occurring in the first place.

What advice or instruction might Paul have given regarding the use of such techniques? Would he have condemned them as idolatrous practices that should be avoided by Christ-followers? Would he have rejected those that required interaction with other gods while permitting the use of more "secular" regimens? Would he have limited his followers to using Christian and/or Jewish healers? What would he have said about prescriptions and treatments that modern Westerners typically disdain as "magical," such as amulets and incantations? If he thought that any of these practices were dangerous or even problematic to his followers, why did he not mention them in his letters?

Finally, there is the question of what kinds of healing regimens Paul might have used to treat his own injuries and illnesses. Paul's letters offer ample evidence that he experienced health problems as a result of his missionary efforts, including many that would have required treatment to promote recovery. The most obvious examples are the "weakness of the flesh" that Paul says was a "trial" to the Galatians (Gal. 4:13-15) and the "thorn in the flesh" for which he prayed for relief in 2 Cor. 12:7-8. Less noticed is the frequent bodily abuse that Paul mentions in his letters, afflictions that would have caused immediate and possibly even lasting injuries to Paul's body. Beatings, whippings, and stonings (2 Cor. 11:23-25; cf. 1 Cor. 4:11) would have opened bloody wounds and caused contusions and fractures that required urgent medical attention, while frequent episodes of hunger, thirst, and exposure to the elements (1 Cor. 4:11, 2 Cor. 11:27, Phil. 4:12) would have increased his susceptibility to more chronic forms of illness, whether directly in the form of deficiency diseases like scurvy, anemia, beriberi, osteomalacia, and pellagra, or indirectly by weakening his body so that it became more vulnerable to infectious diseases like malaria, tuberculosis, and dysentery. Any weakness would have been exacerbated by the extreme conditions of imprisonment in a filthy dungeon (2 Cor. 11:23, Phil. 1:13-14) or floating for days on the open sea (2 Cor. 11:25). It is thus no wonder that Paul describes himself in Gal. 6:2 as carrying "the marks of Jesus" on his body or in 2 Cor. 4:10-11 as "always carrying in the body the death of Jesus" and "being given up to death for Jesus' sake, so that the life of Jesus may be made visible in our mortal flesh." At a minimum, the kinds of physical abuse that Paul endured would have produced permanent scars, and some episodes may even have resulted in lasting disabilities.[53]

What then did Paul do to treat his various illnesses and injuries? Did he use whatever means lay closest to hand, ignoring the religious outlook of the provider,

---

[53] More will be said in Chapter 9 about the possibility of Paul experiencing permanent effects from his sufferings.

or did he insist on being taken to a Christ-follower or Judean for treatment? Did he submit to any and all forms of healing, even those that might today be regarded as "magical," or did he reject techniques that he associated with foreign deities and their followers? Would he have limited himself to spiritual healing and prayers to the God of Israel, or might he have consulted a local physician or a priest of the god Asklepios for advice? Would he have worn an amulet to protect himself from disease-causing spirits or to avert the "evil eye" of an enemy?

The present study attempts to answer these questions. The results will necessarily be speculative since Paul says little or nothing about most of these issues. But we can still formulate intelligent theories about Paul's views and practices by comparing what he does and does not say on the subject with what we know about other people's beliefs regarding sickness and healing, including the opinions of Judeans and Christians other than Paul. The investigation will proceed as follows.

Part I (Chapters 1-6) explores health conditions in the Greco-Roman world and the various systems of care that were available for diagnosing and treating illnesses and injuries.

Chapter 1 examines the nature and extent of illness and injury in Greco-Roman antiquity in an effort to determine what kinds of physical ailments Paul and his followers might have experienced. The inquiry includes a discussion of what modern medical historians and anthropologists have said about how cultural frames affect the way people identify and classify illness and a critical assessment of the benefits and limits of using such methods to examine the past. Attention is also given to what people did to avoid getting sick in the first place.

Chapter 2 begins with an overview of some key ideas from medical anthropology about health care systems and healing, then turns to an examination of Greek and Roman home remedies—those time-tested, family-based practices that individuals and families used to protect or cure themselves from illness and other forms of harm. This system is presented as the foundation for all other forms of health care in the Greco-Roman world.

Chapter 3 examines treatments that scholars have traditionally labeled as "magical." The term "magical" is controversial within the field, so special attention is given to clarifying how it is used here. The remainder of the chapter is devoted to a careful examination of the various healing practices that Greeks and Romans identified (and sometimes vilified) as *mageia*.

Chapter 4 looks at health care practices that were grounded explicitly in religion. Attention is given to the various techniques that Greeks and Romans used to ward off harmful spirits and induce the gods to restore their health in times of sickness, including treatments that were offered at local temples and regional healing centers. The vital role of the Greek healing deity Asklepios is discussed at length.

Chapter 5 explores the rise and influence of Hippocratic medical theories and treatments from the fifth century BCE onward. Both the theoretical and the practical aspects of ancient medical care are addressed, including how physicians were trained, what services they provided to the public, and what conditions they did and did not treat. Attention is also given to the rise of non-Hippocratic schools of medicine that relied on different models of diagnosis and treatment.

Chapter 6 discusses the overlapping and interconnected nature of the four major systems of health care in the Greco-Roman world. Attention is given to the various ways in which each system both drew on and relied upon the others to produce an integrated system of care that included multiple options for maintaining health and treating illness. The freedom of individuals to choose whichever system they preferred or could afford is highlighted throughout.

Part II (Chapters 7–10) investigates ancient Judean[54] and Christian health care practices and their potential significance for the apostle Paul and his followers.

Chapter 7 looks at how Judeans in Paul's day dealt with health problems, including how they viewed and interacted with Greek and Roman health care systems. Scriptural precedents are examined insofar as they might have prescribed or limited what Judeans could do in this area, but the principal focus is on what people actually did in the Second Temple period and the rabbinic era.

Chapter 8 investigates the beliefs and practices of Christians other than Paul regarding health care, including their attitudes toward "pagan" healing methods. The chapter begins with a review of New Testament materials outside of Paul's letters that relate in some way to sickness or healing. The bulk of the chapter is devoted to an exploration of the beliefs and practices of Christians during the first four centuries of the Common Era.

Chapter 9 reviews several possible explanations for Paul's virtual silence on matters of sickness and healing. Three major themes from Paul's letters that might relate to the topic are identified. This is followed by a carefully nuanced reconstruction of what Paul might have done to address his own health problems and what he might have taught his followers to do or not to do.

Chapter 10 explores the possible implications of this study for the success of Paul's mission, including the role that physical healing might have played in his evangelistic program. Sociological analyses of other healing movements are cited to explain what Paul might have meant when he refers to "signs and wonders" and acts of "power" that accompanied his preaching. Paul is then compared with other "freelance religious experts" in an effort to ascertain how his words and actions might have been viewed in relation to his competitors, including why some people followed him and most did not.

One question that will not be addressed in this study is the reality behind the many accounts of miraculous healing that appear in the New Testament and contemporary literature, since the answer is irrelevant to our analysis. As long as people in Paul's day believed that such events were both possible and happened regularly in the world around them, we can assess the potential effects of that belief and any related experiences on the success of Paul's missionary efforts. When therefore one reads in the following pages about acts of healing that most Western readers would dismiss as either impossible (and thus fictitious) or exaggerated, it should be noted that no judgment is being offered about the facticity of these stories. This study focuses on how Paul's mission might have been viewed by potential and actual converts, not the views of modern science.

---

[54] For reasons that I and others have spelled out elsewhere, I find it preferable to render *Ioudaioi* as "Judeans" when referring to the ancient people-group commonly known as "Jews." But I also sympathize with those who insist that this distinctively ethnic translation can be confusing when applied to the unique set of religious beliefs and practices that marked people out as *Ioudaioi*. To avoid this confusion, I will use the traditional terms ("Jewish," "Judaism," etc.) when discussing matters of ideology and praxis and the ethnic labels ("Judean," "Judeans") when referring to the people who held those views. This dual translation strategy will no doubt be deemed confusing by those who champion the consistent use of "Judeans," but adequate translation requires sensitivity to context; it is not a wooden process.

Part I

The Greco-Roman Health Care System

1

Sickness and Disability in the Greco-Roman World

Morbidity Factors in the Roman World

It can be difficult for citizens of modern Western nations to comprehend how vastly different health and sanitation practices were in Greek and Roman cities by comparison with our own and how these practices affected the health of their residents. The research of medical historians is therefore vital for explicating what those conditions were like and the health problems that they presented.

At the most basic level, malnutrition was a persistent threat for all but the upper classes in both the cities and the countryside.[1] Most people lived perilously close to subsistence level, and one bad crop year was enough to leave many without enough food to cover their basic nutritional needs. City residents were not exempt from this danger, since they depended on the neighboring croplands for fresh produce. Even in good years, the seasonal nature of ancient agriculture meant that most crop-based foods were available only at certain times of the year, leading to potential nutritional deficiencies at other times.

Other seasonal changes also played a role in people's health. Insulation against the winter cold was often insufficient, leaving bodies weakened and thus more susceptible to both invasive and endemic illnesses. Certain diseases flared up regularly during the warm summer months, including malaria and gastrointestinal disorders, and epidemics were not uncommon. People were also more likely to move around and interact with others (and thus transfer germs) when temperatures were warm. It should therefore come as little surprise that epitaphs from the era show the greatest concentration of deaths occurring in late summer and early fall.[2]

Poor sanitation, especially in the cities, also contributed heavily to the spread of disease.[3] Human waste was collected in domestic cesspits or thrown into the street,

---

[1] The causes and effects of malnutrition are summarized in Vivian Nutton, *Ancient Medicine* (London and New York: Routledge, 2004), 21–2.

[2] The influence of seasonal factors is discussed in Walter Scheidel, "Disease and Death in the Ancient City of Rome," *Princeton/Stanford Working Papers in Classics* (April 2009): 2–5. An ancient list of illnesses associated with the four seasons can be found in Hippocrates's *Aphorisms* 3.1–23.

[3] Most of the material in this paragraph is taken from Alex Scobie, "Slums, Sanitation, and Mortality in the Roman World," *Clio* 68 (1986): 399–433. According to Scobie, only one of the latrines at a wealthy city like Pompeii shows any sign of ever being flushed with water (409).

where it served as a breeding ground for bacteria and viruses. Many of these pits were located close to kitchens where they increased the risk of contamination. Outside the home, dogs and flies spread germs that they collected from feces, corpses, and the offal of butcher shops. Warm food kept in pots at public food stands offered a fertile environment for germ growth. Public latrines were available, but men (and animals) still relieved themselves freely in the streets and doorways where children played daily. Latrines were rarely cleaned, and the practice of using common sponges to clean oneself afterward provided a ready conduit for the spread of diseases. Urine was used for laundering clothes, and the pots that were employed to carry it through the streets to the fullers' shops were often porous, leaky, and subject to spillage or breakage. Clean, potable water was delivered to cities via aqueducts, but it was easily polluted by germ-bearing insects, animals, slime, and algae. Public baths exposed bathers to all sorts of communicable diseases, and periodic floods spread germs across low-lying areas close to rivers. Several Greek and Roman historians refer to plagues and epidemics that sickened and killed large numbers of people, and Hippocrates (or, more likely, someone writing in his name) wrote an entire seven-book treatise (ἐπιδημίαι) on the topic.[4] In the countryside, wells were often located next to cesspits or rubbish dumps, increasing the possibility of contamination. Human feces were used to fertilize crops, bringing fecal parasites with them.[5]

Broader social developments also played a role in the spread of diseases in the late Hellenistic and early Roman eras. The expansion of the Roman Empire brought new germlines to Greek and Roman cities as Roman soldiers returned from tours in foreign lands and foreign captives were sold as slaves to local farms and households. At the same time, the construction of Roman roads and the establishment of the Pax Romana opened new opportunities for travel and trade both within and beyond the empire. The first century CE in particular saw a rapid increase in urbanization that brought many new residents to the cities,[6] and those at the lower end of the social spectrum usually ended up living in tight quarters on the upper floors of tenement buildings or in dank cellars, or slept on the fetid streets. Sickness would have been hard to avoid under such conditions.

Ancient medical writers were aware that certain types of environments were more conducive to sickness than others, but their theorizing was crude by modern standards. The author of the Hippocratic treatise *On Airs, Waters, and Places* speaks with great confidence about the effects of bad environments on the rise and spread of disease, though many of his specific conclusions are now known to lack merit. Examples of

---

[4] While it is often thought that Roman sanitary practices improved health conditions in cities that adopted them, that belief is not borne out by the evidence. Piers D. Mitchell, director of the Ancient Parasites Library at Cambridge University, recently published a highly detailed study of the archaeological evidence for intestinal parasites in the Roman era. He concluded that Roman sanitation, including the use of public baths, latrines, and aqueducts, did nothing to reduce the incidence of disease-bearing contaminants when compared with earlier periods ("Human Parasites in the Roman World: Health Consequences of Conquering an Empire," *Parasitology* 144 [2017]: 48–58).

[5] S. W. B. Newsom, "Hygiene and the Ancient Romans," *British Journal of Infection Control* 5 (2004): 25; Mitchell, "Human Parasites in the Roman World," 4, 5, 7, 9.

[6] A point noted by Hector Avalos, *Health Care and the Rise of Christianity* (Peabody, MA: Hendrickson, 1999), 4–5. Avalos also mentions the role of the army in spreading disease.

the latter include living north, south, east, or west of the "ideal" climate of Greece; drinking water made from snow or ice; being outside during solstices and equinoxes; and spending too much time on horses. On the other hand, he rightly calls attention to the potentially harmful effects of such factors as high or low temperatures; exposure to marshy, stagnant, or polluted water; and good or bad soil. Other causes cited by ancient authors—evil spirits, the influence of the stars, magical curses, offenses against the gods, the evil eye—are clearly useless for modern analyses of ancient morbidity.[7]

As a result of these and other negative environmental factors, life expectancy in the Roman Empire was low by modern standards, though historians differ over the precise figures. According to William V. Harris, "Almost all students of ancient demography are now agreed that expectation of life at birth was about 25 years."[8] This figure sounds excessively low until we consider that it includes infant and child mortality rates that averaged 30 percent in the first year and 50 percent by age five.[9] According to medical historian Mirko Grmek, bone studies reveal that the average age of death was actually declining in Paul's day from 42.4 years for men and 36.5 for women in the early Hellenistic period to 40.2 for men and 34.6 for women in the Roman imperial era.[10] Of course, many individuals lived well beyond these ages, but the lowness of the numbers for the population as a whole offers clear evidence of the baneful effects of disease on residents of the Greco-Roman world. Life in Paul's day was precarious, and few people would have survived into adulthood without experiencing serious bouts of illness.

---

[7] According to Giuseppe Penso, the Greek philosopher Lucretius (*De rerum natura* 6.1093–1130) is one of the few writers from the ancient world to hint at the existence of germs, followed by the Roman statesman Varro (*Rust.* 1.12.3) (*La Médecine Romaine: L'Arte d'Esculape dans la Rome Antique*, 2 vols [Paris: Les Éditions Roger Dacosta, 1984], 495–6). Medical explanations that trace sickness to problems within the body of the individual will be treated in Chapter 5.

[8] "Popular Medicine in the Classical World," in *Popular Medicine in Graeco-Roman Antiquity: Explorations*, ed. William V. Harris (Leiden and Boston: Brill, 2016), 8. Alex Scobie lists a number of Roman historians who agree with this figure ("Slums, Sanitation, and Mortality in the Roman World," 399). Walter Scheidel, on the other hand, counsels caution in using such figures due to the methodological difficulties that attend the use of epitaphs and skeletal remains to figure ancient mortality rates ("Disease and Death in the Ancient City of Rome," 6).

[9] See the excellent analysis by Nathan Pilkington in "Growing up Roman: Infant Mortality and Reproductive Development," *Journal of Interdisciplinary History* 44 (2013): 1–36. Tim Parkin, drawing on newer studies of infant death rates, recently lowered his estimate of first-year mortality (as proposed in *Demography and Roman Society* [Baltimore: The Johns Hopkins University Press, 1992], 92–3) from 30 to 20 percent. See the discussion in "The Demography of Infancy and Early Childhood," *Oxford Handbook of Childhood and Education in the Classical World*, ed. Judith Evans Grubb, Tim Parkin, and Roslynne Bell (New York and Oxford: Oxford University Press, 2013), 46–50.

[10] *Diseases in the Ancient Greek World*, trans. Mireille Muellner and Leonard Muellner (Baltimore and London: Johns Hopkins University Press, 1989), 104. A more recent study of skeletal remains from Paphos and Corinth (Sherry C. Fox, "Health in Hellenistic and Roman Times: The Case Studies of Paphos, Cyprus and Corinth, Greece," in *Health in Antiquity*, ed. Helen King [London and New York: Routledge, 2005], 59–82) yielded similar figures for Corinth (42.6 for men and 39.6 for women), but lower numbers for Paphos (34.4 for men and 34.6 for women). According to Vivian Nutton (*Ancient Medicine*, 21–2), only 5 percent of those who survived their first year would have reached the age of sixty. Hippocrates's *Aphorisms* 3.24–31 gives a useful list of maladies that Greek physicians associated with different age groups.

Common Ailments

Identifying conditions that facilitated the spread of disease in antiquity is one thing; naming the diseases that afflicted them is quite another. Ancient writings, especially those credited to Hippocrates, are filled with the names of diseases and other medical conditions, and Greek and Latin lexicons give the impression that these words can be easily translated into English and matched with conditions known to modern medicine. But this impression is deceptive.

According to medical anthropologists, terms like "disease," "sickness," and "illness" are rooted in social constructions of health and incapacity that vary from culture to culture.[11] Our modern concept of disease is based on a medical paradigm that categorizes bodily ailments according to an evidence-based, theoretically grounded understanding of biological symptoms and causes. Ancient writers, even those trained as physicians, had at best a limited understanding of such matters. They also held very different ideas about the workings of the human body and the natural world than those that we take for granted in modern Western culture.[12]

For these reasons we cannot simply compile a list of symptoms from an ancient medical treatise or historical work and compare it with a modern list of diseases in the expectation of finding a one-to-one correspondence. Classifications of illness and beliefs about causality vary from culture to culture, as do such basic notions as what constitutes "health" and "sickness." A modern physician who could travel in a time machine to the Greco-Roman world would find all sorts of physical conditions that would qualify as diseases from the standpoint of contemporary epidemiology but were not recognized as such at the time because they were endemic to a society where few people ate balanced, nutritious diets and vaccinations were unknown. The opposite is also true: Greek and Roman literature contains numerous descriptions of conditions

---

[11] The following summary of insights from medical anthropology depends heavily on the work of Hector Avalos (*Health Care and the Rise of Christianity*) and John Pilch (*Healing in the New Testament*), who together have led the way in applying medical anthropology to the field of New Testament studies, though their research has focused primarily on Jesus and the Gospels rather than the apostle Paul. Their influence will also be seen Chapter 2 when the discussion turns to the various means that were used to treat sickness and injury in the Greco-Roman world. Similar points were made around the same time by South African scholar Pieter Craffert, though his work has not received as much attention from American and European scholars (*Illness and Healing in the Biblical World: Perspectives on Health Care* (Pretoria: Biblia Publishers, 1999). See also his later work, *The Life of a Galilean Shaman: Jesus of Nazareth in Anthropological-Historical Perspective* (Eugene, OR: Cascade, 2008), 252–307. All of these authors draw heavily on the classic study by medical anthropologist Arthur Kleinman, *Patients and Healers in the Context of Culture: An Exploration of the Borderland between Anthropology, Medicine, and Psychiatry* (Berkeley: University of California Press, 1980).

[12] Mirko Grmek's caution to modern interpreters is worth citing here: "It is impossible to apprehend correctly the significance of an ancient text concerning a pathological event unless we rid ourselves as completely as possible of the ontological notion of disease embedded in our everyday language.... Diseases exist only in the realm of ideas. They interpret a complex empirical reality and presuppose a certain medical philosophy or pathological system of reference" (*Diseases in the Ancient Greek World*, 1; see the longer discussion in pp. 1–8).

that were defined as illnesses in the ancient world but would not be identified as such today.[13]

Ancient medical theorists also classified bodily dysfunctions differently than modern scientists. For example, fever was viewed as an illness in itself rather than a symptom of deeper bodily disorders. The Romans even had a goddess by the name of Febris who simultaneously embodied and protected her worshippers from this supposed ailment.[14] In a similar way, the Greek word λέπρα, commonly translated "leprosy," actually refers to a variety of skin conditions that may or may not have included what we know today as leprosy, that is, Hansen's disease.[15] The same is true for the Greek word φθίσις, which is usually rendered as "tuberculosis" but could include various other forms of "wasting" sickness.[16] Greek medical treatises also describe ailments whose identity modern medical historians have yet to figure out.

Problems such as these have led medical anthropologists to develop nuanced definitions of terms like "health," "disease," "illness," and "sickness" (as well as "curing" and "healing") to assist them in comparing the various ways in which people identify, conceptualize, and treat health problems across different cultures. To be "healthy" is to be capable of performing the functions necessary for personal maintenance on a daily basis. To have a "disease" is to experience some sort of dysfunction within the human biological system, while being "ill" refers to the sufferer's subjective (and socially conditioned) perception of being unwell. Finally, the term "sickness" describes the sense of meaning that others give to the person's complaint and the roles that the sufferer is expected to perform in a given context.

A similar distinction is made between the words "cure," which means to successfully correct the sufferer's bodily malfunction, and "heal," which involves the reduction or elimination of the socially disvalued states of "illness" and "sickness" and the accompanying restoration of the person to the normal social order. John Pilch summarizes the difference well: "From the perspective of medical anthropology, curing is efficacious when biomedical changes take place; healing is efficacious when the people who seek it say that it is."[17] He goes on to explain that "healing boils down to meaning and the transformation of experience. . . . The life problems may or may not still be present, but their perception is no longer the same."[18]

Such distinctions can seem overly technical and abstruse to people unacquainted with the field, but they do have practical applications. In particular, they help anthropologists to compare how different societies define and manage "normal" and

---

[13] The same is true for many modern societies, as demonstrated by Arthur Kleinman in his tour de force analysis of the competing systems of diagnosis and treatment in twentieth-century Taiwan (*Patients and Healers in the Context of Culture*).

[14] Febris was not the only bodily condition that the Romans associated with a deity; other examples include Morbus (disease), Pestis and Lues (pestilence), Macies (wasting), Tabes (corruption), and Scabies (itching). Particular deities also watched over various parts of the human body, including Angina (throat), Cardea (heart and entrails), Carna (muscles), and Paventia (nerves) (Penso, *La Médecine Romaine*, 39–43). See also Cesidio R. Simboli, *Disease-Spirits and Divine Cures among the Greeks and Romans* (PhD dissertation, Columbia University, 1921), 34–5.

[15] See the discussion in Grmek, *Diseases in the Ancient Greek World*, 152–71.

[16] Ibid., 183–4.

[17] *Healing in the New Testament*, 34.

[18] Ibid., 35.

"abnormal" health without worrying about whether conditions that a society regards as abnormal (e.g., spirit-possession) match any modern definition of a particular disease.[19] They therefore serve as a check on the modernist tendency to view other cultures through the lens of ethnocentrism and biological reductionism. They also give interpreters a way to make sense of ancient stories about the "healing" of a sick person when the actual nature of the physical occurrence seems problematic or even impossible from the standpoint of modern medical science.

This is not to suggest, however, that "sickness" and "health" are entirely subjective categories. Clearly there are abnormal health conditions that can be recognized and categorized as anomalous by members of different social groups who occupy the same or similar epidemiological niches. Malaria is a case in point: its symptoms are similar enough around the world that observers from different cultures could describe their experience and know that they were talking about the same condition even if they used different names for it, had different ideas about what caused it, and treated it differently. Physical malformities such as clubfoot and hunchback are likewise recognized universally as deviations from normal health. Careful attention to how such conditions are described by ancient writers has enabled medical historians to agree on the identity of the majority of health abnormalities that are mentioned in Greek and Roman literature. The key is to avoid using modern epidemiology as a Procrustean bed for classifying ancient diseases.

Medical historians have a wide range of evidence at their disposal to assist them in determining the nature and prevalence of various bodily ailments in the Greco-Roman world, including both literary documents (medical treatises, letters, historical writings, novels, etc.) and non-literary materials (burial inscriptions, statues, mosaics, paintings, medical implements, excavations of treatment centers, traces of drugs and medicines, votive offerings, grave soil, fecal deposits from toilets, and the physical remains of plants, animals, and humans, especially skeletons and teeth).[20] Careful examinations of these materials have identified the following ailments as recurring problems in the world of Paul.[21]

---

[19] These distinctions have proved especially beneficial to New Testament scholars and classicists seeking to understand the historical realities behind ancient "miracle stories." They are less relevant to the present study, however, since the focus here is on how ancient audiences understood sickness and healing without regard to the validity of their perceptions (i.e., what "really happened" from a modern medical standpoint). I will therefore use the terms "disease," "illness," and "sickness" somewhat interchangeably in the pages that follow, unless indicated otherwise. The same is true for "curing" and "healing."

[20] See Grmek, *Diseases in the Ancient Greek World*, 2, and the broader discussions in Craffert, *Illness and Healing in the Biblical World*, 3–8, and Ralph Jackson, *Doctors and Diseases in the Roman Empire* (Norman and London: University of Oklahoma Press, 1988), 7–10. For a helpful survey of the methods and sources used in modern paleoepidemiology, see Efthymia Nikita, Anna Lagia, and Sevi Triantaphyllou, "Epidemiology and Pathology," in *A Companion to Science, Technology, and Medicine in Ancient Greece and Rome*, ed. George L. Irby (New York: Wiley-Blackwell, 2016), 465–82.

[21] This list combines observations from a number of sources, including Grmek, *Diseases in the Ancient Greek World*, 36–48, 57–89, 122–71, 183–96, 254–81, 334–55; Jackson, *Doctors and Diseases in the Roman Empire*, 23–4; Penso, *La Médecine Romine*, 245–512; Nutton, *Ancient Medicine*, 23–35; Craffert, *Illness and Healing in the Biblical World*, 10–16; Scobie, "Slums, Sanitation, and Mortality in the Roman World," 421–2; Nikita et al., "Epidemiology and Pathology," 465–82; Estee Dvorjetski,

Infectious diseases	Internal maladies	Skeletal/skin problems	Mental conditions[a]
Tuberculosis	Cancers/tumors	Spinal deformities	Mania
Malaria	Organ infections	Herniated disks	Depression
Typhoid fever	Anemia	Sciatica	
Rheumatic fever	Gout	Osteoarthritis	
Diphtheria	Bladder/kidney stones	Hunchback	
Pneumonia	Gangrene	Clubfoot	
Pleurisy	Ophthalmia/blindness	Rickets	
Dysentery	Glaucoma	Broken bones	
Cholera	Deafness	Dislocations	
Hepatitis	Epilepsy	Tooth decay	
Common cold	Menstrual problems	Psoriasis	
Herpes	Stomach worms	Skin infections	
Mumps	Colic	Skin ulcers/abscesses	
Conjunctivitis	Ulcers	Scabies	
Tetanus	Scurvy		
Salmonella	Asthma		
	Constipation		
	Hemorrhoids		

[a] According to Chiara Thumiger ("The Early Greek Vocabulary of Insanity," in Harris, *Mental Disorders*, 62–70), the Hippocratic treatises use fifty different words to refer to various forms of mental illness, but only the two listed here have any settled meaning apart from "phrenitis," the symptoms of which she never describes. Jouanna ("Typology and Aetiology") reaches a similar conclusion.

Of these conditions, the most common appear to have been tuberculosis (described by Mirko Grmek as "a serious but not necessarily mortal disease that is banal, ubiquitous, and well known"),[22] malaria, rheumatic fever, cancerous tumors, gout, various infections and fevers, anemias, ophthalmia, bladder stones, and osteoarthritis. Fractures, dislocations, and other bodily injuries were also a normal part of life, especially among soldiers and farmers. Epilepsy is mentioned often in the literature, but this is probably due to its unusual symptoms rather than its frequency. Several common modern diseases are unattested in ancient records and may not have existed in the Greco-Roman world, including measles, chickenpox, rubella, scarlet fever, syphilis, gonorrhea, rheumatoid arthritis, and polio. Degenerative diseases also appear rarely due to the relative shortness of most people's lives.[23]

"Medicinal Hot Springs and Healing Spas in the Graeco-Roman World," in *Leisure, Pleasure and Healing: Spa Culture and Medicine in Ancient Eastern Mediterranean* (Leiden: Brill, 2007), 84–5; Robert Garland, *The Eye of the Beholder: Deformity and Disability in the Graeco-Roman World* (London: Bristol Classical Press, 2010), 123–38; François P. Retief and Louise Cilliers, "Tumours and Cancers in Graeco-Roman Times," in *Health and Healing: Disease and Death in the Graeco-Roman World* (Bloemfontein, South Africa: Publications Office of the University of the Free State, 2005), 200–12; and Jacques Jouanna, "The Typology and Aetiology of Madness in Ancient Greek Medical and Philosophical Writing," in *Mental Disorders in the Classical World*, ed. W. V. Harris (Leiden and Boston: Brill, 2013), 98–118. Among the ancient sources, Hippocrates's *Aphorisms* is a particularly rich source of data regarding the maladies encountered by ancient physicians.

[22] *Diseases in the Ancient Greek World*, 193.
[23] On the latter point, see Nutton, *Ancient Medicine*, 23–4.

In the absence of modern medical knowledge and treatments, many of these conditions would have been painful, debilitating, and even fatal.[24] Those that were chronic in nature would have left their victims with periodic or ongoing bouts of sickness that hindered their ability to perform ordinary bodily functions and thus to maintain their livelihoods. Even minor infections could lead to lymphatic problems, peritonitis, necrosis, and eventually death. Most congenital problems were viewed as untreatable, forcing those with severe conditions to rely on the aid of family members or to beg for a living. Those with hardy constitutions may have avoided any lasting consequences from illness or injury, but even they would have been concerned to maintain their health against the many forces that conspired to afflict them. Life was unpredictable, illness ubiquitous, and treatments unreliable. Even the sturdiest of people could not hope for a life free from physical ailments.

The Quest for Health and Healing

Given the human proclivity for avoiding or eliminating pain and suffering and the necessity of physical exertion for all but the elites to eke out a meager living, health was a vital concern for everyone in the ancient world. This was especially true for the laboring masses in both the cities and the countryside who toiled from sunup to sundown to keep food on the table and a roof over their heads. Such people could not afford to lose work time due to illness or injury.[25] The consequences could be both physically and financially debilitating, especially for those who were permanently disabled or developed serious mental disorders.[26]

Health was also a persistent concern of the wealthy elites. Rebecca Flemming highlights the frequency with which health is commended in ancient Roman literature, appearing as a subject of prayer and thanksgiving in letters, a topic for hymns and

---

[24] Unlike many modern doctors, ancient physicians were willing to admit that certain conditions were beyond their ability to cure, including birth defects, congenital illnesses, and internal cancers. Religious healing centers, on the other hand, reported miraculous cures even for these conditions. See Garland, *Eye of the Beholder*, 123–5; Retief and Cilliers, "Tumours and Cancers in Graeco-Roman Times," 209; John Scarborough, "The Pharmacology of Sacred Plants, Herbs, and Roots," in *Magika Hiera: Ancient Greek Religion and Magic*, ed. Christopher A. Faraone and Dirk Obbink (New York and Oxford: Oxford University Press, 1991), 141; and Bronwen L. Wickkeiser, "The Appeal of Asklepios and the Politics of Healing in the Greco-Roman World" (PhD dissertation, University of Texas, 2003), 35–46.

[25] Plato (*Rep* 3.406c-d) describes well how the precarious existence of the poor compelled them to seek quick cures: "For all well-governed peoples there is a work assigned to each man in the city which he must perform, and no one has leisure to be sick and doctor himself all his days.... A carpenter ... when he is sick expects his physician to give him a drug which will operate as an emetic on the disease, or to get rid of it by purging or the use of cautery or the knife. But if anyone prescribes for him a long course of treatment with swathings about the head and their accompaniments, he hastily says that he has no leisure to be sick and that such a life of preoccupation with his illness and neglect of the work that lies before him isn't worth living. And thereupon he bids farewell to that kind of physician."

[26] On the prevalence, diagnosis, and treatment of mental disorders in the ancient world, see the essays in Harris, *Mental Disorders in the Classical World*.

toasts at social gatherings, and a basis for analogies and metaphors in speeches.[27] Unlike the poor, they could afford to pay physicians to care for them when their health was threatened, and they could travel to regional healing centers for treatment if their ailment was beyond the power of the local physician to cure.[28] They also had the knowledge and resources to protect themselves and their environs from known causes of illness, and they possessed a great deal of popular lore about how to keep their bodies healthy.[29] Yet even they recognized that money could not buy health; sickness was a troubling and often fatal fact of life that could never be fully avoided.

Of course, modern germ theory was unknown to ancient Greeks and Romans, and the idea that sickness could spread through contact with bodily fluids or objects used by the sick person was only dimly understood. But those who studied the subject did recognize that certain kinds of environmental conditions and personal behaviors were often associated with sickness or health, and they took various precautions that they believed would minimize the former and maximize the latter.

Some of these precautions affected the city as a whole. When planning a new aqueduct, Roman engineers were careful to find an unpolluted source of water (as far as they could determine such matters), and their practice of channeling the water into settling tanks provided closed spaces where many bacteria would have died.[30] The use of elaborate fountains to aerate the water where it entered the city would also have served to mitigate the formation of algae and scum in the water supply. Larger cities had sewers to carry away the polluted rainwater that ran through the streets after a storm, though this was done mainly to remove excess water rather than to control the spread of sickness. Civic officials were charged with overseeing the water supply and sewer systems, including their cleanliness, while maintenance teams watched over the integrity of the aqueducts and cleaned them as needed.[31] Public baths, which were fed by the aqueduct system, were also cleansed periodically, and the practice of regular bathing and anointing doubtless kept down the spread of disease outside the baths, though the baths themselves provided a ready venue for the spread of germs.[32] Public latrines theoretically served to limit human waste to a controlled facility, but they were

---

[27] *Medicine and the Making of Roman Women* (Oxford: Oxford University Press, 2000), 63–4. The same was true in the sphere of religion: "The quest for health was one of the most urgent personal demands made upon the deities by people living in the Roman Empire" (Case, *Experience with the Supernatural in Early Christian Times*, 229).

[28] "Medical tourism" was quite common among elite Greeks and Romans, with the larger healing centers operating somewhat like nineteenth-century European spas where the wealthy gathered to "take the waters." More will be said about this in Chapters 4 and 5. For a fictionalized account of such a journey to the sanctuary of Asklepios at Pergamon in western Turkey, see Christopher D. Stanley, *A Rooster for Asklepios* (Buffalo: Amelia Press, 2020), and *A Bull for Pluto* (Buffalo: Amelia Press, 2020).

[29] The first three chapters of Aulus Cornelius Celsus's *De medicina* (early first century CE) are dedicated to this topic. As an encyclopedist, he summarizes popular views rather than offering his original thoughts on the subject. Similar ideas can be found in the Hippocratic Corpus and other ancient writers.

[30] See Newsom, "Hygiene and the Ancient Romans," 25, and Jackson, *Doctors and Diseases in the Roman Empire*, 43–53.

[31] As described by Ido Israelowich, *Patients and Healers in the High Roman Empire* (Baltimore: Johns Hopkins Press, 2015), 125–8.

[32] Scobie, "Slums, Sanitation, and Mortality in the Roman World," 425–6.

not very effective since neither Greeks nor Romans were aware that such products could spread disease.[33] Property owners were required by law to remove filth from around their homes and businesses, but how far this was actually done is unknown.[34]

At a more personal level, Greeks and Romans engaged in a variety of activities that they believed could protect them from sickness. Among the wealthy elites, regular exercise at the gymnasium helped to maintain the fitness and health of the body, while the practice of eating a regular and varied diet served a similar purpose.[35] Those who experienced illness also had the resources to follow a more specialized diet if it was prescribed by a physician and the freedom to rest and recuperate while their slaves carried on the business of the household. On top of this, their spacious houses allowed them to segregate the sick from contact with others, thus limiting the spread of germs.

The poor masses, by contrast, had no such options. They had to push their ailing bodies until work became impossible, and their diets, sorely limited in both variety and nutrition, would have left them more susceptible to illness. Their cramped and dirty living quarters would likewise have made it hard for them to protect themselves and their families from contamination by communicable diseases. Many would have had difficulty paying the fees demanded by physicians, leaving them to rely on self-care and folk remedies or else to deteriorate into disability or death.[36]

Both rich and poor also used various ritual practices to protect themselves from sickness. In a world where virtually everyone believed that divine beings played a role in sickness and healing, it was vitally important to keep beneficent divinities on your side and avert the maleficent ones. Both public officials and individuals offered sacrifices, prayers, and offerings at local temples (especially the temple of Asklepios) to preserve or restore the health of the petitioners.[37] Prayers, rituals, and incantations were also used to avert evil spirits, especially at key moments such as pregnancy, birth, puberty, and returning home from travels.[38] The wearing of protective amulets, which Cesidio Simboli describes as "the most universal means of preventing disease," was widely

---

[33] For more on these latter points, see Ann Olga Koloski-Ostrow, *The Archaeology of Sanitation in Roman Italy: Toilets, Sewers, and Water Systems* (Chapel Hill: University of North Carolina Press, 2015).

[34] Scobie, "Slums, Sanitation, and Mortality in the Roman World," 418.

[35] Of course, the well-documented tendency of Roman elites to overeat would have mitigated the effectiveness of these efforts for many individuals.

[36] The problem of physicians' fees for the poor has been noted by many researchers—see Avalos, *Health Care and the Rise of Christianity*, 28–30; Kollman, *Jesus und die Christen als Wunderttätter*, 366–73; Flemming, *Medicine and the Making of Roman Women*, 68–9; Plinio Prioreschi, *A History of Medicine*, Vol. 2, *Greek Medicine* (Lewiston/Queenston/Lampeter: Edwin Mellen Press, 1994), 651–2. Even the Asklepian healing sanctuaries required small fees, the details of which are described in Maria Elena Gorrini and Milena Melfi, "L'archéologie des cultes guérisseurs," *Kernos* 15 (2002): 258–64. As a result, most of the poor would have had to settle for the kinds of self-care and folk treatments discussed in the next chapter.

[37] Emma J. Edelstein and Ludwig Edelstein, *Asclepius: Collection and Interpretation of the Testimonies*, with a new introduction by Gary B. Ferngren (Baltimore and London: Johns Hopkins University Press, 1998), 1.182–4.

[38] On the power of evil spirits to produce illness and the use of rituals to avert them or counteract their effects, see Simboli, *Disease-Spirits and Divine Cures among the Greeks and Romans*, 13–44. On the use of incantations, see Kee, *Medicine, Miracle and Magic in New Testament Times*, 102–3. More will be said on both of these subjects in Chapters 2 and 3.

accepted and prescribed by both physicians and folk healers.[39] Various materials were worn on different parts of the body depending on the type of evil that one wished to avert. Talismans of various types were also used for this purpose. According to Gerald Hart, "Coins with a portrait of Asclepius were the most convenient and economical talisman and might be perforated for suspension from a necklace or bracelet. The wealthy wore rings, brooches and pendants made from jewels into which the magic symbol had been cut in cameo or intaglio format."[40] At least some Jews are known to have copied the divine name onto various objects for the same purpose.[41]

No matter what people did to protect themselves from sickness, however, none could wholly avoid its dreaded touch. Knowing that it was inevitable, they did not despair when it arrived. Instead, they turned to one or more of the many resources and practices that were available to help people deal with illness. These resources will be examined in the next four chapters.

---

[39] The quote comes from Simboli, *Disease-Spirits and Divine Cures among the Greeks and Romans*, 73. For more on the use and contents of amulets, see Ludwig Edelstein, "Greek Medicine in Its Relation to Religion and Magic," in *Ancient Medicine: Selected Papers of Ludwig Edelstein*, ed. Owsei Temkin and C. Lilian Temkin, trans. C. Lilian Temkin (Baltimore and London: Johns Hopkins University Press, 1967), 232–5; Scarborough, "The Pharmacology of Sacred Plants, Herbs, and Roots," 120, 135. Jews and Christians used them as much as "pagans" did—see Georg Luck, *Arcana Mundi: Magic and the Occult in the Greek and Roman Worlds* (Baltimore and London: Johns Hopkins University Press, 1985), 19; Naomi Janowitz, *Magic in the Roman World: Pagans, Jews and Christians* (London and New York: Routledge, 2001), 57; Gideon Bohak, *Ancient Jewish Magic: A History* (Cambridge: Cambridge University Press, 2008), 121–2, 370–4. More will be said on this subject in Chapters 2 and 3.

[40] Gerald D. Hart, *Asclepius, the God of Medicine* (London: Royal Society of Medicine Press, 2000), 104.

[41] Bohak, *Ancient Jewish Magic*, 117–19.

2

Home Remedies

The Problem of Western Bias

When people today hear the words "health care system," most of us think immediately of the complex array of physicians, nurses, hospitals, and other facilities that are involved in the delivery of modern Western medicine or the financing system (generally taxes or insurance) that is used to pay for such services, or both. Some might also include so-called alternative therapies (dietary supplements, meditation, acupuncture, etc.) in their definitions, but few would seriously question the dominant role of medical science in defining, diagnosing, and treating illness. Even fewer would think to include religious practices such as faith healing, prayer, and fasting in their understanding of "health care," and only a tiny minority would regard such New Age techniques as crystal healing, foot reflexology, iridology, or aura manipulation as reliable methods for treating sickness and maintaining health, much less prefer them to standard medical care.

This hegemony of the biomedical model of health care over Western thinking about sickness and health can make it difficult for people who have lived their entire lives under such systems to imagine a world in which no single model of health care predominates, but a diverse array of beliefs and practices compete for influence and mutual interpenetration and borrowing are common. This is the health care environment in which Paul and his communities lived, thought, and acted.

Four broad systems of health care were available to treat illness and injury in the Greco-Roman world: (a) *home remedies*, a category that encompasses a wide range of self-care and familial treatments that served most people as the first line of defense when health was threatened; (b) "magical" *treatments*, a controversial label for a series of protections and remedies that relied on ritualized words and actions to manage the effects of unseen forces upon the sick person; (c) *religious healing*, a diverse set of practices designed to move divine beings to restore the sufferer to health, ranging from personal prayers and vows to familial and communal sacrifices to lengthy stays at a regional sanctuary; and (d) *medical treatment*, an organized system of observation-based theories and practices that laid the foundation for modern Western biomedicine.

This fourfold schema is deceptive, however, insofar as it suggests the existence of four distinct systems of health care delivered by different types of practitioners, as when a person suffering from back pain today might choose between applying a heating pad or consulting an orthopedist, a chiropractor, or an energy healer. In reality, there were serious disagreements over both theory and praxis within each of these systems of health care, along with significant overlaps and borrowings among their practitioners. Physicians and priests included traditional remedies and "magical" cures in their treatments; folk healers performed religious or "magical" rituals to imbue their prescriptions with sacred power; and priests and "sorcerers" adopted ideas, language, and techniques from medical providers. Proponents of all four models argued on occasion that their modes of treatment were better or more effective than others, but there was no societally shared preference for one system over the others such as we see today.

This is important to keep in mind as we try to imagine what Paul and other first-century Christ-followers might have done to maintain their health and to treat illnesses and injuries when they occurred. If we are not careful, the modern Western bias in favor of scientific modes of health care might lead us to presume without evidence that the early Christian community shared our preference for medical over folk and religious treatments, while the negativity of modern science toward "magical" remedies might cause us to reject the possibility that Paul and his followers used such methods. Similar cautions are required when dealing with religious modes of treatment: modern Christian ideas concerning the exclusivity of monotheism could lead us to suppose that the early Christ-followers would have rejected out of hand any techniques associated with "pagan" deities or the manipulation of unseen spiritual forces and so overlook the substantial evidence that Judeans and Christians in the post–New Testament era made regular use of such practices.[1] In short, we must make a serious effort to lay aside our modern biases regarding what qualifies as legitimate or spurious forms of health care if we hope to develop a credible estimation of what Paul and his followers might have thought and done to protect their health and care for the ill and injured in their midst.

Insights from Medical Anthropology

An effective counterbalance to Western prejudices concerning health care can be found in the work of medical anthropologists who have performed cross-cultural analyses of health care systems around the world. Instead of presupposing the superiority of Western medicine, they engage in a sympathetic study of how different societies define health, sickness, disability, and similar terms and what techniques and institutions they use to maintain health and remove sickness.

The seminal figure in this area is Arthur Kleinman, who analyzed how health care was viewed and practiced in Taiwan in the 1970s. His goal was to create a comprehensive description of the island's health care system as it actually functioned, without privileging one element or viewpoint over another. Writing from a social-scientific perspective, Kleinman defined "health care system" as a set of "socially organized responses to disease that constitute a special cultural system . . . anchored in particular

---

[1] The evidence for this point is laid out in Chapters 7 and 8.

arrangements of social institutions and patterns of interpersonal interactions."[2] Such a system typically includes, among other features, "patterns of belief about the causes of illness; norms governing choice and evaluation of treatment; socially-legitimated statuses, roles, power relationships, interaction settings, and institutions."[3]

Kleinman distinguished three overlapping sectors of health care that he claimed were present in all societies: (a) the popular sector, which offers "lay, nonprofessional, non-specialist types of care" by the patient, the family, or other social relations; (b) the professional sector, embodied in "the organized healing professions," including both Western and indigenous modes of treatment; and (c) the folk sector, which comprises both sacred and secular healing by the hands of a "non-professional, non-bureaucratic, specialist" (e.g., shaman, herbalist).[4] He also described five core clinical functions that all health care systems provide for individuals and societies: (a) the cultural construction of illness as a psychosocial experience that requires particular interventions; (b) the creation of general criteria to guide people in assessing the seriousness of their problem and evaluating options for treatment; (c) the provision of names and explanations for particular illnesses; (d) the prescription of treatments for those illnesses; and (e) the management of therapeutic outcomes that result from these treatments, whether good or ill.[5]

Other medical anthropologists have refined and expanded on Kleinman's work, but his theories and models remain foundational to research in this area. Historians of Greco-Roman antiquity and early Christianity have also drawn on Kleinman's insights and language to analyze ancient health care systems, including William V. Harris, Vivian Nutton, and Olympia Panagiotidou in the field of classics and Hector Avalos, John Pilch, and Pieter Craffert in the discipline of New Testament studies.[6] The latter group has produced a number of creative studies that use Kleinman's approach to analyze the health care system of first-century Palestine and the social position and healing activities of Jesus.

When it comes to Paul and his (predominately gentile) followers, on the other hand, the work of Kleinman and other medical anthropologists has received little attention.

---

[2] *Patients and Healers in the Context of Culture*, 24. Hector Avalos, who relies heavily on Kleinman, puts it more clearly: "A health care system may be defined as a set of interacting resources, institutions, and strategies that are intended to maintain or restore health in a particular community" (*Health Care and the Rise of Christianity*, 19).

[3] *Patients and Healers in the Context of Culture*, 24.

[4] *Patients and Healers in the Context of Culture*, 50–9; applied to Taiwan, 60–70. The distinction between popular and folk healers is not always clear in Kleinman, a point noted by several of the contributors to Harris, *Popular Medicine in Graeco-Roman Antiquity*. The problem arises from the fact that his definition of the folk sector ("methods that are transmitted and put into practice by healers not officially approved by the state or by the 'orthodox' medical profession" [*Patients and Healers in the Context of Culture*, 59]) relies on slippery notions of social approval. More will be said herein about the difficulties that arise from trying to apply Kleinman's categories to the ancient world.

[5] Ibid., 71–82.

[6] For an accessible collection of studies by classical scholars, see Harris, *Popular Medicine in Graeco-Roman Antiquity*. For the New Testament authors cited here, see the notes in Chapter 1. Other scholars in both fields have used terms like "folk healer" and "health care system" when talking about matters of sickness and healing in the ancient world, but a review of their discussions reveals that they are drawing on popular understandings of these terms rather than the technical sense in which they are used by medical anthropologists like Kleinman.

The same is true for the broader topic of health care among the early Christ-followers outside of Palestine. Several reasons can be posited for these lacunae, but the most obvious is the dearth of attention to the subject by New Testament authors. The only non-Gospel texts that speak specifically about procedures that were used to maintain health or procure healing are (a) the miraculous healings in the book of Acts; (b) Paul's references to the *charisma* of healing in 1 Corinthians 12 and the care that he received from the Galatians in Gal. 4:14-15; (c) Paul's prayer in 2 Cor. 12:8-9 that he might be rescued from his "thorn in the flesh"; (d) the commendation of wine as a treatment for stomach problems in 1 Tim. 5:23; (e) the brief description of a prayer-centered healing ritual in Jas 5:14-16; and possibly (e) the metaphorical reference to eye-salve in Rev. 3:18.[7] The handful of other texts in which sickness or injury is mentioned (1 Cor. 11:30, 2 Cor. 6:5, 2 Cor. 12:23-25, Phil. 2:25-30, 2 Tim. 4:20) say nothing about how the ailment was treated. Much has been made of the reference to "Luke the physician" in Col. 4:14, but the passage says nothing about whether Luke used his skills to treat Paul, the Colossians, or any other group of Christ-followers.

Based on this limited evidence, all that we can say with certainty is that the earliest Christians relied on prayer to the God of Israel (including the hope of a miraculous cure), ordinary home remedies, and nursing care to treat illnesses and injuries. But given what we know about the nature and extent of physical ailments in the Greco-Roman world, the variety of means that were available to treat them, and the nature of health care systems in general (as theorized by medical anthropologists), this conclusion leaves too many questions unanswered.[8] In particular, it tells us little about how early Christ-followers made sense of sickness or how they decided what kinds of home remedies or other treatments were and were not acceptable for members of their exclusivist movement. If they had been taught by leaders like Paul to avoid virtually the entire system of health care that they had followed for their entire lives due to its association with "pagan" deities, we would expect such a radical demand to be mentioned somewhere in the New Testament. What we encounter instead is silence.

Arguments from silence are, of course, notoriously weak, but in this case the total absence of any call to avoid certain types of health care in favor of others is telling, especially when the authors show no such hesitation in demanding the cessation of other practices that gentile audiences would have viewed as normal and harmless in their pre-Christian days, including premarital and extramarital sex, eating meat offered to non-Israelite deities, advancing one's own honor at the expense of others, or retaliating when wronged. The contrasting lack of instruction about appropriate and inappropriate health care practices, even those associated with "pagan" deities, is puzzling if this was indeed a matter of concern within the early Christian community.

In view of Paul's silence on the subject, the burden of proof would seem to rest on anyone who would contend that the early Christ-followers rejected all but the limited range of health care options that are explicitly mentioned in the New Testament.

---

[7] The references to healing in Heb. 12:13, 1 Pet. 2:24, and Rev. 13:3, 13:12, 22:2 are clearly metaphorical and are too general to draw any conclusions about actual care for the sick. A rare article that makes at least indirect use of anthropological approaches to health care is Martin C. Albl, "'Are Any among You Sick?' The Health Care System in the Letter of James," *JBL* 121 (2002): 123–43.

[8] Many of these questions are laid out in the Introduction and need not be repeated here.

A more reasonable starting point would be to presume that Paul and his followers employed the same methods of health care as their non-Christian peers unless we find evidence (or at least strong arguments) to the contrary. The fruitfulness of this presumption will become apparent later when we consider its implications for Paul's theology and practice, including whether there were any limits to the types of health care that he and his followers were willing to use.[9] First, however, we must develop a better understanding of the types of treatment that were available to Paul and his audiences.

Framing the Conversation

As we noted earlier, Kleinman claimed that all health care systems include three different sectors of activity to which people can turn to address their health concerns: the popular sector, the professional sector, and the folk sector. When we attempt to apply this model to Greco-Roman health care, however, we run into immediate difficulties.

The professional sector would seem to be the easiest to identify, as it consists of providers who have undergone some type of formal training to care for the sick and are therefore honored by others as having special expertise in this area. Physicians trained in Hippocratic medicine are the most obvious members of this sector. But would ancient audiences have classified physicians as more "professional" than other care providers? The Greco-Roman health care system included a broad array of practitioners who had been carefully trained in the arts of their discipline, including root-cutters, midwives, exorcists, drug-makers, diviners, dream interpreters, and others. All of these healers, including physicians, were educated in a similar manner through hands-on instruction by a family member or apprenticeship with a local practitioner, not in a formal school setting.[10] None of them received any formal accreditation or licensing at the end of their training—professional success or failure depended on their ability to find customers who would pay for their services. To single out one of these categories of healers as "the organized healing professions" to the detriment of the others is both anachronistic and tendentious.

Admittedly, some of the Hippocratic texts and elite authors like Pliny the Elder do make an effort to frame physicians as the only legitimate healers while deriding their rivals as magicians, charlatans, and quacks. But this kind of verbal jousting was a

---

[9] This and other questions regarding Paul's beliefs and practice regarding health care will be examined in Chapter 9.
[10] The term "schools of medicine" as used by ancient authors refers to various combinations of theory and praxis that were accepted, taught, and used by physicians, not to a physical space where they were trained. Some of these schools were associated with a (real or mythical) founder, such as Hippocrates or Herophilos, while others were named after key elements of their doctrine (e.g., Methodists, Pneumatists). Physicians were trained individually or in small groups by a practicing physician who instructed them in the system of treatment that he himself employed, with little or no regard for competing approaches. A few were trained at healing centers like the ones at Pergamon, Cos, or Carura in Asia Minor. Most medical education was performed at the patient's bedside, not in a formal class setting. For more on ancient schools of medicine, see Chapter 5.

standard feature of the partisan rhetoric by which medical providers sought to establish their credibility and attract followers from other practitioners; it does not reflect shared social norms.[11] Clearly the many people who sought cures from non-medical healers did not view them in this jaundiced light. A historically sensitive application of Kleinman's model would require that we class all of the disparate varieties of trained healers under the heading of "the organized healing professions" in order to distinguish their work from the informal care provided by friends and family members. But such a categorization would be so broad as to be useless, and the dividing lines between "professional" and non-professional types of healing would still be unclear in many cases.[12]

Similar problems surround efforts to distinguish between "popular" and "folk" healers. Part of the trouble arises from the difficulty of defining professional healers—we can't effectively categorize some providers as "popular" or "folk" if we have no clear means of distinguishing them from the ones that we label "professional."[13] Even if this were not a problem, however, the theoretical distinction that Kleinman sets up between popular and folk healers is hard to maintain for Greco-Roman society. The key difference between them, according to Kleinman, is the nature of the provider: popular healing is delivered by "non-professionals" while folk healing is done by "healers not officially approved by the state or by the 'orthodox' medical profession."[14] But as we have noted, no category of healers can be properly called "the 'orthodox' medical profession" in Greco-Roman antiquity, nor was there any formal state or medical authority that "officially approved" healers of any type. In short, Kleinman's categories do not work for Greco-Roman antiquity.

Rather than trying to categorize healers according to their mode of training and level of societal recognition as Kleinman does, we should look for categories that reflect the social realities of the world that we are studying—in short, we should apply an "emic" rather than an "etic" approach.[15] Yet even here the distinctions are less clear than we might like, since the various forms of Greco-Roman healing shared common historical roots and borrowing was common. But the fuzziness of the boundaries does not prevent us from seeing that Greek and Roman authors recognized four different spheres of healing, each of which was represented by a distinct set of providers and practices.

---

[11] For more on this point, see Chapter 5.
[12] Where, for example, would we class a man like Cato, who makes the paterfamilias responsible for tending to the ailments of his family and animals and offers detailed prescriptions for the use of cabbage as a healing agent in *Agr.* 156–8? Clearly he was trained by someone (his own father?), and he seeks to pass on his knowledge to other elite landowners through his writing.
[13] Classical scholar William V. Harris also recognizes this problem: "'Popular medicine' and 'folk medicine' . . . are problematical categories, especially in societies such as those of the classical Greeks and Romans in which there were professional healers but no 'professions' in a modern sense" ("Popular Medicine in the Classical World" 2). A similar judgment can be found in Laura M. Zucconi, *Ancient Medicine: From Mesopotamia to Rome* (Grand Rapids, MI: Eerdmans, 2019), 7, who points to the influence of Western colonial thinking on the development of the categories.
[14] Kleinman, *Patients and Healers in the Context of Culture*, 59.
[15] In the social sciences, an "emic" approach works from the perspective of the people being studied while an "etic" approach relies on models developed outside the group. The former approach seeks to explicate how the subjects themselves view reality while the latter privileges the observer's experience and frame of reference.

The oldest mode of treatment was what we might call "home remedies," a variegated mix of experience-based healing techniques that range from dietary regimens and natural medicines to religious rituals such as prayer and sacrifice to the use of charms, incantations, amulets, and similar practices that modern observers have often labeled as "magical." For the most part these remedies would have been performed by the individual or family members, though local practitioners could have been consulted in doubtful cases. Age and gender played a role as well, with older people serving as stores of traditional knowledge and women and men experiencing different problems that required different types of care. In short, the native healing practices of Greeks and Romans (and the indigenous peoples whose lands they conquered) resembled what we see in traditional cultures around the world.

Over time, three different but overlapping systems of health care emerged out of these time-tested remedies, each relying on a different set of practitioners. One system involved the use of ritualized words and actions to manipulate invisible forces that were believed to permeate the visible world and affect the fates of humans for good (as in healing) or ill (as in curses). The Greeks labeled these techniques *mageia* due to a popular belief that they originated with Persian ritual experts called *magi*, but their use in health care has deep roots in traditional Greek and Roman practices.[16] The negative image that the term "magic" carries today can be traced to the creators and defenders of Hippocratic medicine, who beginning in the fourth century BCE derided "magical" health care as irrational, ineffective, and potentially dangerous.[17] Despite these attacks, *mageia* grew into a highly developed art in Greco-Roman antiquity with its own view of reality, its own recognized practitioners, and its own techniques. Healing was only one of its concerns, but many people relied on it for cures.

A second system of health care that played a vital role in home care but developed over time into a more organized regimen was religious treatment. Offering prayers, vows, and sacrifices to the gods in solicitation or acknowledgment of their benefits was a standard element of Greek and Roman life, but illness or serious injury made human dependence upon the divine more pressing, especially when other modes of treatment proved ineffective. Any god or goddess could be approached for healing, but certain deities were believed to have a special interest in curing the sick. The preeminent healing deity was the Greek god Asklepios, whom the Romans appropriated under the name of Aesculapius. Every town or city had its temple of Asklepios where people could present offerings and sacrifices to the god, while the larger temples also offered treatment advice and opportunities for dream interpretation after a night of ritualized sleep at the temple. Regional healing sanctuaries offered similar services at a more advanced level, together with many of the services associated today with health spas (baths, gymnasia, massage, etc.). Oral and written reports of both mundane and miraculous cures circulated widely throughout the Greco-Roman world, reinforcing people's faith in the efficacy of religious modes of treatment.

---

[16] More will be said on these points in Chapter 3.
[17] Recent concerns about the use of "magic" and "magical" as categories for social analysis will be discussed in Chapter 3.

The third system of health care that arose out of traditional healing methods was medicine. The traditional originator of medical treatment was Hippocrates, who developed his system of diagnosis and treatment out of training that he had received at the healing sanctuary of Asklepios on the island of Cos in southwestern Asia Minor in the late fifth century BCE. Others before him had put forward theories about the nature of the body and how to care for it, but he appears to have been the first to work out a rational system of theory and practice that could be taught and applied by others to treat illness and injury with a degree of consistency and success. Most of the treatment regimens that he and his followers prescribed—dietary changes, heating or cooling, exercise, baths, medications—were derived from traditional healing practices, but Hippocrates and his followers organized them into a more coherent and reliable system. They also pared away many of the religious and "magical" elements from traditional health care, though they did not wholly reject either system, especially for treating conditions that their methods were unable to cure. Other schools of medicine arose over time that disagreed with major elements of Hippocratic theory and practice, but they all followed his experience-based approach to health care. This mindset is what distinguished practitioners of medicine from "magical" and religious healers, regardless of which school they represented.

This fourfold classification of ancient health care into home-based, "magical," religious, and medical systems is more consistent with the historical evidence and more useful for analyzing the health practices of the early Christ-followers than the tripartite system developed by Kleinman and his disciples. The fruitfulness of this schema will become apparent as we examine each of these systems in more detail, beginning with home remedies in the present chapter and moving on to "magical," religious, and medical healing in Chapters 3–5.

Home Remedies

One of the truisms of writing social history is that one must learn to read between the lines and against the grain of elite literary sources to uncover what can be known or reasonably guessed about the experiences of ordinary women and men in the distant past. This is certainly the case with regard to what people did at home to treat illness and injury. Such mundane practices rarely attracted the attention of elite authors, and virtually no one among the rural or urban masses was literate enough to compose texts that might offer information on the subject. Archaeological records are also less useful here than otherwise since home care required no special buildings and few implements that might be distinguished as such in the archaeological record. Vivian Nutton describes the problem well: "The fact that the great majority of our evidence comes from the major cities, most notably Rome, has distorted our perceptions of what medicine was like in Antiquity for most people. . . . The medicine of the countryside, with its knowledge of local plants and herbs, appears fitfully across the centuries."[18]

---

[18] *Ancient Medicine*, 314.

Still, there are enough references and hints in elite literature to give us at least a broad sense of what home health care was like in the Greco-Roman world. One type of evidence comes from literary depictions of practices that were rejected and disparaged by elite authors. Many of these practices are associated with ordinary people and can thus be assumed to reflect traditional modes of care. A second source of information is elite references to healing techniques that the author assumes to be well known and accepted, especially those involving substances and practices that would have been readily available to the general public (medicinal applications of common plants and foods, techniques for setting broken or dislocated bones, instructions for handling difficult pregnancies, etc.). Finally, we find occasional mentions by elite authors of practices that were used in the countryside where traditional home remedies were more likely to be preserved. Some of these latter references can be confirmed or supplemented by inscriptions found in rural religious sanctuaries, a popular resort for ordinary people seeking healing.[19]

A review of these sources reveals that home health care in the Greco-Roman world involved treatments that correspond broadly with the three broad systems that we identified earlier: "magical," religious, and medical.[20] In practice, however, the categories were routinely blurred: an ordinary food item like wine or eggs might be taken as a cure with or without the recitation of a charm or incantation, or prayers might be offered to a healing god while creating or putting on an amulet. All three modes of care appear to be equally ancient and equally utilized, an observation that undermines all efforts to prioritize one over another. We can categorize the various remedies for the sake of analysis, but we must keep in mind that these distinctions are modern ones that would not have been apparent to the people who were using them.

Quasi-Magical Cures

Our investigation begins with a time-honored method of treatment that could be performed on its own or in conjunction with other remedies: the use of charms, incantations, amulets, and similar practices to influence or manipulate suprahuman forces that were believed to have a role in causing, enhancing, or averting sickness or injury. Such practices are often labeled "magical" because they recall the techniques used by people trained in the skills of *mageia*, which will be explored in Chapter 3.[21]

---

[19] An illuminating study of rural inscriptions in Asia Minor can be found in Angelos Chaniotis, "Illness and Cures in the Greek Propitiatory Inscriptions and Dedications of Lydia and Phrygia," in *Ancient Medicine in Its Socio-Cultural Context*, ed. Ph. J. van der Eijk, H. F. J. Horstmanshoff, and P. U. Schrijvers (Amsterdam and Atlanta: Editions Rodopi, 1995), 323–44.

[20] William Harris includes a wide range of practices and providers in his study of "popular" Greco-Roman healing: prayers, spells, amulets, herbs, minerals and gems, wonder-workers, dreams, healing centers, astrologers, and (less commonly) exorcisms and oracles ("Popular Medicine in the Classical World," 53–61). Vivian Nutton observes similarly that healing techniques were basically the same among Greek and Roman rural residents, consisting of a mix of herbs, chants, prayers, and charms ("Roman Medicine, 250 BC to AD 200," in *The Western Medical Tradition, 800 BC to AD 1800*, ed. Lawrence I. Conrad, Michael Neve, Vivian Nutton, Roy Porter, and Andrew Wear [Cambridge: Cambridge University Press, 1995], 39).

[21] The term is also used in a more derogatory sense to reflect a perceived resemblance to the intentionally deceptive techniques used by modern "magical" entertainers to trick gullible

But "quasi-magical" is a more appropriate term, since we are focusing here on practices that could be performed by ordinary people who had not been trained in the arcane systems of knowledge and practice that came to be known as *mageia*.

Both "magical" and "quasi-magical" forms of health care are rooted in the belief, common in traditional societies, that ritualized words or actions can channel or even compel invisible forces to help or harm humans. Some cultures view these forces as impersonal and immanent within the material world, while others characterize them as personal (and often divine) beings whose presence and powers can be enlisted by humans who possess the requisite skills. Beliefs such as these were endemic to the Romans, who saw suprahuman presences and powers all around them and relied heavily on rituals as a means of regulating their effects on daily life. But similar ideas and practices can also be found among the Greeks and the various indigenous peoples of the Mediterranean region, so there is nothing distinctively Roman about this mode of care.

As with other aspects of popular health care, the full extent of these remedies is unknown since they attracted little attention from Greek or Roman authors. But the evidence is sufficient to enable us to identify three broad categories of quasi-magical health care that were practiced at all levels of society and thus would have been available to Paul and his followers: the recitation of oral formulae, the performance of ritualized actions, and the wearing of protective objects. The Greek vocabulary in all of these areas is varied and inconsistent, and the literary and archaeological material that has survived tells us more about the practices of the elites than the uneducated masses. But there are enough references in ancient sources to confirm that such activities were common, even if we cannot always be sure what form they took.

(a) The use of *oral formulae* is expressed in English translations by such words as "charms," "spells," and "incantations." Efforts to draw clear distinctions among the various Greek terms as they are used in magical literature have reached widely varying conclusions, and the problem is even more acute for lay usage.[22] When studying health care, however, fine distinctions are less important since the manner in which oral formulae were deployed is fairly clear: some were recited to prevent illness from occurring (including countering the effects of curses), while others were used to cure it.

The use of healing incantations by Greeks is attested as early as Homer, who in *Od.* 19.455-58 describes the sons of Autolykos reciting a spell over Odysseus's leg to staunch the bleeding of a wound that he had received during a hunt (ἐπαοιδῇ δ' αἷμα κελαινὸν ἔσχεθον).[23] In the classical era, Plato speaks of Socrates having learned from a Thracian physician a cure for headache that involved the utterance of an incantation (ἐπῳδὴ) in

---

audiences into believing that something unnatural or even supernatural has occurred before their eyes. This usage will be discussed further in Chapter 3.

[22] For two different views on the subject, see Richard Gordon, "The Healing Event in Graeco-Roman Medicine," in van der Eijk et al., *Ancient Medicine*, 363–76, and Stephen Skinner, "Refining the Definition of Amulet, Phylactery, Charm, Lamen and Talisman as They Appear in the *PGM* and the Grimoires," an unpublished paper posted online at https://www.academia.edu/34736473367. Gordon does not address "spells" in his study, while Skinner does not discuss "incantations."

[23] Noted by Plinio Prioreschi in *A History of Medicine*, Vol. 1, *Primitive and Ancient Medicine* (2nd edn; Omaha, NE: Horatius Press, 1996), 38.

conjunction with the application of a particular leaf (*Charm*. 155b-e). "Without the charm," insisted Socrates, "there was no efficacy in the leaf" (*Charm*. 155e). Elsewhere Socrates (via Plato) cites as common knowledge the fact that midwives use both drugs and incantations to stimulate or alleviate the labor pains of a pregnant woman (*Tht*. 149c-d). The frequent polemics against charms and spells in the Hippocratic treatises (fourth century BCE to second century CE) underline how popular such practices were among the people whom Greek physicians sought to cure. The earliest parts of the *Papyri Graecae Magicae* (*PGM*) (fourth century BCE to fifth century CE) offer similar evidence for Hellenistic and Roman Egypt, though the length and complexity of their formulae make it unlikely that they were recited in their current form by ordinary people.

Among the Romans, spells and incantations were used from early times to influence the many invisible forces that people encountered in their daily lives.[24] They were especially popular for protecting and healing people and animals from illness, together with prayers and herbal remedies. Britta Ager lists some of the purposes for which incantations were prescribed by the Roman agronomists:

> to promote the growth of seeds and crops, to avert mildew and sickness, to cure crop and animal disease when it occurs, to avert pests and storms, to affect the offspring of animals and the produce of trees and vines, to protect the harvest once it is gathered, to avoid weeds, kill bugs, and generally to smooth the farmer's troubles through the year.[25]

Cato the Elder (second century BCE) is often cited as an example of how these ancient incantations might have been used to procure healing.

> If you have a dislocation of any sort, it will be healed by this incantation [*cantio*]. Take a green reed four or five feet long, split it down the middle, and have two men apply it to your hips. Begin the incantation [*cantare*], "motas vaeta daries dardares astataries dissunapiter," until they come together. Wave a knife over them. When they have met and are touching each other, take the reed in your hand and cut it short on both right and left sides. Bind the reed-pieces to your dislocation or fracture and it will heal. Even so, use the incantation on a daily basis. Or, for a dislocation, you can use this one: "huat haut haut istasis tarsis ardannabou dannaustra."[26]

---

[24] Incantations are mentioned as early as the fifth century BCE in the Twelve Tables, an early codification of Roman law—see Elizabeth Ann Pollard, "Charms, Spells, Greece and Rome," in *The Encyclopedia of Ancient History*, ed. Roger S. Bagnall, Kai Brodersen, Craige B. Champion, Andrew Erskine, and Sabine R. Huebner (Malden, MA: Wiley-Blackwell, 2013), 1444.
[25] "Roman Agricultural Magic," 50.
[26] *Agr*. 160; English translation by Daniel Ogden, *Magic, Witchcraft, and Ghosts in the Greek and Roman Worlds: A Sourcebook* (Oxford: Oxford University Press, 2002). The meaning of the words in the chants is unknown. Whether they represent the corruption of originally meaningful words or the kind of nonsense syllables that appear in many later incantations is unclear.

Of course, Cato was a wealthy landowner and not a rural peasant, but the uniqueness of this cure by comparison with others in the same treatise suggests that he had learned it from someone on his farm rather than a fellow elite Roman.

Varro, another Roman patrician who wrote on agriculture (first century BCE), mentions a quasi-magical healing ritual for curing foot pain that includes chanting the following incantation twenty-seven times while fasting: "I am thinking of you, cure my feet. The pain go in the ground, and may my feet be sound." The chant was to be accompanied by touching and spitting on the ground, though the details are not specified.[27] Pliny the Elder refers twenty-three times to the use of healing incantations in his *Natural History*, including thirteen that are simple enough to have been used by ordinary people.[28] Most involve words to be recited while harvesting, preparing, or applying an herbal remedy.[29] Soranus of Ephesus (early second century CE) warns midwives against allowing "a dream or omen or some customary rite" to distract them from the practices that they were trained to follow (*Gyn.* 1.4). The term "customary rites" probably included the kinds of spells and incantations that were commonly used to ensure safe delivery.[30]

More examples could be cited from these and other authors, but all point to the same conclusion: the use of oral formulae to avert sickness and induce healing was universally popular in Greco-Roman antiquity even after Hippocratic medicine came to be widely accepted. The link between the two systems was encapsulated in a frequently repeated maxim: "When the art of the physician fails, everybody resorts to incantations."[31]

How exactly such oral formulae were thought to work is never explained, apart from the general belief that sacred words correctly recited can move the gods to act.[32] Pliny's

---

[27] *Rust.* 2.27 (Loeb translation, 1934). An older translation by F. H. Belvoir (1918; posted online at https://en.wikisource.org/wiki/Res_Rusticae_(Country_Matters)) limits the incantation to the latter part of the text quoted above: "May the earth keep the malady, May good health remain here." The Latin text is ambiguous. Varro credits the cure to the first-century BCE author Saserna, whose writings are now lost. Though he disparages Saserna for including such irrelevant material in a work on agriculture, he never states clearly what he thinks of the remedy.

[28] The incantations are listed and discussed by Patricia Gaillard-Seux, "Magical Formulas in Pliny's Natural History: Origins, Sources, Parallels," in *"Greek" and "Roman" in Latin Medical Texts*, ed. Brigitte Maire (Leiden: Brill, 2014), 201–23. Cf. Ager, "Roman Agricultural Magic," 5: "Unlike most surviving curses or, especially, the often very elaborate spells in the surviving papyrus handbooks, even someone who was illiterate could use this magic."

[29] For example, "Begone, cantharides [a skin condition], for a savage wolf seeks your blood" (27.100). In seven cases the instructions include reciting the name of the person for whom the plant is being gathered or the disease that it is meant to cure, or both. In ten cases the incantation is accompanied by some sort of ritualized action, including four where the remedy was to be worn as an amulet. Six passages preserve the wording of an incantation (24.176, 24.181, 26.93, 27.100, 27.131, 28.42), including two that mention the name of a deity (e.g., "Apollo tells us that a plague cannot grow more fiery if a naked maiden quench the fire," 26.93). Whether such explicitly religious chants might have been avoided by Paul will be discussed in Chapter 9.

[30] On the use of spells and incantations in connection with delivering a baby, see Wainwright, *Women Healing/Healing Women*, 39, citing Plato *Tht.* 149a-150c.

[31] E.g., Diodorus fr XXX, 43, Plutarch, *De fac.* 920b; cited in Edelstein, "Greek Medicine in Its Relation to Religion and Magic," 245.

[32] Speaking from an "etic" perspective, David Frankfurter observes that "the concept of 'charming' revolves around a culturally-specific belief that vocal and musical sounds in themselves have a persuasive effect on people, animals, and things, and that there exist particular verses or tunes that

discussion of the question in *HN* 28.10-21 is instructive. He begins by distinguishing between the opinions of the gullible public and those of the critically minded elites regarding incantations, claiming that "all our wisest men reject belief in them, although as a body the public at all times believes in them unconsciously" (28.10). But then he goes on to cite numerous examples from both past and present experience that compel him to admit that "there is power in ritual formulas" and that the gods can indeed be moved by properly formed and recited words (28.13-14). The popularity of this belief is evident in his assertion that people are "always on the lookout for something big, something adequate to move a god, or rather to impose its will on his divinity" (28.19-20). Such inconsistencies in a Roman author should not surprise us; as Vivian Nutton has rightly observed, the Roman approach to healing was utterly practical, with little or no theoretical foundation.[33] But Pliny does testify clearly to the popularity of spells and incantations among the "gullible public."

(b) *Ritualized actions* also played an important role in quasi-magical cures, whether performed alone or in conjunction with oral formulae. Many of these actions were associated with the harvesting of plants to be used in healing, while others were designed to protect people from getting sick by averting dark powers that might damage their health. Still others were used to channel healing power to people who were already sick. All of these activities are rooted in the common ancient belief that ritual acts can influence the behavior and effects of invisible forces that pervade the visible world, bringing weal or woe to humans. Pliny's observation is typical: "It is clear that scrupulous actions, even without words, have their powers."[34] Combining them with incantations can make them even stronger: the sacred words give power to the acts (and protection to the actor), while the actions create the channel by which the powers reach their targets.

Numerous examples can be cited from both Greek and Roman sources of people using ritualized actions to protect or restore health to people or animals. On the protective side, the Greek philosopher Theophrastus (fourth century BCE) commended the hanging of squill plants outside of a home to keep away evil spirits.[35] The practice appears to have been popular, as it was repeated centuries later by the Roman authors Dioscorides and Pliny the Elder (first century CE).[36] A similar effect can be achieved,

---

concentrate that effect" ("Spell and Speech Act: The Magic of the Spoken Word," in *Guide to the Study of Ancient Magic*, ed. David Frankfurter [Leiden and Boston: Brill, 2019], 613–14).

[33] Vivian Nutton, "Healers in the Medical Marketplace: Towards a Social History of Graeco-Roman Medicine," in *Medicine in Society: Historical Essays*, ed. Andrew Wear (Cambridge: Cambridge University Press, 1992), 37. The use of incantations continued well into the Christian era, as is evident from the frequent condemnations of the practice by both patristic writers (Wendt, *At the Temple Gates*, 198; Gary B. Ferngren, *Medicine and Religion: A Historical Introduction* (Baltimore, MD: Johns Hopkins University Press, 2014), 83; Evelyn Frost, *Christian Healing*, 2nd edn [London: A. R. Mowbray, 1949], 99, 101, 106) and medical writers like Galen and Soranus (Nutton, "Roman Medicine, 250 BC to AD 200," 55).

[34] *HN* 28.24.

[35] *Hist. pl.* 7.13.4. Theophrastus attributes most of his knowledge about gathering plants to root-cutters and drug sellers, whose methods were deeply rooted in traditional practices.

[36] Dioscorides, *De mat. med.* 2.171.4, Pliny *HN* 20.39; noted by Ella Faye Wallace, "The Sorcerer's Pharmacy" (PhD dissertation, Rutgers University, 2018), 24–5.

according to Dioscorides, by laying branches of buckthorn across windows and gates.[37] Both plants were readily available to people in the country.

A different type of protective ritual can be seen in a prescription for avoiding eye trouble that Pliny claims has been tested and observed by many people, an expression that likely refers to a traditional remedy that has been tried with success by members of his own class. One should first remove all bands from one's body (shoes, rings, etc.), then pluck the bud of a bitter pomegranate tree using only the thumb and forefinger, then brush one's eyes with it lightly before swallowing it without touching the teeth. If done properly, this ritual will prevent eye trouble for a full year (*HN* 23.110). Similar results can be achieved by tying the two middle fingers of the right hand together with a linen thread (*HN* 28.42) or rubbing the body with a mixture of breast milk taken from both a mother and her daughter (*HN* 28.73).[38]

On the curative side, the Roman patrician Columella (first century CE) commends a treatment for sick sheep that involves burying a sick animal upside down at the entrance to the sheepfold and driving the other sheep over it so that their sickness will pass to the one buried in the ground.[39] Similar rituals of transference are mentioned several times in Pliny's *Natural History*, as when he suggests laying a duck or a newborn puppy on the stomach or chest of a person suffering from intestinal problems so that the illness can pass into the animal, which then dies (30.61, 30.64).[40] Numbers, which were widely believed to have mystical properties, also play a role in many healing rituals, such as Pliny's recommendation for carrying a heliotrope plant three times around the bed of a person sick with tertian ("third-day") fever and then placing the plant under the patient's head (*HN* 22.60).[41]

Other curative rituals are concerned with regulating how and when plants are picked and handled so as to preserve or enhance their healing powers. Numerous examples could be cited from both Greek and Roman sources, though it can be hard to discern which recommendations reflect traditional practices and which represent the more refined arts of the *rhizotomai* (root-cutters) that will be discussed in Chapter 3.

---

[37] Dioscorides, *De mat. med.* 1.119. He introduces this prescription with the words, "It is said," which is generally taken as a reference to a traditional practice.

[38] The health-giving power of mother's milk is noted by many ancient medical authorities (Pliny cites over twenty uses for it) and probably reflects a belief held at all levels of society. Tying the fingers together with linen requires no special materials and thus could well go back to traditional practices.

[39] *Rust.* 7.5.17. Cited by Ager, "Roman Agricultural Magic," 51.

[40] The ritual with the puppy is more elaborate; it must be done for three days, and the puppies must be suckled with milk from the patient's mouth. Pliny described both cures as *mirum* ("wonderful," "extraordinary," "strange"), a term that he applies elsewhere to "marvels" that he finds credible, as in 3.88 where he describes the nightly fires of Mount Etna (though cf. 30.143, where he adds "if it is true" when speaking of a prescription for an aphrodisiac). He distinguishes these cures from the foolish prescriptions of the Magi, who claim that applying bat's blood to the belly will protect a person from colic for an entire year (30.64). A similar distinction of terminology can be seen in 24.99 when he shifts from discussing plants that are *mirabiles* to those that are *magicae*. According to Patricia Watson, such distinctions generally indicate that Pliny is drawing on folk cures—see "Animals in Magic," in *Magic in Greece and Rome*, ed. Lindsay C. Watson (London and New York: Bloomsbury, 2019), 128–30.

[41] An alternate prescription in the same passage reflects the same principle: mixing four heliotrope seeds into a drink for a person with quartan ("four-day") fever and three seeds for tertian ("three-day") fever. The latter remedy is also cited by Dioscorides in *De mat. med.* 4.190.

The precise ritual to be used varies from plant to plant: examples include harvesting the plant at night during a specific cycle of the moon; drawing circles around the plant using a tool made from a particular kind of metal; dancing around the plant naked (or wearing special clothing) while chanting prayers or incantations; standing upwind or downwind of the plant while picking it; naming the person or condition for which the plant is being harvested; removing the plant with a specific hand and holding it in a certain way; watching out for a particular bird that might cause harm to those harvesting the plant; and placing a sacred offering into the hole left by extracting the plant.

A couple of examples that might reflect traditional practice are instructive.[42] Pliny the Elder, after praising the medicinal effects of mistletoe, states that "some superstitiously believe" that the effect of the medicine is stronger if one gathers it "from the hard-wood oak at the new moon without the use of iron, and without its touching the ground." Picking the plant in this way and carrying it on one's person can cure epilepsy or help a woman to conceive (*HN* 24.12).[43] Elsewhere he describes a ritual for preparing the wild mallow plant (very common in the Mediterranean region) for use on scrofulous sores: its root must be dug up before sunrise and wrapped in fresh wool from a ewe that has given birth to a ewe lamb, without letting it touch the ground (*HN* 20.29). Scribonius Largus, writing around the same time as Pliny, offers a less detailed ritual for picking holy vervain or sharp trefoil (both common plants) for medicinal use: "It is fitting to note them on the day before, and to draw a circle around them with the left plow-ear, setting down some fruits, and on the day after, at sunrise, to pick them with the left hand, to hold them thus bound" (*Comp.* 108). Given Scribonius's persistent skepticism of "magical" remedies, such a prescription must surely reflect traditional practices.[44]

Still other rituals concern the time and manner in which healing substances are to be applied. To cure warts, for example, Dioscorides states that "some people" (indicating a non-professional source) touch the tip of each wart with a different chickpea at the time of the new moon, then wrap the peas together in a linen cloth and throw it out, believing that the warts will fall off as a result.[45] To cure boils, according to Pliny, "they say" (a common reference to popular traditions) that one should take nine grains of barley in the left hand and trace a circle three times around the boil with each one, then throw the grains into the fire and the boils will disappear (*HN* 22.135). Elsewhere Pliny cites as common knowledge the practice of applying saliva to incipient boils while fasting in order to prevent them from growing (28.36). These and many other texts

---

[42] An excellent (though somewhat dated) source regarding the various rituals that were recommended for picking, handling, and preserving plants used in healing is Armand Delatte, *Herbarius: Recherches sur le Cérémonial Usité chez les Anciens pour la Cueilette des Simples et des Plantes Magique*, 3rd edn (Brussels: Palais des Académies, 1961).

[43] When Pliny says words like "some superstitiously believe," he is citing a traditional treatment of which he is skeptical.

[44] Commenting on Scribonius's work, Ella Faye Wallace observes that "plant-picking traditions seem to have been normalized in Rome to the point that they were not considered a Greek or otherwise foreign import (which would likely condemn them to the category of *magia*), but rather an acceptable Italian practice" ("Sorcerer's Pharmacy," 117).

[45] *De mat. med.* 2.104. Noted by Lindsay C. Watson in *Magic in Greece and Rome*, 109.

show that ritualized actions played a vital role in traditional Greek and Roman health care systems.

(c) A third type of quasi-magical health treatment that was especially popular in the ancient world was the wearing of *amulets*. Naomi Janowitz gives a helpful, though rather broad, definition of amulets: "Amulets are any objects used to directly mediate between divine forces and a particular individual or place. They work by bringing some type of physical representation of the supernatural force into direct physical contact with the person/animal/place for which aid is sought."[46] In most cases they were worn on the body, whether hung around the neck or tied to the body part that was suffering from sickness, but amulets could also be laid on top of a sick body or placed in close physical proximity to the sick person without direct physical contact (under the pillow, beneath the bed, etc.).

According to Cesidio R. Simboli, amulets were "the most universal means of preventing disease" in Greco-Roman antiquity, employed by people at all levels of society across every region.[47] "Amulets were ubiquitous and their use largely uncontroversial," agrees Justin Meggitt. "Those who rejected the use of amulets to protect themselves from disease were sufficiently eccentric as to be considered mad.... To judge from the archaeological record, almost everyone carried an amulet to aid digestion and ward off such things as fever."[48] Even the skeptical were known to resort to them in times of extremity: "As an infection festered or a fever lingered, even the sternest critics of traditional or 'superstitious' remedies turned to the application of amulets."[49]

Amulets could be either protective (warding off evil powers that might cause harm) or curative (removing illness and restoring a state of wholeness). Some were highly elaborate, consisting of images and inscriptions engraved on gems or metal sheets (including silver and gold), but most were simple and easy to make from available materials (plants, animal parts, minerals, etc.).[50] Some were prepared using spells and incantations that were believed to imbue them with power to heal or prevent sickness, while others were made from substances whose healing powers were regarded as inherent, especially materials that were used in other forms to treat illness.[51]

The use of amulets in health care actually predates the coming of the Greeks and Romans. Roy Kotansky has traced their presence among the Egyptians, Phoenicians,

---

[46] *Magic in the Roman World: Pagans, Jews and Christians* (London and New York: Routledge, 2001), 57.
[47] *Disease-Spirits and Divine Cures among the Greeks and Romans*, 73.
[48] Justin J. Meggitt, "Did Magic Matter? The Saliency of Magic in the Early Roman Empire," *JAH* 1 (2013): 176 n. 45.
[49] Roy Kotansky, "Incantations and Prayers for Salvation on Inscribed Greek Amulets," in Faraone and Obbink, *Magika Hiera*, 107.
[50] The more elaborate forms will be discussed in Chapter 3, since most of them had to be prepared by specialists.
[51] Roy Kotansky provides numerous examples of amulets being accompanied by incantations in "Incantations and Prayers." Regarding the uninscribed type, Jerry Stannard observes that "a large number of common plants were thought to provide security by being carried or worn on one's person as a pendant, knot, or amulet" ("Medicinal Plants and Folk Remedies in Pliny, 'Historia Naturalis.'" *History and Philosophy of the Life Sciences* 4 (1982): 22).

and Mesopotamians, and earlier examples have been found in prehistoric burials.[52] Among the Greeks, uninscribed amulets (those made from plain materials without words or pictures) are known from Homer onward, while inscribed amulets appear for the first time in the classical era. The history is similar for the Romans, where simple amulets were a standard part of the healing repertoire from ancient times, though the inscribed form did not reach their heyday until the second to fifth centuries CE.[53] The growing influence of Hippocratic medicine did little to undermine their popularity; in fact, it is not uncommon to see medical writers listing amulets as one of several modes by which a healing substance might be applied to a patient.[54] Medical writers from the authors of the Hippocratic Corpus (fourth to second centuries BCE) to rational Roman physicians like Celsus (late first century CE) and Galen (second century CE) agreed that amulets were effective, though they disagreed over why they worked and how they should be used.[55]

Among ancient authors, Dioscorides and Pliny the Elder have the most to say about the use of amulets in healing. A few examples from each author will illustrate the rich variety of materials used as amulets and the broad range of ailments to which they were applied. All of these examples use substances and methods that were readily available to ordinary people.[56]

Dioscorides writes as a medical expert. His *De materia medica*, which describes over 600 plant and animal substances that could be used to treat a broad range of ailments, became the key textbook on the subject until the Renaissance. His work contains at least twenty-five prescriptions for amulets, including the following recipes.[57]

---

[52] "Textual Amulets and Writing Traditions in the Ancient World," in Frankfurter, *Guide to the Study of Ancient Magic*, 508–31.

[53] Kotansky, "Textual Amulets," 537–47; Matthew W. Dickie, *Magic and Magicians in the Greco-Roman World* (London and New York: Routledge, 2001), 125–6.

[54] Archaeological finds also confirm the use of gems and other amulets in medical practice—see Véronique Dasen and Árpád Nagy, "Gems," in Frankfurter, *Guide to the Study of Ancient Magic*, 435. According to these authors, amulets were used primarily to treat mysterious internal sicknesses, particularly those of the uterus and stomach, and not common ailments like toothaches and fractures ("Gems," 439–42).

[55] Nutton, "Roman Medicine, 250 BC to AD 200," 55; Harris, "Popular Medicine in the Classical World," 13–14; John Scarborough, *Roman Medicine* (Ithaca: Cornell University Press, 1969), 120; Danielle Gourevitch, "Popular Medicines and Practices in Galen," in Harris, *Popular Medicine*, 264–9; Paul T. Keyser, "Science and Magic in Galen's Recipes (Sympathy and Efficacy)," in *Galen on Pharmacology: Philosophy, History and Medicine*, ed. Armelle Debru (Leiden: Brill, 1997), 176. As we will see in Chapters 7 and 8, similar admissions can be found among Jewish and Christian authors.

[56] Britta Ager highlights how many of these amulets (and other treatments) appear to have been created and used by ordinary people before being taken up into elite literature. Her observations regarding Columella could be applied to many ancient authors. "Where did Columella learn to make an amulet to cure a shrew-bite in cattle?" she asks. "Ultimately, much of the lore on veterinary medicine, fertilizers, amulets, bug repellants, and so forth which the agronomists record must come from the countryside.... Although the agronomists occasionally imply that much of their advice originated with such people, their works show a continuing effort to launder humble knowledge through natural philosophy and make it the exclusive possession of the educated" ("Roman Agricultural Magic," 150–1).

[57] Paul Jonathan Harms, "The Logic of Irrational Pharmacological Therapies in Aretaeus of Cappadocia, Scribonius Largus and Dioscorides of Anazarbus" (PhD dissertation, University of Calgary, 2010), 199, 216–21.

- To treat a bite from a rabid dog, tie a canine tooth from the dog to the victim's arm in a small pouch (2.47).
- To cure quartan fever, place the web of a particular type of spider into a pouch and hang it from the arm (2.63).
- To relieve a toothache, tie a root from the pepperwort plant (described as "a familiar little herb") around the sufferer's neck (2.174).
- For inflammation of the groin, wear hare's foot trefoil (which "grows in garden plots") suspended on the body (4.17).

Pliny, unlike Dioscorides, makes no pretense to being an expert on medical matters. The dozens of amulets that he describes in his *Natural History* are part of an encyclopedic effort to catalog the entire natural world, including the benefits that humans have derived from its varied contents (plants, animals, minerals, etc.). Some of his prescriptions are similar to those cited by Dioscorides, involving the simple attachment of an object to the body, while others require elaborate ritual actions to make them effective. Some examples from the latter category will show why amulets are often classed under the heading of "magic" rather than medicine.[58]

- To cure scrofulous sores, dig up the root of a quince tree with the left hand after first drawing a ring around the tree and stating the purpose for which the root is being dug and the name of the patient, then apply it as an amulet (23.103).
- To prevent excessive menstruation, break off a branch of a newly budded mulberry tree at full moon without letting it touch the ground and tie it on the woman's upper arm (23.138).
- To keep away night fevers, wrap a couple of strangury bugs in a piece of wool stolen from shepherds and attach it to the left arm. For day fevers, wrap them in a red cloth (29.64).
- To ease childbirth, tie the sloughed-off skin of a snake to the loins of the laboring woman, but make sure to take it away immediately after delivery (30.129).

As with medicinal plants, there is nothing in any of these quasi-magical remedies that could not have been performed by an illiterate peasant or a poor city-dweller, and there is ample evidence that such treatments were in common use at this level of Greek and Roman society. But it would be wrong to limit such methods to the ignorant poor; the fact that they are commended by elite authors as effective modes of self-treatment implies that elite audiences embraced such remedies as well. Elite opinion was divided over the more elaborate techniques use by experts in *mageia*, as we will see in the next chapter, but this should not be taken as a rejection of all "non-rational" cures. Quasi-magical remedies were a vital part of the healing repertoire at all levels of Greek and Roman society, including people who joined the Christ-movement.

---

[58] The examples cited here are all ones that Pliny appears to accept as valid, excluding those that he rejects as foolish superstitions of the Magi (more on this in Chapter 3). The detailed instructions for preparing amulets in the Greek magical papyri will also be treated in Chapter 3.

Religious Cures

As medical historian Gary Ferngren notes, "Medicine and religion have had a close association throughout history, one that can be traced back to the earliest human attempts to heal the human body and to understand the meaning of illness."[59] This is as true for Greeks and Romans as for any other people: efforts to move gods, spirits, or other invisible powers to preserve or restore health are pervasive from earliest times in both cultures. Gods or spirits (including *daimones*) were believed by many to cause sickness and disability, and it was vital to maintain their favor in order to prevent or remove illness.

As in most cultures, interaction with the gods by Greeks and Romans included both individual and collective rituals and practices. Since the present chapter deals with healing at the individual and household level, the following discussion will be limited to these practices.[60] Most of the ways in which Greeks and Romans appealed to the gods regarding health have parallels in other cultures, but a few are more distinctive and thus require additional comment.

(a) The most obvious and universal mode of seeking divine assistance was *prayer*. Literature from Greco-Roman antiquity can give the impression that all prayers followed prescribed language and modes of address, but human experience shows that people in the real world do not always adhere to such strictures, especially when faced with life-threatening illness. There is no reason to think that Greeks and Romans were an exception to this pattern. But it is also true that interactions with the divine were highly regulated in both Greek and Roman cultures, so even spontaneous prayers would have tended to follow traditional models.

Greek and Roman prayers followed similar patterns. Since the gods were not necessarily paying attention or favorably disposed to individual humans, it was necessary to solicit their favor by invoking their names, titles, qualities, and so on at the beginning of the prayer. Next came the purpose for which the god was being invoked—in this case, a petition for healing—followed by various reasons for the prayer to be granted. Reasons might include the petitioner's piety, the god's beneficence and/or honor, an offering to be presented in conjunction with the prayer or in the future, or assurances of future devotion. The prayer would usually conclude with a more general evocation of the deity's favor. Redundancy and pleonasm of expression were common in Roman prayers, as was an emphasis on following precise words and forms.[61] If all was done correctly, the god was expected to act, though the expectation was not as automatic as is sometimes portrayed; Greek and Romans were keenly aware of the fickleness of the gods.

Vows also played an important role in many prayers for healing. In a vow, the sick person (or the person praying for them) promises to perform a particular act if

---

[59] *Medicine and Religion*, 1.
[60] Modes of healing that involve interaction with institutional or collective forms of religion, including visits to Asklepian sanctuaries, will be treated in Chapter 4.
[61] Summarized from James B. Rives, *Religion in the Roman Empire* (Malden, MA: Blackwell, 2007), 23–8, and Frances Hickson Hahn, "Performing the Sacred: Prayers and Hymns," in *A Companion to Roman Religion*, ed. Jörg Rüpke (Malden, MA: Wiley-Blackwell, 2011), 235–41.

the requested benefit (healing in this case) is received. The use of vows in prayer is modeled on the patronage system, where exchanges of benefits and services between inferiors and superiors were a standard element of social practice. The vow might be framed in general terms or include specific conditions that the god must fulfill for the vow to become binding. Usually it was some sort of cultic sacrifice or offering that was promised, but people were free to offer whatever they thought would move the god to act.

(b) Ritual *offerings* also played a role in ancient Greek and Roman appeals for healing. While it was theoretically possible to pray anywhere, both Greeks and Romans emphasized the value of praying in front of household images of the gods. While there were differences between Greek and Roman practice, families in both cultures gathered regularly in front of a household shrine that was associated directly or indirectly with the hearth where food was prepared and a fire was kept burning at all times. Here the head of the household offered ritualized prayers for the health and prosperity of the family, coupled with small gifts of food, wine, incense, and other materials, to the household deities. In Greek homes, these offerings were made by dropping the items into the hearth fire or (in the case of wine) onto the floor. In Roman homes, the shrine included one or more small altars and offering plates onto which the offerings were placed.

In Greek homes, Zeus and Hestia (goddess of the hearth) were the chief recipients of household worship and thus the gods to whom daily prayers for healing were most likely to be directed. In Roman households, daily devotion was directed to the Lares and Penates (guardians of the family and the pantry), Vesta (the Roman equivalent of Greek Hestia), and the male ancestral spirit of the household, known as the "genius." Small statuettes of other gods were also included in the shrine according to the preference of the *paterfamilias* and the needs of the family. In times of sickness, he might add an image of Apollo or his son, the healing god Asklepios (or Aesculapius as he was known to the Romans) to the display and present special prayers and offerings to this god as part of the family ritual.[62]

(c) Another type of religious healing activity that was used occasionally at the household level was *divination*. Divination was the art of discerning messages from the gods through the observation of signs and omens, such as the flight or birds or the entrails of a sacrificed animal. Literary sources speak mostly about divination as a public ritual, especially in the case of Rome, but divination was also used by ordinary people to interpret unusual phenomena or to seek divine assistance with perplexing problems.

With regard to sickness, the most common form of divination was the interpretation of dreams. Both popular and official opinion viewed dreams as a channel of divine communication; the challenge was to determine which ones should be taken as

---

[62] As Vivian Nutton has observed, "It is misleading to talk of 'healing gods' as if they formed a distinct category, for one could direct a prayer for assistance with health problems to any god one wished" (*Ancient Medicine*, 273–4). The vital role of Asklepios in institutional forms of religious health care will be discussed in Chapter 4.

revelatory and how they should be interpreted.[63] People who claimed to be able to interpret dreams did a thriving business, but even those who could not afford such services sought to learn from their dreams the causes and potential cures of their own or a family member's sickness. Ideally they hoped to have a god—especially Asklepios or his daughter Hygieia—visit them in a dream and provide an instantaneous cure.[64] But gods were also known to reveal the hidden causes of sickness and/or what should be done to cure them. Even rationalist physicians accepted this revelatory function of dreams and used them in their practice.[65]

(d) *Purifications and aversive rituals* were also used on occasion by ordinary Greeks and Romans as a way of removing the causes of sickness and procuring healing. Much of the evidence is indirect, but both were common enough to receive mention.

According to Ido Israelowich, "Pollution and purification were inherent features of the Greco-Roman health-care system."[66] Certain illnesses were thought to be sent by the gods as punishments for ritual pollution, especially epilepsy, and various ritual purifications were prescribed to deal with them.[67] Such ideas were common in both Greek and Roman cultures before the rise of Hippocratic medicine, and they remained influential among the illiterate masses even after they were largely rejected as *superstitio* by the elites in favor of the more rational explanations offered by the Hippocratic tradition.[68] Some forms of ritual purification could be performed by the householder, such as sprinkling water, burning incense, hanging squill or black hellebore around the house, or performing an appropriate incantation.[69] Others required a specialist of the type that will be described in Chapter 4. The popularity of these professional purifiers

[63] As Giuseppe Penso observes, "Tous les peoples anciens, sans exception, ont-ils attribué aux songes une origine divine, et l'inteprétation des songes a toujours été une partie essentielle de la science des devins" (*La Médecine Romaine*, 59). Scholars are divided over what to make of these dream reports. As John S. Hanson has observed, "Whether or not these literary reports [of dreams] have a historical basis is in most cases an irresolvable question. The accepted mode of narrating a dream or vision determines the memory or imagination of dreamers and literati alike. As a result, it is difficult to move from the literary level to actual experience" ("Dreams and Visions in the Graeco-Roman World and Early Christianity," *ANRW* 23.2.1400-01). William V. Harris, drawing on modern studies of dreams, lays out a set of criteria for assessing whether a dream report is likely to be rooted in actual experience or created out of whole cloth (*Dreams and Experience in Classical Antiquity* [Cambridge, MA and London: Harvard University Press, 2009], 105–6).

[64] As Ido Israelowich notes, "Inscriptions and literary reports testify that the appearance of a deity in a dream bearing a command was common in the dream experience in the Graeco-Roman world" (*Society, Medicine and Religion in the Sacred Tales of Aelius Aristides* [Leiden and Boston: Brill, 2012], 76.) Artemidorus's *Oneirocritica*, the oldest surviving dream-interpretation manual, has a long section on how to interpret the appearance of various gods in dreams (2.33–9), an indication that his elite readers were familiar with such experiences (noted by ibid., 84). Reports of dreams involving instant cures are known mainly from healing centers rather than private households. More will be said about this in Chapter 4.

[65] More will be said about this in Chapter 5.

[66] Ibid., 46.

[67] On epilepsy, see Garland, *Eye of the Beholder*, 126–7.

[68] Cf. Edelstein, "Greek Medicine in its Relation to Religion and Magic," 219; Dale B. Martin, *Inventing Superstition: From the Hippocratics to the Christians* (Cambridge, MA and London: Harvard University Press, 2004), 27–54.

[69] On the ritual uses of squill, see John Michael Chase, "Notes on Squill in Antiquity," in *Miroirs de la mélancholie*, ed. H. Cazes and A.-F. Morand (Paris: Hermann, 2015), 29–48. The use of black hellebore in purification is described in Dioscorides, *De mat. med.* 4.162.4. Cato relates a ritual for purifying farmland, including averting sickness, that involved sacrifices and prayers (*Agr.* 141).

despite the ridicule of the elites shows the continuing power of such beliefs among the masses.[70]

Rituals of aversion presuppose that sickness is caused by some sort of external power that must be driven off before the person can be restored to health. Most people agreed that at least some illnesses were caused by jealous or vengeful gods,[71] but Greeks and Romans also recognized the reality of dark or evil spirits in the world that sought to harm humans. Among the Greeks, the Nosoi and Keroi were the chief culprits, while the Romans linked deities with a host of illnesses, including Febris (fever), Macies (Wasting), Tabes (Corruption), Scabies (itching), and many others. *Daimones* could also be cited as a cause, though this idea was less common.[72]

Both cultures developed rituals to prevent such powers from causing harm or to eliminate their baneful effects. Amulets played an important role on the prevention side, as did ritualized gestures like spitting or holding up the hand in a "fig sign" (closed fist with the thumb protruding between the first and second fingers). Ritual purifications were also used to cleanse a place or a sick body from evil influences. Prayers and incantations were recited both to drive away harmful spirits and to enlist the aid of good ones, and exorcistic rituals were also performed on occasion, though these were more common among Jews and Christians.[73] Other aversion rituals required the presence and skills of a specialist, whether a *magus* or a priest, as we will see in Chapters 3 and 4.[74]

Quasi-Medical Cures

The final mode of treatment used by ordinary people in antiquity consisted of quasi-medical cures that could be administered in the home using readily available materials.[75] Several treatises have survived from Greek and Roman authors around the time of Paul that describe the many medicinal substances that were used by physicians and ordinary people to treat illnesses and injuries, including works by Pedanius

---

[70] The practice continued even among the early Christians—Did. 3:4 warns against being a "purifier" due to its links with idolatry.
[71] As Dale Martin observes, the more philosophically minded elites rejected this idea as "superstition" due to their belief that gods could not do evil, but such ideas did not filter down to the masses (*Inventing Superstition*, 54–78).
[72] On the mixed views of *daimones* in the ancient world, see Martin, *Inventing Superstition*, 98–107, 158–9; Luck, *Arcana Mundi*, 163–5. Still useful on the subject of divine causality is the rather dated study by Simboli, *Disease-Spirits and Divine Cures among the Greeks and Romans*. Other people were also believed to able to cause illness by casting an "evil eye" upon a victim, but this is not a specifically religious cause, so it is better dealt with in the next chapter.
[73] Exorcists are included in the list of quasi-professional experts who formed part of the Greco-Roman healing system by Vivian Nutton, "Medicine in the Greek World, 800-50 BC," in Conrad, *Western Medical Tradition*, 16; Gordon, "The Healing Event in Graeco-Roman Medicine," 363; and Ferngren, *Medicine and Religion*, 38–9. Heidi Wendt observes that Celsus includes exorcism among the skills that certain Egyptians are hawking in the marketplace, while Philostratus credits the same skill to Apollonius of Tyana (*At the Temple Gates*, 83, 126–7).
[74] Aversive techniques are a central preoccupation of the Greek magical papyri (*PGM*), while sacrifices sometimes played a similar role in the traditional temple system.
[75] The term "quasi-medical" is used here to distinguish these traditional practices from the more developed theories and methods used by practitioners who had been formally trained in medical modes of healing.

Dioscorides, Aretaeus of Cappadocia, Scribonius Largus, Aulus Cornelius Celsus, and Pliny the Elder. More information on the subject can be gleaned from other medical writers, including the Hippocratic Corpus, Soranus of Ephesus, Galen, and others.[76]

Mingled together with the many arcane and/or expensive remedies described in these texts are cures involving such common foods as wine (a virtual cure-all in antiquity), eggs, milk, cheese, cabbage, and bread. Virtually every culinary herb is said to have some kind of curative power, and the same is true for a variety of wild plants that would have been well known to anyone who had spent much time in the countryside. In fact, Pliny asserts that "illiterate country-folk" know more about healing herbs than do physicians.[77] Prescriptions are given for a broad range of illnesses and injuries affecting every part of the body—Celsus and Scribonius even catalog their treatments according to the affected body part for easy reference, as does Pliny in a less systematic way. Remedies are not limited to plants—substances taken from animals and even humans (hair, menstrual blood, bath scrapings, etc.) are also cited as cures. Some of these non-herbal treatments involve exotic animals or rare materials, but many involve materials that were readily available to ordinary people (dung, hair, suet, blood, etc.).[78]

Multiple cures are offered for virtually every ailment, particularly those that were common. Dioscorides lists over 120 substances that could be used to treat different types of abdominal troubles, including such common kitchen items as oregano, mint, celery, and olive oil. Pliny identifies nearly fifty cures for eye problems (an affliction that many scholars think Paul may have experienced based on texts like Gal. 4:15 and Gal. 6:11), including the juice of wild onions or cabbage, pounded roots of anise or dill, parsley mixed with honey, and bread dipped in wine. He also lists dozens of substances that could be applied to abrasions, wounds, and inflammations (problems that we know Paul had to address because of the beatings and whippings that he mentions in his letters), including bread sopped in vinegar, crushed radishes mixed in honey, garlic ground up in oil, and lettuce leaves pounded with barley.[79]

---

[76] The oldest surviving treatise on the medicinal use of plants is book 9 of Theophrastus's *Historia Plantarum*, which was written in the late fourth to early third centuries BCE and covers the medicinal properties of roughly sixty plants. The Hippocratic Corpus (fourth century BCE to second century CE) mentions more than 300 substances (mostly plants) that were used to treat various illnesses. By the first century CE that number had exploded to 600 in Dioscorides's *De materia medica* and 900 in Pliny the Elder's *Natural History*. Historical surveys of the Greek pharmacological tradition can be found in Plinio Prioreschi, *A History of Medicine*, Vol. 3, *Roman Medicine* (Omaha: Horatius Press, 1998), 228–45, and Keyser, "Science and Magic in Galen's Recipes (Sympathy and Efficacy)," 178–85. A thorough analysis of the pharmacological material in the Hippocratic Corpus that distinguishes traditional self-help remedies from professional medicine can be found in Laurence M. V. Totelin, *Hippocratic Recipes: Oral and Written Transmission of Pharmacological Knowledge in Fifth- and Fourth-Century Greece* (Leiden: Brill, 2008).

[77] HN 25.16; cf. 29.2–3, where he laments how "things ready to hand and appropriate have become obsolete in medical practice." Pliny places so much stock in the healing power of plants that he is willing to credit "much truth" to the most incredible of stories—see his comments in *HN* 25.13–15. Pliny concludes his review with the statement that "most authorities hold that there is nothing that cannot be achieved by the power of plants" (*HN* 25.15). Jerry Stannard summarizes Pliny's analysis with the observation, "It was the exceptional plant that did not serve in some medicinal capacity" ("Medicinal Plants and Folk Remedies in Pliny, 'Historia Naturalis,'" 10).

[78] Pliny devoted the whole of books 28–30 to remedies made from the bodies of animals and humans.

[79] Pliny's longest discussions of eye treatments are in *HN* 25.142–64, 28.167–72, and 30.117–32, but additional cures are scattered throughout his work, as are those for wounds and abrasions. Celsus

While many of these cures are fairly innocuous by modern medical standards (setting aside the question of whether they worked), others involve beliefs and practices that readers informed by Western medicine would consider ill-founded or superstitious, or both. Celsus, for example, relates a remedy for strep throat that involves burning a nestling swallow that has been preserved in salt and mixing the ashes with hydromel (a drink made of fermented honey and water) as a curative draught. The traditional origin of this remedy is evident both from his introduction ("I hear it commonly said") and from his comment that the practice "has considerable popular authority" despite being absent from medical books.[80] Pliny includes many such remedies in his *Natural History*, even when we omit the ones that he disparages as the tricks of the Magi. A quick review of books 20-32, where he surveys the medicinal uses of various plant and animal substances, reveals the following quasi-medical cures that anyone could have performed.

- To draw pus out of scrofulous neck sores, apply a mixture of pitch and barley meal boiled in the urine of a prepubescent child (24.39).
- To stop the fits of an epileptic, spit on them (28.36).
- To eliminate swelling of the groin, tie the big toe to the one next to it (28.42).
- To cure runny eyes, mix a mother's milk (preferably from a woman who has given birth to a boy) with an egg white and apply it to the forehead on a piece of wool (28.73).
- To treat conjunctivitis, swallow the dung of a she-goat covered in wax during a full moon (28.170).

No special skills or implements were required to prepare any of these remedies, nor any notable expense—the ingredients were readily available to anyone living in the countryside, though poorer city-dwellers might have found some of them unaffordable.[81] Knowledge about which remedy to use for what condition and how

---

lists nearly twenty substances that can be used to stanch bleeding, twenty for wounds, and six for swelling (*Med.* 5.1–2). Most of his prescriptions are not on Pliny's list, and many involve materials that would not have been readily available to ordinary people. Pliny's list is cited here as a better reflection of popular remedies.

[80] *Med.* 4.7. He also claims in the same passage that one can prevent the onset of this condition by eating a nestling swallow every day for a year.

[81] Cato the Elder, writing for his fellow elite landowners some 250 years before Paul, recommends a variety of natural remedies in his treatise on agriculture, including mixtures made from pomegranates, wine, honey, marjoram, and especially cabbage, which can be combined with other items to cure a wide range of ailments (*Agr.* 114–15, 122–3, 126–7, 156–7). Jane Draycott, writing about Cato's medical recipes, notes that "the ingredients required are all those which he either explicitly states were cultivated within his *hortus*, or were likely to have been" ("Literary and Documentary Evidence for Lay Medical Practice in the Roman Republic and Empire," in *Homo Patiens: Approaches to the Patient in the Ancient World*, ed. Georgia Petridou and Chiara Thumiger [Brill: Leiden, 2106], 435). Britta K. Ager's comments about Pliny's appropriation of traditional knowledge are valid for a wide range of elite authors: "Pliny remarks that many plants with useful properties remain unknown to science, although country dwellers know them; although the agronomists occasionally imply that much of their advice originated with such people, their works show a continuing effort to launder humble knowledge through natural philosophy and make it the exclusive possession of the educated; or, more charitably, to improve on traditional knowledge with modern science" ("Roman Agricultural Magic", 150–1).

it should be applied would have been passed on orally among family members and friends as part of the popular health care lore that can be found in every society. Similar channels would have been used to transmit prescriptions for managing such common bodily conditions as broken bones, dislocated joints, and complicated pregnancies. More difficult cases might have required the assistance of an outside expert such as a bone-setter or midwife, but most would have been managed within the home by family members. All of these practices are paralleled in other traditional societies.

Conclusion

As we have seen in this chapter, the health care systems of Greco-Roman antiquity were complex and multifaceted. Three distinct systems of treatment were available to people seeking expert assistance with preserving or restoring their health: "magical," religious, and medical forms of healing. Each mode had its own set of providers, its own theories regarding the causes of sickness, and its own prescriptions for treating and removing illness. There were overlaps among them, to be sure, but the differences were clear enough for people to distinguish them and choose which one best suited to their needs.

None of these systems, however, arose in a vacuum. All have deep roots in traditional home-based methods of health care that predated and prefigured the more systematized forms of care and continued to be used alongside them. Such traditional methods of healing were passed on orally from parents to children and served as the first line of treatment at all levels of society. For the many who could not afford to consult an expert, they were the only system of care.

Given the current consensus that the earliest Christ-followers came primarily from the lower end of the socio-economic scale, we can reasonably assume that their beliefs and practices regarding health care would have resembled those described in this chapter. If this is so, it raises questions about whether affiliation with the Christ-movement necessitated any changes in this area. Were they told to abandon their belief that some sicknesses were caused by jealous gods or harmful spirits? Did they have to stop wearing amulets and reciting spells to protect themselves from illness? Were they warned against eating or applying substances that had been prepared using "magical" rituals and incantations? Were prayers to Asklepios no longer allowed? Should they ignore him if he appeared to them in a dream with instructions about how they could be cured?

In short, what health care activities did people have to give up in order to demonstrate the validity of their commitment to Christ? If significant changes were required, why do we hear nothing about it in the letters of Paul or any of the other documents that were eventually included in the New Testament? Is it mere happenstance, or is it possible that Paul and his fellow leaders failed to reflect on these questions? If their silence is intentional, what might this say about their ideas regarding the parameters of acceptable behavior for Christ-followers? Does their praxis in this area tell us anything about their theology?

These are important questions that should be kept in mind as we turn to examine the three major types of health care providers that would have been available to members of Paul's congregations both before and after they became Christ-followers. Which of these practitioners might Paul have deemed acceptable for his followers and which not? Which ones might he have used to address his own health care needs? Would he have approved some of their practices and not others? What did other Jews and Christ-followers think and do in this area? These and similar questions will be investigated in Part II of this study (Chapters 8–10).

3

"Magical" Treatments

Why "Magical"?

Using the term "magic" to designate a particular set of beliefs and practices in the Greco-Roman world—practices that included certain forms of healing—has become so controversial in recent years that some justification must be offered for its retention here.

There is no question that the term "magic" has been misused in modern times as an Orientalizing Western designation for the "Exotic Other," a category that has deep roots in Western notions of cultural and racial superiority.[1] It is equally evident that modern scholarly discourse about "magic" was polluted from the start by Protestant prejudices against *ex opere operato* rituals (the product of historic conflicts with Catholicism) and modernist denigration of beliefs and practices that were judged primitive and irrational by comparison with modern scientific worldviews. The latter judgment was fortified by an uncritical reading of Greek and Roman authors, who routinely deride practitioners of *mageia* as quacks, charlatans, and frauds.[2] Reconstructing the actual beliefs and practices of such people after centuries of calumny and neglect can be challenging, to say the least.

Some interpreters despair of the attempt, insisting that all efforts to reconstruct "magic" as a historical practice are misguided. As they see it, the presence of "magic" and "magicians" in the ancient world is a literary illusion; the terms *mageia* and *magos* are polemical labels employed by ancient elites to disparage any foreign, secret, or nonofficial practice that they viewed as a threat to institutional authority. Such labels were designed "to discourage and control marginal ritual practices through belittlement, scary exaggeration. . ., silencing, and even trials, executions, and

---

[1] Brief historical surveys of modern studies of magic can be found in Derek Collins, *Magic in the Greek World* (Malden, MA: Blackwell, 2008), 1–26; Bernd-Christian Otto and Michael Stausberg, ed., *Defining Magic: A Reader* (Sheffield: Equinox, 2013), 1–12, 194–6; and Peter Schäfer, "Magic and Religion in Ancient Judaism," in *Envisioning Magic: A Princeton Seminar and Symposium*, ed. Peter Schäfer and Hans J. Kippenberg (Leiden: Brill, 1997), 19–26. Richard Horsley is also helpful on how the concept of "magic" is rooted in Western colonial encounters with beliefs and rituals that were viewed as "primitive" (*Jesus and Magic: Freeing the Gospel Stories from Modern Misconceptions* [Eugene, OR: Cascade Books, 2014], 88–9). So also Christopher I. Lehrich, "Magic in Theoretical Practice," in Otto and Strausberg, *Defining Magic*, 220–8.

[2] More will be said on this point later in the chapter.

lynchings."[3] Scholars can investigate "magic" as an elite intellectual construct—"part of a flexible and evolving vocabulary for ritual practices (and their specialists) that some cultural institutions or movements deem ambiguous or even illegitimate"[4]—but to speak as if there were people practicing "magic" in the ancient world (including "magical" healing) is to reify a discursive category. All efforts to reconstruct them are doomed to failure.

Other scholars argue that the term "magic" should be abandoned because of its perceived fruitlessness as a category for cross-cultural analysis. From its earliest days, the cross-cultural study of "magic" has been riddled with ambiguities and conflicts regarding the content, boundaries, and coherence of the term. The confusion is especially apparent in controversies over how to distinguish "magic" from religion and science.[5] Bernd-Christian Otto and Michael Strausberg offer a stark summary of the current research environment: "There is no unanimously agreed academic definition of 'magic,' nor any shared theoretical language—and apparently not even any agreement on the range or type of actions, events, thoughts or objects covered by the category."[6] David E. Aune voices a similar judgment at the end of a lengthy critical survey of recent scholarship on the subject: "The varied ways in which the term is used means that 'magic' cannot function as a properly scientific term. The English word 'magic' and its cognates . . . is burdened by far too much connotative baggage to be useful in historical study."[7] Jonathan Z. Smith speaks for many who have struggled to bring order out of this scholarly chaos: "I see little merit in continuing the use of the substantive term 'magic' in second-order, theoretical, academic discourse. . . . For any culture I am familiar with, we can trade places between the corpus of material commonly labeled 'magical' and corpora designated by other generic terms (e.g., healing, divining, execrative) with no cognitive loss."[8]

These are weighty concerns, to be sure, and they must be taken seriously by anyone who wants to talk about "magic" as a social phenomenon in Greco-Roman antiquity. But they are by no means fatal to the present enterprise. Most of the problems cited earlier can be traced to a persistent scholarly quest for macro-level explanations at the expense of micro-level analysis.

The modern study of "magic" began over a century ago when scholars like E. B. Tylor and James Frazer attempted to construct from Western observations of "primitive" societies a cross-cultural category of "magical" (i.e., "non-rational") thinking that led pre-scientific peoples to develop ineffectual rituals to manipulate nonexistent invisible forces in an effort to control their environment. The modernist and Eurocentric value-judgments embedded in this enterprise were rejected long ago by Western scholars of "magic," but only recently have interpreters acknowledged that the very act of

---

[3] Horsley, *Jesus and Magic*, 93. This view is laid out more fully by David Frankfurter, "Introduction," in Frankfurter, *Guide to the Study of Ancient Magic*, 29–35.
[4] Frankfurter, "Introduction," 29.
[5] A good critical summary of these debates can be found in David E. Aune, "'Magic' in Early Christianity and Its Ancient Mediterranean Context: A Survey of Some Recent Scholarship," *Annali di storia dell'esegesi* 24 (2007): 229–94.
[6] *Defining Magic*, 1.
[7] Aune, "Magic," 293.
[8] Jonathan Z. Smith, "Trading Places," in Meyer and Mirecki, *Ancient Magic*, 16.

searching for examples of "magic" in a given culture reflects certain *a priori* judgments about the existence, content, markers, and importance of a cross-cultural category called "magic." Why, they ask, should this or that unusual belief or practice be lumped together with others from the same or different cultures and labeled as "magic"? What is gained from making such cross-cultural generalizations, and what is lost? Do they help us to better understand local cultures, or do they merely obfuscate? Who benefits and who loses in these comparative studies?

These and similar questions have led to a growing scholarly consensus that studies of "magic," if they are to be performed at all, should focus on a single society or culture with a view to explicating its particular understanding and experience of "magic" rather than beginning with a pre-formulated category of "magical" beliefs and practices and looking for examples that fit the definition. But this definition of the scholarly task still leaves unanswered the question of what should be construed as "magic" in such a localized study. Two different answers have been put forward by scholars who have grappled with this question.

One solution is to use insights from traditional studies of "magic" as a guide for identifying localized expressions of broader cross-cultural patterns. Bernd-Christian Otto and Michael Strausberg coined the phrase "patterns of magicity" to describe what this approach seeks to uncover. Practices that might signify the influence of "magic" in a society include ascribing efficacy to specific words uttered in ritual sequences; associating power with particular signs, objects, or places; believing that humans can control or harm other people through the use of rituals; ascribing miraculous powers to certain people; and similar patterns of thought and action.[9] David Frankfurter sounds similar themes when he opines that the category of "magic" "highlights for our scholarly scrutiny features of materiality, potency, or verbal or ritual performance we might not otherwise appreciate as part of a culture's religious world, or aspects of the social location of ritual practices we might not otherwise appreciate."[10] Such observations are useful insofar as they call our attention to cross-cultural patterns that might otherwise be overlooked, but questions remain about whether classifying these patterns as examples of "magic" undermines the effort to understand their meaning and function within the local culture.

A second solution that has garnered significant support among scholars relies on a functional definition of "magic." Under this approach, "magic" is a social construct reflecting the judgment of people in power that certain beliefs and practices are culturally deviant or inappropriately practiced. Kimberly Stratton's definition is typical: the term "magic" refers to "culturally specific ideas about illegitimate and dangerous access to numinous power."[11] In this definition, the category of "magic" has no fixed

---

[9] *Defining Magic*, 11.

[10] "Ancient Magic in a New Key: Refining an Exotic Discipline in the History of Religions," in Frankfurter, *Guide to the Study of Ancient Magic*, 13–14.

[11] "Magic Discourse in the Ancient World," in Otto and Strausberg, *Defining Magic*, 245. A similar definition is offered by Paul T. Keyser: "Magic may be usefully defined as 'excluded practices depending for their effect on forces or powers in the world beyond human understanding.' The contrast is at once with technology: 'accepted practices based on powers within human understanding,' and with religion: 'accepted practices depending on powers beyond human understanding'" ("Science and Magic," 175).

content, since cultures have different ideas about what counts as "illegitimate and dangerous" knowledge or behavior. Societal out-groups are a common target for such labeling, but it can also be a tactic for mitigating the influence of ritual experts whom the authorities believe are misappropriating or misusing public symbols, objects, or rituals by divorcing them from their culturally accepted setting and employing them for private purposes. In both instances, the labeling of certain people and practices as "magical" can have serious social consequences by identifying them as suitable targets for control and sanction, whether verbal, relational, or penal.[12] To study "magic," then, is to identify those beliefs and practices that a given society categorizes as "magical" and to describe the consequences that arise from such classifications, including who benefits and who suffers from these constructions.

This solution is more flexible than the first one, but it is too narrow and rigid to account for all of the evidence. Critics have pointed out that "magic" is not always an ascriptive term applied by outsiders; it can also be a category of self-definition. This is especially true for Greco-Roman antiquity where, as Einar Thomassen rightly observes, "The evidence from literature, curse tablets and the magical papyri leaves no doubt that there actually existed in all periods of antiquity individuals who saw themselves as practising what society at large called *mageia*, *goeteia*, etc." He goes on to remark that in this era, "the category of magic is not merely the expression of an ideological prejudice against 'the other'; it was also a profession and a practice understood by its practitioners as being something different from the official cult of the gods."[13] David Lincicum agrees, noting that "it seems clear . . . from a myriad of texts that the practitioners themselves were aware of doing something different in adjuring a spirit than in praying to God and that such actions were subject to varying social judgments."[14]

So where does this leave us? In the first place, these observations suggest that we should avoid broad, cross-cultural generalizations about the nature and qualities of "magic" and focus instead on how Greeks and Romans understood the term and where practitioners of "magic" fit into their social world.[15] In short, we should adopt an "emic," rather than an "etic," methodology for analyzing our data.[16] The task is clearer in the

---

[12] Stratton, "Magic Discourse in the Ancient World," 248.
[13] "Is Magic a Subclass of Ritual?" in *The World of Ancient Magic: Papers from the First International Samson Eitrem Seminar at the Norwegian Institute at Athens May 4–8, 1997*, ed. David R. Jordan, Hugo Montgomery, and Einar Thomassen (Bergen: Paul Astroms, 1999), 57.
[14] "Scripture and Apotropaism in the Second Temple Period," *Biblische Notizen* 138 (2008): 64.
[15] The investigation will be broadened later to include Judeans and Christians, who of course were influenced by Greek and Roman ideas (Chapters 8–10).
[16] Kimberly Stratton explains this point well: "It is only this emic approach that will illuminate how, when and why a particular practice or person is labeled magic in a specific context and what that reveals about larger social dynamics in the society being considered. Applying the label magic to practices that meet modern definitions of magic (i.e., contrasted with contemporary notions of science or religion) but are not regarded as magic by ancient observers obfuscates our understanding of what magic meant and how it operated (or did not operate) in that culture" ("Magic Discourse in the Ancient World," 248). At the same time, we must acknowledge with Yuval Harari that it is impossible to maintain an absolute barrier between emic and etic approaches since all interpretation begins with assumptions about what we are looking for and what we find must always be interpreted ("Ancient Israel and Early Judaism," in Frankfurter, *Guide to the Study of Ancient Magic*, 141–2).

case of Greeks and Romans than for some other societies since there is no question that "magic" played a role in ancient social discourse—the Greek word *mageia* and its Latin derivative *magia* appear often in their respective literatures. But we do need to be careful about presuming that Greeks and Romans held identical views about "magic" and its practitioners. Only historical research can tell us if that was the case.

Secondly, we must keep in mind the often polemical nature of the term "magic" in both Greek and Roman usage and avoid equating rhetoric with social reality. Much of the extant literature paints "magic" and "magicians" in a negative light, but these are the views of the elites, not those of ordinary people. As Heidi Wendt observes, "Most writers are more interested in denouncing them as charlatans or inculpating them in some mishap than they are in accurately describing their teachings and practices or explaining their appeal."[17] The fact that elite authors felt compelled to speak so forcefully against these practices suggests that *mageia/magia* was popular with the masses, a fact that some authors grudgingly admit. Their writings can help us to understand the kinds of activities that upper-class citizens defined (and in most cases rejected) as "magic," but we should not assume that ordinary townspeople and farmers held similar opinions. What the elites regarded as "magical" healing techniques, for instance, might have appeared to the masses as no different than other ritual modes of healing.

Finally, we must learn what we can about the various Greek and Roman healing experts who defined their work in "magical" terms, including what kinds of services they offered, who used them, and why.[18] Most of this information will come from counter-readings of elite literature, but there is also a limited amount of archaeological evidence that can be applied to this purpose. Investigating how these people viewed and practiced their trade can give us a counterweight to the prejudiced views of the elites. The importance of this observation will become apparent later when we discuss the health care options that would have been available to Paul and his congregations, since virtually all of his converts hailed from the lower levels of society.

"Magic" in the Greco-Roman World

The history of the term "magic" in Greco-Roman antiquity is long and colorful, and only the high points can be noted here.[19] The noun μάγος (pl. μάγοι) entered Greek

---

[17] *At the Temple Gates*, 4.
[18] Since this study is concerned with healing practices, our investigation will be limited to people who offered services in this area. Other forms of "magic"—prosperity, curses, love charms, and so on—will be left to the side.
[19] For more thorough treatments of the subject, see Janowitz, *Magic in the Roman World*; Dickie, *Magic and Magicians in the Greco-Roman World*; Fritz Graf, *Magic in the Ancient World*, trans. Franklin Philip (Cambridge and London: Harvard University Press, 1997); "Excluding the Charming: The Development of the Greek Concept of Magic," in Meyer and Mirecki, *Ancient Magic*, 30–42; and James B. Rives, "Magus and Its Cognates in Classical Latin," in *Magical Practice in the Latin West*, ed. R. L. Gordon and F. Marco Simón (Leiden: Brill, 2010), 53–77. The following summary draws heavily on their narratives.

literature through Herodotus (484–425 BCE),[20] who used the plural form to designate both a tribe of the Medes (*Hist.* 1.101) and members of a Median priestly class who served the Persians by reciting chants, offering sacrifices, reading omens, pouring libations, conducting funeral rites, and interpreting dreams (*Hist.* 1.107, 1.120. 1.128, 1.132, 1.140, 7.19, 7.37, 7.43, 7.113, 7.191). In all but one instance (1.132) he portrays them as advisers who traveled with the king and not as religious officials serving local communities. Only once does he speak of them using anything like "magical" skills to influence the powers of nature, when they cause a storm to cease by offering sacrifices to the gods and chanting spells (7.191). A similar picture of μάγοι is given by two other ancient authors who were familiar with the Persians, Xenophon (430–354 BCE) and Aristotle (384–322 BCE).[21] There is little in these early references that would distinguish Persian μάγοι from any other official ritual experts in antiquity (e.g., priests, augurs), and virtually nothing that would qualify them as practitioners of "magic."

So where did the common Greek and Roman image of μάγοι as dangerous performers of dark arts come from? As we saw in Chapter 2, many of the practices that would eventually be classified as "magic" (μαγεία)—chants, spells, purifications, exorcisms, amulets, etc.—were employed from hoary antiquity by ordinary Greeks and Romans as mechanisms for coping with the vagaries and uncertainties of life.[22] We can now add to that picture the fact that such rituals were not only performed by members of the family; various types of ritual experts were also available from ancient times to address problems that exceeded the competency of the household to manage. Some lived in the local community, while others traveled from place to place as their services were needed. Some were women, especially in small villages and hamlets where the practice of midwifery included the use of spells, amulets, and other rituals to protect both mother and baby from the power of evil spirits.[23] Many plied their trade in rural areas, but we also find references to ritual experts who wandered from door to door in the cities offering their services to anyone who could pay.

By the first century CE, some of these traditional forms of ritual expertise had evolved into what we might, for lack of a better term, call "disciplines" or schools of practice that offered different services to the general public. Some oversaw the digging and harvesting of plants for medicinal use, while others compounded these plants into medicines and sold them in the agora. Some were experts in the chanting of spells and incantations, while others specialized more narrowly in curses or exorcisms. Some created amulets or carved gems to avert evil spirits, while others concocted potions to

---

[20] The validity of an earlier (sixth-century BCE) reference by the philosopher Heraclitus of Ephesus is disputed for two reasons: it appears to portray them as a Greek phenomenon, and it is only known from a brief comment by Clement of Alexandria some 700 years later.

[21] Xenophon mentions them twice (*Cyrop.* 8.1.23, 8.3.11). Aristotle's views are known only from later authors quoting a lost book that he is said to have written on the Magi. The texts are laid out at https://www.ancientmedicine.org/home/2018/3/11/aristotles-lost-book-on-magic.

[22] Matthew Dickie, an expert on ancient magic, confirms this observation: "Many of the techniques and practices that were later held to constitute sorcery were in existence in the Greek-speaking world long before there is any sign of the emergence of magic as a distinct category of thought" (*Magic and Magicians in the Greco-Roman World*, 22).

[23] Much work has been done on this topic in recent years; see Dickie, *Magic and Magicians in the Greco-Roman World*, 79–81, 91–3, 108, 131–4.

elicit love, avert jealousy, or stir up hatred. Some divined the future through dreams and omens, while others performed rituals to appease the gods or ensure good fortune. Some even claimed to be able to control the forces of nature. Most learned their skills through apprenticeship or residence with an existing practitioner.[24] Some were literate and thus able to learn from (often secret) books as part of their education, but most relied on oral and experiential instruction.[25]

More will be said later about the practitioners in this list whose skills included healing. First, however, we must address the broader question of why so many of these traditional practices came to be lumped together and defined negatively as μαγεία and what effects (if any) such a categorization might have had on their marketability. Two social and intellectual movements contributed heavily to giving "magic" a bad name: Greek philosophy and Hippocratic medicine.[26]

Philosophy and Magic

Plato typifies the philosophical disdain for "magic." Writing some fifty years after Herodotus introduced Persian μάγοι to the Greek world, he speaks critically about a class of "beggar priests and diviners" who "go to the doors of the rich man and persuade him that the gods have provided them with a ***power based on sacrifices and incantations***." He summarizes their appeals as follows: "If he himself, or his ancestors, has committed some injustice, they can ***heal it with pleasures and feasts***; and if he wishes to ruin some enemies at small expense, he will injure just and unjust alike with certain ***evocations and spells***. They, as they say, persuade the gods to serve them" (*Rep.* 364b–c, highlights mine).[27] He goes on to say that they

> present a babble of ***books by Musaeus and Orpheus***, . . . according to whose prescriptions they busy themselves about their ***sacrifices***. They persuade ***not only private persons, but cities as well***, that through ***sacrifices and pleasurable games*** there are, after all, deliverances and purifications from unjust deeds for those still living. And there are also ***rites for those who are dead***. These, which they call initiations, deliver us from the evils in the other place; while, for those who did not ***sacrifice***, terrible things are waiting. (*Rep.* 364e–365a, highlights mine)

Two broad conclusions can be drawn from this passage. First, the highlighted phrases show that these "beggar priests and diviners" were in fact ritual experts who taught that the gods could be placated and their punishments averted by performing appropriate

---

[24] For more on this point, see Graf, *Magic in the Ancient World*, 4–5; Luck, *Arcana Mundi*, 15–16.

[25] On the latter point, see Dickie, *Magic and Magicians in the Greco-Roman World*, 67, 98. On the secrecy that surrounded "magical" books, Fritz Graf offers the following observation: "Given the largely esoteric nature of ancient magic, to which most often one could have access only after undergoing initiatory rites, these books were no doubt transmitted in closed circles, from master to disciple, from father to son" (*Magic in the Ancient World*, 4–5).

[26] The chief proponent of this interpretation is classical philologist Fritz Graf, whose work has been taken up by many others. See especially *Magic in the Ancient World*, 30–5.

[27] This and the following quotations are drawn from Allan Bloom's translation, *The Republic of Plato*, 2nd ed. (New York: Basic Books, 1991).

rituals, including sacrifices, incantations, spells, feasts, games, sacrifices, and rites for the dead. There is nothing unusual about this list; every act on it could be found in the civic cult. Even the verbal rituals that Plato mentions—spells, incantations, and curses—have parallels in the language of civic prayers and imprecations against public enemies and violators of cultic sites.[28]

What makes these people problematic is their status as "freelance religious experts" who claim to have an influence with the gods that exceeds that of the civic cult.[29] It is highly unlikely that such self-appointed experts would ever have succeeded in persuading the Athenian authorities to follow their advice, but the very audacity of their effort would have evoked opposition from the elites. Their use of esoteric books also troubles Plato, though he does not say why. At a minimum, such concerns reveal a division in the ranks of the literati regarding the sources and proper application of cultic power, a division that threatened the unity of the city and the authority of the officials who guided its affairs.[30] The ability to interpret such books also gave their users an almost numinous authority in the eyes of the illiterate masses, a fact that would have elicited charges of *hubris* and demagoguery from the educated elites.

Plato's second reason for objecting to these private ritual experts is theological: his opponents' insistence that rituals can manipulate or even compel the gods to forgive sins or inflict harm upon humans is immoral and unworthy of the divine dignity (*Laws* 933 AB, 10.909 AB). Plato had similar concerns about the poets, whom he proposed to exclude from his ideal republic to prevent them from corrupting civic virtue with their scandalous tales about the gods. Other philosophers shared Plato's repugnance at the way the gods were depicted in poetry and popular drama, but their alarms were ignored by the masses whose ideas were much closer to those of the wandering priests. This division of opinion is yet another reason for both the popularity of these "freelance religious experts" and the negative way in which elite authors like Plato portrayed them.

---

[28] When framing the laws of his ideal city, Plato proposes strict penalties for those who use sorceries, incantations, and spells to harm others: death if the person is a diviner (μάντις) or soothsayer (τερατοσκόπος) (i.e., a professional ritual expert) or financial payments if the person is a layman (*Laws*, 933a–934a). Fear of personal harm is one of the persistent anxieties about *mageia* in the Greek and Roman world.

[29] This felicitous term serves as the central organizing concept in Heidi Wendt's analysis of wandering religious experts (including the apostle Paul) in her book *At the Temple Gates*. Cf. Frankfurter, "Magic," 726: "Magic is not the misuse or misunderstanding of these [ritual] materials but simply their use outside of their institutional setting as potent symbols of an authoritative tradition." Einar Thomassen makes a similar point, arguing that the privatization of rituals in a "magical" context upsets the normal ritual balance between individuals and the collective and thus opens the door to antisocial activity in a way that public rituals do not ("Is Magic a Subclass of Ritual?," 63–5).

[30] Matthew Dickie highlights the importance of books in the trade of the soothsayer and the authority that inhered in those who could interpret them in a mostly illiterate society: "The stock-in-trade of the successful soothsayer of the entrepreneurial type was characteristically his possession of a book or books of oracles. .... The possession of a book of oracles invested its possessor with power and authority" (*Magic and Magicians in the Greco-Roman World*, 68). He goes on to observe that "most soothsayers were probably not respected. They seem to have been thought of as sharp operators and not as respectable members of society," that is, as quacks or charlatans (70). The relevance of these observations for Paul will become clear in Chapters 9 and 10.

Plato does not use the term μάγοι to describe these experts,³¹ but his account of their activities is virtually identical to what later authors include under that heading. His preferred term for such activities is γοητεία, an older label that became virtually synonymous with μαγεία in popular usage. Derived from the Greek word for "lament," γοητεία invariably carries a negative connotation in elite usage, as reflected in its usual English translation as "sorcery." The noun γόης, referring to a person who practices γοητεία, appears often in company with words like ἀλαζών ("imposter, charlatan") and ἀγύρται ("vagabond") that further underline its negative valence. Other words that formed part of the same complex include μάντις (diviner), ἐπῳδός (chanter), θαυματοποιός (wonder-worker), and φαρμακεύς (drug-maker). Judging by the surviving literature, whatever distinctions may have existed among these terms in ancient times had been largely lost by the classical era.³²

If we broaden our review of Plato to include these additional words, we find even more negative judgments against those who practice such crafts. In *Rep.* 598d and *Soph.* 234c he depicts them as artful deceivers of the young and simple-minded who puff them up with false knowledge, while in *Rep.* 602d and *Soph.* 235a he insists that they offer only a poor imitation of the truth. In *Rep.* 601b and 607c-d he compares their work with the subtle deceptions of the poets, while in *Soph.* 241b he classes them with "false-workers" and sophists. In *Symp.* 215c-d he speaks ironically of Socrates "bewitching" his hearers with his words to the point that they become irresistible, while in *Rep.* 608a he speaks of true knowledge as a "countercharm" to the charms of poetry.³³ In short, he claims that the practitioners of γοητεία follow the same false and deceptive path as the poets and Sophists: they appeal to the non-rational faculties of the soul as opposed to the philosopher's rational quest to illuminate the soul with truth.³⁴

In summary, Plato criticizes the practitioners of "magic" on three grounds: (a) they work outside the established cult and so threaten the stability of the city; (b) they hold a faulty view of the gods, whom they believe can be manipulated to do their bidding;

---

31 Plato's use of the μαγ- word group is limited and diverse. When describing the training of the heir to the Persian throne (*Alc.* 122a), he refers to the μαγεία of Zoroaster in a way that reveals an awareness of its original meaning. In *Rep.* 572e, by contrast, he uses the noun μάγοι in a figurative sense that implies a negative valuation of the category. Finally, in *Stat.* 280e he uses the related word μαγευτικός ("magical") in conjunction with ἀλεξιφάρμακα, a plural noun that can mean "antidotes," "remedies," or "charms." This association suggests that he was aware of the early link between μαγεία and healing. The latter two texts are discussed by Shaily Shashikant Patel in her 2017 PhD dissertation from the University of North Carolina, "Magical Practices and Discourses of Magic in Early Christian Traditions: Jesus, Peter, and Paul," 66–7.

32 Matthew Dickie's summary reflects the common judgment: "Although there are indications that *goetes, epodoi, magoi* and *pharmakeis* originally pursued quite distinct callings, there is no indication when the terms are first encountered in the fifth century that they refer to specialized forms of magic. The terms seem, so far as their denotation goes, to be interchangeable" (*Magic and Magicians in the Greco-Roman World*, 14; cf. Collins, *Magic in the Greek World*, 60–1).

33 References from Elizabeth Belfiore, "Epode, Elenchus and Magic: Socrates as Silenus," *Phoenix* 34 (1980): 128.

34 The same idea is found several decades before Plato in Gorgias's *Encomium to Helen* 10, where he describes how μαγεία καὶ γοητεία (used here as a hendiadys) lead the soul into error in the same way that an incantation (ἐπῳδή) removes pain and brings pleasure: by conversing only with the δόξα ("opinion") of the soul and not with its νοῦς ("reason").

and (c) they appeal to human emotions rather than to reason as they seek to entice others into their errors.

Medicine and Magic

Plato does not mention healing as one of the services offered by the ritual experts that he opposes, but criticisms relating to "magical" forms of healing can be found in some of the medical writings from the early followers of Hippocrates. Examples are scattered throughout the literature, but the concerns are stated most forcefully in *De morbo sacro* (*On the Sacred Disease*), which is also one of the earliest treatises in the Hippocratic Corpus, dating from around the time of Plato (400 BCE).

The "sacred disease" that forms the focal point of this treatise is what we today call epilepsy. It was regarded as sacred by many Greeks who viewed its sudden onset and violent manifestations as signs that the person's body had been temporarily taken over by some sort of suprahuman spirit, whether a god or a *daimon*. Writing against this view, the author of *De morbo sacro* insists that this disease is no more sacred than any other. His point is not that divine causality of disease should be rejected but rather that all diseases have divine origins since everything that exists is imbued with divinity. But divinity works through the elements of the natural world, in this case a hereditary defect in the brain that is exacerbated either by internal changes in cranial fluids or by external shifts in the wind-patterns.[35] Nothing can be done about the defective brain, but the physician can temper the illness by applying the same regimen as with other illnesses, such as, regulating the internal and external influences on the brain.[36]

The novelty of this diagnosis is apparent from the energy with which the author seeks in Chapters 2 and 3 to refute both the popular belief in divine causality and the treatment regimens of those who held this view. He rails against these traditional practitioners, whom he describes as "the magicians, purifiers, charlatans, and quacks of our own day, men who claim great piety and superior knowledge" (μάγοι τε καὶ καθάρται καὶ ἀγύρται καὶ ἀλαζόνες, ὁκόσοι δὴ προσποιέονται σφόδρα θεοσεβέες εἶναι καὶ πλέον τι εἰδέναι).[37] He attributes their diagnosis and treatment of the disease to a combination of ignorance and trickery: "Being at a loss, and having no treatment which would help, they concealed and sheltered themselves behind superstition, and called this illness sacred, in order that their utter ignorance might not be manifest." He describes their prescriptions—incantations, ritual purifications, abstinence from baths and certain foods, avoidance of black robes and goatskins, refraining from putting one hand or foot on top of the other—in mocking tones, accepting only their culinary practices as potentially helpful. Just as he earlier listed μάγοι first among the

---

[35] The explanation, which sounds quite logical in view of ancient understandings of the body, occupies the bulk of the treatise (chapters 6–20 out of 21 chapters).
[36] The author does not specify any particular treatments, but rather presumes in chapter 21 that the physician knows and can apply general Hippocratic prescriptions regarding the regulation of bodily fluids and external influences.
[37] Except for καθάρται, these are the same words that we encountered in Plato, though more prominence is given here to μάγοι. English translations are taken from the Loeb edition by W. H. S. Jones.

practitioners, so he mentions them again when he summarizes their treatment regimen as "purifications and magic arts" (οἷός τε περικαθαίρων ... καὶ μαγεύων).

Like Plato, the author accuses these practitioners of impiety for thinking that their own acts can manipulate the gods to do their bidding, whether by healing or more spectacular feats: "They profess to know how to bring down the moon, to eclipse the sun, to make storm and sunshine, rain and drought, the sea impassable and the earth barren" (4.1-4). Such claims are impious since they imply either that the gods do not exist or that they lack the power to act apart from human efforts (4.8-9). The same criticism applies to their diagnostic system, which the author lampoons in a famous piece of satire (4.21-34).

> If the patient imitate a goat, if he roar, or suffer convulsions in the right side, they say that the Mother of the Gods is to blame. If he utter a piercing and loud cry, they liken him to a horse and blame Poseidon. Should he pass some excrement, as often happens under the stress of the disease, the surname Enodia is applied. If it be more frequent and thinner, like that of birds, it is Apollo Nomius. If he foam at the mouth and kick, Ares has the blame. When at night occur fears and terrors, delirium, jumpings from the bed and rushings out of doors, they say that Hecate is attacking or that heroes are assaulting.[38]

Whether these verses reflect actual diagnostic practices or hyperbolic extrapolations from the healers' teachings is unclear, but the author's disapproval of both their theories and their practices could hardly be clearer. Such "magical" modes of healing, he insists, are impious and ineffectual; if anyone is ever healed by them, it is due to the ordinary working of natural forces and not their absurd ritual acts. They claim to have superior knowledge, but in reality they are simply covering up their own ignorance and deceiving others. In short, they are incompetent frauds.[39]

The Ancient Discourse of Magic

Despite their obvious differences, Plato and the author of *De morbo sacro* shared one vital social fact: both were trying to carve out a niche for their theories in a society where the vast majority of people thought differently than they did about the nature of the universe and how people ought to live within it. Those of us who were nurtured in Western or Western-influenced cultures where Greek philosophy and modern medicine have been persistently valorized can easily forget that men like Plato and Hippocrates were not speaking for the majority of people in their society but were rather a small group of elite males pioneering a new intellectual and social path that

---

[38] While such diagnoses might seem ludicrous to us, they would have found a ready audience among the masses since, as Dale Martin observes, "The assumption that gods and other superhuman beings (such as daimons) may be vengeful or jealous or cause disease was shared by most people around the ancient Mediterranean throughout antiquity" (*Inventing Superstition*, 54).

[39] The polemical nature of these claims will become especially apparent in Chapter 5, where we will see physicians approving many of the practices that are elsewhere classified as magic, such as incantations, amulets, purifications, and dream interpretation.

challenged deeply held beliefs and accepted practices. This was true even for their fellow elites; as Fritz Graf has noted, "There were those Athenian citizens of the upper classes who believed in the efficacy of magic and who therefore used the services offered by the seers and begging priests; and the vast majority of Athenians must have shared their attitude."[40] Dale Martin agrees: "There is simply no evidence that the majority of people in the ancient Mediterranean ever gave up most of the ideas and behaviors labelled 'superstitious' by the philosophers."[41]

As with all such movements, success required them to distinguish their ideas from the broader culture, a task that involved not only arguing for the superiority of their worldview but also deprecating long-established ideas and practices. One of their strategies was to forge a negative category of "magic" out of a diverse set of opposing practices to serve as a foil for their views. Such "discourses of alterity" rely on overgeneralization, caricature, hyperbole, and even lying to overturn accepted norms.[42] Labeling their opponents as μάγοι and their practices as μαγεία was a key weapon in this strategy, since both terms recalled the ritual experts (μάγοι) of the hated and recently defeated Persians.[43] Tactics like these are a common though regrettable practice of many new social movements, including those in antiquity.

In view of these circumstances, we should not presume that the depictions of "magicians" and their practices that we encounter in the writings of Plato and Hippocrates (and their successors) are either representative or historically accurate. As we will see later in this chapter, the evidence that we possess regarding the actual beliefs and practices of the people whom they attacked shows that they were neither. Instead, we should regard their ideas as part of a broader discourse of "magic" that emerged in the fifth century BCE and dominated the thinking of elite intellectuals in both Greek and Roman societies for many centuries until it was taken up and Christianized by the early church.[44]

What was included in this discourse? Classical historian Matthew Dickie, after surveying a broad variety of evidence from the writings of Greek historians, dramatists,

---

[40] "Excluding the Charming," 34.
[41] *Inventing Superstition*, 228.
[42] The term comes from Kimberley Stratton, "Magic Discourse in the Ancient World," 247. Stratton relies heavily on the work of Michel Foucault when discussing the agonistic nature of magical discourse. Cf. Dickie, *Magic and Magicians in the Greco-Roman World*, 20.
[43] As Ella Faye Wallace observes, "It is a well-established trope of the classical tradition to claim that practices considered unsavory or heretical are external and foreign to one's own people" ("Sorcerer's Pharmacy," 81). For more on this point, see Otto and Strausberg, *Defining Magic*, 16; Graf, "Excluding the Charming," 36; Janowitz, *Magic in the Roman World*, 9. Pliny the Elder claims that the μάγοι of his own day are the heirs of an oral tradition that originated when various Greeks traveled to Persia to learn the lore of the Persian priests (*HN* 30.8–10), but this is pure speculation on his part.
[44] Matthew Dickie devotes two lengthy chapters to a historical analysis of "magic" in the Roman world and another to its appropriation and regulation by Christians in the first three centuries CE (*Magic and Magicians in the Greco-Roman World*, 135–262). Of special interest for this study is his observation that the view of "magic" in Horace's Fifth Epode (first century BCE) "is essentially Plato's conception of magic with the addition of the idea that magic is an essentially misguided attempt to defeat the ordinary course of nature" (135).

poets, medical writers, and others, offers the following summary of the claims and practices that they attribute to "magical" practitioners.[45]

> *Magoi* hold out the promise of prolonging life. They also practise incantations and purifications. The incantations they intone in their purificatory rituals are characterized by barbaric and unintelligible sounds. *Goetes* and *epodoi* offer initiation into ecstatic mystery-rites *(teletai)*. *Magoi* are able through the techniques they employ to bring about the disappearance of persons. They are also able, through engaging in a mystery-rite *(telete)*, to pull the moon out of the sky, cause the sun to disappear and effect alterations in the weather.

Elsewhere he adds that they use love-potions and incantations to attract or repel potential lovers and that they operate in secrecy.[46]

Much of this material is the product of hearsay and dramatic license, but drama has to have some basis in reality in order to be understood, even if that reality exists only in people's minds. Most likely there were people in the Greek world who claimed the power to do most of these things, but their claims and activities were viewed quite differently by the elites, who generally embraced the worldview of the philosophers and physicians, and the masses, who did not.

Whether this discourse also had social consequences is unclear. No laws were passed against "magic" until the Roman imperial era, and even then they were rarely enforced.[47] The few cases that are recorded involve members of the elite class, not the broader populace. Practitioners who worked at the lower end of the social pyramid (the vast majority) performed their rites with little concern for legal or social sanction except for the rare occasion when a member of the local elite was accused of using their services to curse or harm another member of their class or when a Roman official or an unruly mob felt the need to reduce foreign influences in the city.[48] It was not uncommon for elite citizens to dabble in "magical" lore and practices, and if we include people like root-cutters and amulet-makers in our idea of "magic," we can affirm with certainty that the elites made regular use of "magical" services. An urbane Roman like Pliny the Elder could even undertake a semi-serious inquiry into the subject without suffering any evident social consequences.[49] As far as we know, however, few members

---

[45] *Magic and Magicians in the Greco-Roman World*, 33. Dickie's full argument for the fifth century BCE origins of the discourse of "magic" is laid out in pp. 27–43.

[46] *Magic and Magicians in the Greco-Roman World*, 36–9.

[47] The term *magia* does not appear in Roman literature until the late Republican period, when its connotations are entirely negative. As Daniel Ogden observes, "For all that that magic spread over the entire world, it is presented as fundamentally external and antithetical to Roman culture" (*Magic, Witchcraft, and Ghosts in the Greek and Roman Worlds*, 44; cf. Dickie, *Magic and Magicians in the Greco-Roman World*, 135–41).

[48] For details, see Dickie, *Magic and Magicians in the Greco-Roman World*, 142–60. Ancient sources speak of three instances when astrologers and magicians were expelled from Rome—in 33 BCE, 16 CE, and 68 CE (Dickie, *Magic and Magicians in the Greco-Roman World*, 185–6).

[49] The highly negative portrait of *magi* that we see in Pliny's writings would have insulated him from any immediate charges of sympathy with their practices, but the fact that he describes so many of their treatments for his readers and approves practices that are similar to theirs suggests that their influence on him was greater than he admits.

of the educated elite ever seriously practiced the magical arts, so those practitioners who relied on books must have passed the skill of reading from father to son.[50] In any event, the negative discourse of magic appears to have had little social impact except at the elite level, where it marked certain people and practices as targets for censure without precluding the use of their skills.

"Magical" Healers

So what kinds of health care experts should be included in a survey of "magical" healing? What criteria should be used to identify them? Should we focus on the providers themselves or on the practices that they employed? Were certain practitioners regarded as "magical" per se, or did people's assessments of them vary according to the skills that they applied in a given situation?

One possible criterion for differentiating "magical" healing from other methods of treating illness is whether the practitioner claims to be able to manipulate or even compel suprahuman forces to do his or her bidding by the skilled application of words and rituals. The classic scholarly belief that this is a sine qua non for distinguishing "magic" from religion has been properly criticized by investigators who have demonstrated that it does not apply to all cultures and that similar ideas have been held in many societies (including those of the Greeks and Romans) with regard to non-magical rituals.[51] But the fact that such claims fail as universal norms does not mean that they are invalid for the cultures that we are studying here. The belief that properly performed rituals can move the gods to act was a staple of both Greek and Roman religion, whether civic or personal, so we need not worry that we are imposing external standards if we find them holding similar ideas about "magical" healing rituals.[52] In fact, there is ample evidence from ancient authors that this is precisely what they thought was happening when people performed acts of μαγεία or γοητεία and that at least some practitioners made such claims for themselves.

Both Plato and the author of *De morbo sacro* accuse their opponents of advertising their power to move the gods. In *Rep.* 364b-c, Plato paraphrases them as saying that "the gods have provided them with a power based on sacrifices and incantations" and that "they ... persuade the gods to serve them." Similar claims appear in *Morb. sac.* 4, where the author charges μάγοι and others with asserting that they "know how to bring down the moon, to eclipse the sun, to make storm and sunshine, rain and drought, the sea impassable and the earth barren ... by rites or by some cunning or practice." A bit later he clarifies that they do these things "by magic and sacrifice" (μαγεύων τε καὶ θύων). All of these forces that the μάγοι allegedly claimed to manipulate were

---

[50] Matthew Dickie can cite only three elite Romans who are known to have practiced "magical" arts (*Magic and Magicians in the Greco-Roman World*, 162–8). The majority of practitioners would have learned "the rudiments of reading and the tricks of their trade" from an older master to whom they were apprenticed (68).
[51] David E. Aune critiques this and other classic theories of magic in "'Magic' in Early Christianity and Its Ancient Mediterranean Context," 229–94.
[52] This in fact is the view that people like Plato and the Hippocratic school were seeking over overturn.

traditionally thought to lie under the control of the gods. Thus if the author's report is to be believed, the μάγοι were asserting that they could override even the power of the gods with their rituals.

At the other end of our chronological spectrum, Pliny the Elder (late first century CE) has a lot to say about the healing claims and practices of the *magi* in his *Natural History*, particularly in books 28 and 30. Many interpreters have noted how Pliny repeatedly denounces what he calls the "fraudulent lies" of the *magi*, ridiculing their remedies while at the same time commending many cures that modern readers would class as "magical."[53] Several times he refers to the supposed powers of the *magi* to compel divine action. Nero's interest in their art, according to Pliny, was driven by his desire "to issue commands to the gods" (30.14). Elsewhere he observes that "there is indeed nobody who does not fear being spell-bound by imprecations" (28.19). The power of spoken charms (*carmina*) is so commonly accepted that people are "always on the look-out for something big, something adequate to move a god, or rather to impose its will on his divinity" (28.20). Similar effects can be achieved through ritual acts: "Scrupulous actions, even without words, have their powers" (28.24). Some practitioners are so imbued with these powers that mere contact with their bodies can bring healing (28.30-31).

Between Plato and Pliny lies a mountain of evidence affirming the belief that ritual words and actions properly performed can channel divine power and benefits to humans.[54] Thus we would not be amiss to conclude that the ability to deploy such power for the benefit of others is a necessary, but not sufficient, criterion for identifying certain healing techniques as "magical."

The reason why we cannot rely solely on this criterion is that similar statements could also be made about religious modes of healing, as we will see in Chapter 4. We therefore need additional criteria to differentiate these two systems of health care. A promising place to look is the writings of Plato that we examined earlier. As we saw, Plato is concerned not only about the impiety and deceptiveness of his opponents but also by the fact that they present themselves as religious experts who operate outside of the civic cultus, marketing their own versions of traditional public rituals as effective tools for addressing the religious needs and interests of individuals. Some of them claim (according to both Plato and the author of *De morbo sacro*) that their rituals enable them to perform miraculous deeds that are beyond the reach of traditional, community-oriented forms of religion. Similar reports can be found in many other authors.

If we strip away Plato's value-judgments, what we find is a useful distinction between "magic" and "religion" that would have resonated with many Greeks and

---

[53] This ambivalence appears most fully in Pliny's oft-quoted observation about the nature of *magia*: "Frivolous and lying as it is, it still bears, however, some shadow of truth upon it" (*HN* 30.17). As Georg Luck rightly observes, "He dislikes and distrusts professional magicians as a class and calls them 'frauds' and 'charlatans,' and yet he seems to admit, almost grudgingly, that there are certain things they know and can do" (*Arcana Mundi*, 39).

[54] Confirmation that this was an important element of popular thinking about "magic" can be seen in the *Apologia* of Apuleius, written a century later than Pliny. In the course of answering the charge that he had used magic to entice a wealthy widow to marry him, he remarks that "the common herd" defines a magician as "one who by communion of speech with the immortal gods has power to do all the marvels that he will, through a strange power of incantation" (26.6, Butler translation).

Romans: "religion" is rituals performed in public by recognized authorities to serve the public good, while "magic" is rituals performed in private (even secretly at times) by self-approved experts to serve the needs of individuals.[55] If we apply this to health care, "magical" healing would be the performance of rituals by self-appointed experts in a private setting with the intent of moving the gods or other powers to remove an illness and restore a sick person to health. The precise nature of the rituals is irrelevant—they could be distinctive or similar to those used in the public cult. What marks them as "magical" is their private application and the nonofficial status of the person who performs them.[56]

This last point leads to one final clarification regarding what will be considered "magical" healing for the sake of this study. Just as many of the rituals employed by "magical" healers were drawn from the public cultus, so also many of them are more complex and refined versions of traditional home remedies. Taken together, these similarities make it impossible to identify a particular set of practices as uniquely "magical."[57] The difference between traditional and "magical" forms of healing lies not in the treatments that they offer but in the fact that the former are performed by friends and family members (i.e., amateurs) while the latter are performed by trained experts. The types and amounts of training that these experts received varied widely, but it was apparently sufficient for their tasks, if we judge by their popularity.

Scholars of ancient magic have identified a variety of health care practitioners whose modes of treatment might qualify as "magical" under the criteria laid out earlier. Plinio Prioreschi lists "root-sellers (*rhizotomoi*—root-cutters), drug-sellers (*pharmacopolai*), itinerant sellers of charms and purifications, . . . and, finally, magicians and other charlatans."[58] Vivian Nutton speaks in one passage of "wise women, magicians, druggists, faith healers, and quacks," while adding "bird-diviners, prophets, astrologers, and number mystics" in another place and "root-cutters and exorcists" in a third.[59] Richard Gordon divides them into five categories: diviner-healers, root-cutters, purifiers, exorcists, and sorcerers.[60]

---

[55] The word "public" here includes the family, where religion is the performance by the (normally male) head of the household of established rituals to secure the favor of the gods for both the family and the city.

[56] David Frankfurter's cross-cultural definition of "magic" is applicable here: "magic" is "the ritual or material context in which a Great Tradition (that may or may not be associated with living cults or temples) is interpreted by a ritual expert, located in time and space, and linked with particular circumstances, e.g., a rivalry, an illness, a fear—that is, mediated into the immediate circumstances of the Local Tradition" ("Magic as the Local Application of Authoritative Tradition," in Frankfurter, *Guide to the Study of Ancient Magic*, 725).

[57] One might reasonably ask, then, why I have chosen to retain the term "magical" to describe the healing practices discussed in this chapter. The simple answer is that no obvious replacement exists; every substitute that has been proposed is equally problematic. "Magic" is a term that is native to Greeks and Romans, not an imported category. As long as we are careful to clarify what ancient users meant by it, we are adhering to the recommendations of anthropologists that we should focus on the views and categories of particular cultures and avoid cross-cultural generalizations.

[58] *History*, 2.639–40.

[59] "Healers in the Medical Marketplace," 53, 56; "Medicine in the Greek World, 800-50 BC," 16.

[60] "The Healing Event in Graeco-Roman Medicine," 363. Gordon adds that there are numerous subtypes of each category, a stipulation that shows his awareness of the complexity of the task.

Gordon's categories are more precise than the somewhat makeshift lists of Prioreschi and Nutton, but his inclusion of purifiers and exorcists in his list is problematic in that it combines two related, but methodologically distinct, modes of practice. Purification and exorcism presuppose divine causality of sickness and prescribe rituals for manipulating gods or *daimones* to cease their affliction of the patient. To use modern terms, their system of diagnosis and treatment is self-consciously "religious." Divination, root-cutting, and sorcery, on the other hand, involve the application of practical skills that may or may not include efforts to influence personalized divine beings. The two systems overlap, to be sure, but they are different enough to raise questions about whether the apostle Paul would have regarded both in the same light. For this reason the present chapter will focus exclusively on practices in the second category, while purification and exorcism will be treated with other modes of religious healing in Chapter 4.

Diviner-Healers

The term "diviner-healers," unlike the other categories in Gordon's list, is not quite an "emic" label. Ancient authors refer to various types of diviners (μάντεις) and healers (ἰατροί), but the combined form ἰατρόμαντεις appears only three times in Greek literature, never with reference to a person who practices both medicine and divination.[61] But the artificial construction can be forgiven in this case since Gordon's intent appears to be to focus attention on a subclass of the broader category of diviners, those whose work is associated in some way with the treatment of illness or injury.

(a) In the broadest sense, a *diviner* is someone who discerns the will of the gods by using rituals. While the term can be applied to official cult practitioners such as oracles (Greek) and augurs (Roman), it most often refers to people who use their skills to serve individuals rather than a temple, army, or city.[62] People consulted them when they wanted to know things that lay beyond normal human perception, such as why something was happening to them, how they could improve their fate, or what choices they should make regarding the future. Elite authors criticized them for misleading people and wandering from place to place in search of fees, but the validity of these criticisms is hard to assess. Most interpreters seem to think that they contain nuggets of truth about how some private diviners operated. But these criticisms did not prevent members of the elite from using their services from time to time.[63]

Scattered references in Greek and Roman literature suggest that at least some μάντεις applied their skills to the treatment of illness. Two broad types of "diviner-healers" can be discerned: those who offered direct, divinely inspired guidance to sick

---

[61] This point has been persuasively argued by William V. Harris in "*Manteis* and Medicine," *Menemosyne* 73 (2020): 21–35.

[62] This is not to say that μάντεις served only individuals—for a masterful survey of Greek divination that includes ample material on the various uses of divination in public life, see Matthew Dillon, *Omens and Oracles: Divination in Ancient Greece* (London and New York: Routledge, 2017).

[63] The evidence suggests that most elites probably began by consulting physicians, then moved on to dream-readers, diviners, seers, spell-casters, and other "magical" practitioners if the physicians were unable to cure them. See Harris, "Popular Medicine in the Classical World," 40–2, 48–9, 57–8; Dickie, *Magic and Magicians in the Greco-Roman World*, 193–201.

people regarding the diagnosis, treatment, or prognosis of their conditions and those who interpreted dreams for the same ends.[64]

The corpus of data from Greek sources regarding the first type of μάντις is limited, as William V. Harris has recently shown.[65] But there are enough references to indicate that such people did indeed exist in both the classical and Hellenistic eras. Several are said to have served their cities by ending plagues, and Harris thinks it likely that "every city and many armies periodically suffered from epidemics severe enough to have caused the consultation of *manteis*."[66] They also served individuals: Harris cites texts from Hippocrates (*Virg.* 36-40), Thucydides (2.47), and Polybius (33.17) that speak of individual Greeks consulting them about personal illness and following their advice.[67] This evidence is invaluable since all three authors voice skepticism about the practice.

The importance of divination to the Romans is well known, but its use in the private treatment of illness is not. Our best source is Galen (second century CE), who often compares himself to a μάντις and regards μαντική (divination) as an art comparable to medicine.[68] In *HVA* 1.15 he speaks of two freelance diviners who predicted the outcome of an illness by observing the flights of birds, while in *Praen.* 3.7 he observes that some Romans have credited the success of his prognostications to divination, implying that diviners were known for making such predictions.[69] Whether Roman diviners made recommendations regarding treatment is unknown. But Roman authors mention the presence of Greeks practicing all sorts of magical arts in Rome during the late Republican and early imperial periods, and it seems reasonable to suppose that their number included Greek diviners who treated illness.[70]

As for what exactly these μάντεις did, the evidence is sparse. Plato indicates that their practices included purifications and fumigations and that their prescriptions included drugs and purgations.[71] Other Greek sources suggest that they offered

---

[64] A similar distinction is made in Cicero's treatise *De Diviniatione*, where the two modes of divine revelation are "frenzy" and dreams.
[65] See Harris, "*Manteis* and Medicine."
[66] On plagues, see Ibid., 26.
[67] Ibid., 28.
[68] A helpful discussion can be found in Peter Van Nuffelen, "Galen, Divination, and the Status of Medicine," *Classical Quarterly* 63 (2014): 337-52. Galen's view is hardly idiosyncratic; it has deep roots in the Hippocratic Corpus, where *Epistle* 15.33-6 states, "The medical arts and the mantic arts are of the same lineage, since these are two children of one father, Apollo" (cited by Lisa Raphals, "Divination and Medicine in China and Greece: A Comparative Perspective on the Baoshan Illness Divinations," *East Asian Science, Technology, and Medicine* 24 [2005]: 94).
[69] Van Nuffelen, "Galen, Divination, and the Status of Medicine," 340-4. "For Galen," says Van Nuffelen, "divination is as 'rational' as medicine (in that it relies on principles and knowledge), but not as accurate and powerful in matters of health" (342). Juvenal, as we might expect, is more skeptical, speaking mockingly of a woman consulting an astrologer about "the lingering death of her jaundiced mother" (*Satires* 6.563-4).
[70] As Matthew Dickie observes, "Men and women from the Greek East who were peddlers, soothsayers, jugglers, conjurors and even magicians will have been familiar figures" in the Roman world from the late third century BCE (*Magic and Magicians in the Greco-Roman World*, 126). Dickie presents a wide range of materials relating to the presence and activities of wandering freelance diviners in Greek and Roman societies, including the important role of women, but little of it relates to healing (*Magic and Magicians in the Greco-Roman World*, 128-9, 156-63, 233-9).
[71] *Laches* 198d and *Cratylus* 405 a, cited by Harris, "*Manteis* and Medicine," 30. He also notes a passage from Theophrastus (*HP* 9.10.4) that suggests a connection with drug prescriptions.

divinely inspired guidance regarding treatment, which typically involved some sort of ritual act to placate the divine power that had caused the illness.[72] By the Roman era some were predicting the future course of an illness, as noted by Galen, but whether this was a new development reflecting the well-known Roman concern for divining the future or a continuation of Greek practices is uncertain.[73] The plays of Plautus mention diviners going door to door offering to help people with their problems, but it is not clear whether sickness is included.[74] A clearer example can be seen in Juvenal's derisive reference to a woman "lying in bed ill" who consults an astrologer about "the hour appropriate for taking food" (*Satires* 6.580-81). Galen mentions the use of books by a μάντις to support his prognosis regarding the future course of an illness, a practice that accords well with what we know about diviners in general, but their tendency toward secrecy and the vagaries of time have left us with little knowledge about what such books contained or how they were used.[75]

In short, while it is hard to reconstruct their social settings and activities, there is ample evidence to indicate that freelance diviners used their skills in both Greek and Roman contexts to address the health care needs of the populace in a way that fits our definition of "magical" treatment.

(b) The importance of *dream interpretation* as a mode of health care is well documented in both Greek and Roman sources. It was accepted as a method of treatment in all three health care systems that were available to Paul and his congregations: "magical," religious, and medical.[76] The interpretation of dreams by cultic experts and physicians will be discussed in Chapters 4 and 5; the focus here is on how they were used by freelance diviners.

The idea that dreams are a channel for communication from the gods goes back to hoary antiquity for both Greeks and Romans. Physicians and philosophers who sought to redefine them as a product of mental or bodily processes were fighting a losing battle even among the elites, some of whom consulted regularly with diviners whom they kept as clients to advise them and interpret their dreams.[77] Even the skeptical were known to resort to dream interpreters when other channels of healing failed, as Plutarch observed in *De facie* 920b: "Those who are ill with chronic diseases and do

---

[72] Harris, "*Manteis* and Medicine," 30, citing evidence from the oracle at Dodona. The observation about divine causality and treatment comes from Leanne McNamara, who points to Herodotus's call to build a shrine to the Furies in *Hist.* 5.149 and Hippocrates's statement in *Virg.* 36-40 about dedicating clothing to Artemis ("'Conjurers, Purifiers, Vagabonds and Quacks'? The Clinical Roles of the Folk and Hippocratic Healers of Classical Greece," *Iris: Journal of the Classical Association of Victoria* 16-17 [2003-4]: 15-16).

[73] Some of the language in the Hippocratic treatises suggests that Greek diviners might have engaged in prognosis, but there is no direct evidence (Harris, "*Manteis* and Medicine," 29). According to Leanne McNamara ("'Conjurers, Purifiers, Vagabonds and Quacks'?," 18), "There is no indication that sufferers tended to ask oracular *manteis* for a prognosis and, in addition, it is likely that the practitioners themselves preferred to avoid predicting the future course of an illness."

[74] Noted by Dickie, *Magic and Magicians in the Greco-Roman World*, 156-7. Wandering diviners were also present in the countryside, as both Cato (*Agr.* 5.4) and Columella (*Rust.* 1.8.5-6) feel compelled to warn their farm managers against consulting them (ibid., 184-5).

[75] Ibid., 67-73.

[76] It was also used in a less systematic way by ordinary people as an element of traditional home health care, as we saw in Chapter 2.

[77] Dickie, *Magic and Magicians in the Greco-Roman World*, 186-94.

not succeed by the usual remedies and the customary diet turn to purifications and amulets and dreams."

If we ask where and how ordinary people found diviners to interpret their dreams, we run into the same problem that we noted earlier regarding the paucity of our sources. The Roman playwright Plautus (254-184 BCE) associates the practice with women who for a fee interpret dreams, prophesy, and look for signs in the entrails of animals or the sky.[78] Matthew Dickie describes a class of wandering men who put on shows in the public square that included prophecies, necromancy, dream interpretation, and conjuring tricks. He notes how Artemidorus, in the Preface to his *Oneirocritica* (late second century CE), states that he learned to interpret dreams from μάντεις who offered their skills in the agoras and at religious festivals in the cities of Greece, Asia Minor, and Italy.[79] The geographic breadth of his references underlines their popularity, though he also notes that many people (presumably members of his own class) thought poorly of them. "Chaldeans," a term that could refer to virtually any astrologer from the East,[80] were especially famous for working as diviners and dream interpreters, and the same was true for Judeans.[81] In short, dream interpreters were usually marginalized people translating messages from the gods on a freelance basis outside of the traditional cultic system, a fact that is sufficient to explain why Roman authorities acted against them from time to time.[82]

As for how dreams were used in the treatment of sickness, the evidence suggests that practitioners applied the same interpretive techniques that they used with any other dream. Most of the dreams that a freelance interpreter encountered would have been the spontaneous products of a night's sleep at home and not the carefully managed environment of an Asklepian healing center.[83] The magical papyri speak of spells that could be used to promote diagnostic dreaming, but how far such practices were used in the time of Paul is unclear.[84] Interpreters scrutinized every detail of a dream—who was involved (including divine beings), what they looked like, what they did, where it took place, what resulted from the action, and so on—in an effort to discern clues or patterns that revealed the underlying cause of the illness, what should be done to treat it, and what type of outcome to expect. They also probed the background and personal characteristics of the dreamer, such as occupation, health, status, habits, and age. There

---

[78] Ibid., 162–8.
[79] Ibid., 230–1, 236–9. In the prologue to his *Oneirocritica*, Artemidorus criticizes "those who are haughty-faced and look down their brows" at the dream-interpreting μάντεις and stigmatize them as "beggars, sorcerers, and buffoons" (προίκτας καὶ γόητας καὶ βωμολόχους).
[80] On the diverse meanings of "Chaldeans," see Dickie, *Magic and Magicians in the Greco-Roman World*, 106–8, 150, 153, 157. With regard to healing, Dickie suggests that "it is possible that some of them emerged from the ranks of the priests expert in conducting healing and exorcistic rituals who continued to be a presence in Babylonia under the Seleucids" (107).
[81] According to Juvenal, "The Jews will sell you whatever dreams you wish for the tiniest copper coin" (*Satires* 6.542-7). On Jews more generally, see Wendt, *At the Temple Gates*, 88–9. Josephus prided himself on his ability to interpret dreams—see Bohak, *Ancient Jewish Magic*, 85.
[82] On the various expulsions of Chaldeans, Judeans, and other types of "magicians" from the city of Rome, see Dickie, *Magic and Magicians in the Greco-Roman World*, 107–8, 118–19, 147–51.
[83] The latter will be described in some detail in Chapter 4. The *Sacred Tales* of Aelius Aristides (117–81 CE) is a particularly rich source of diagnostic dreams and their interpretation, but his interactions are with physicians and Asklepian priests, not freelance diviners.
[84] Graf, *Magic in the Ancient World*, 107.

was no common system for decoding dreams, so different interpreters could reach very different judgments regarding the meaning and implications of the same report using the interpretive system that they had been taught.[85]

For the most part it seems that dream interpreters saw themselves as occasional advisers and not as active managers of a person's illness. The distinction is clear in book 4 of the Hippocratic treatise *On Regimen*, which lays out a medical approach to dream interpretation that the author claims is superior to that of the μάντεις. According to the author, "They [μάντεις] give no instruction how to take precautions, but only recommend prayers to the gods. Prayer indeed is good," he avers, "but while calling on the gods a man should himself lend a hand" (4.87).[86] Artemidorus's *Onerocritica*, written in the second century CE, gives a similar impression: certain types of dreams can signal the impending onset of sickness or whether a sick person will recover or die, but nothing is said about potential remedies except for one passage where he casts doubt on the validity of prescriptions received in dreams and recommends the study of medicine for that purpose (4.22).

In summary, the interpretation of dreams was a vital element of the ancient healing enterprise, whether performed by freelance diviners, religious functionaries, or physicians. Dreams were regarded as messages from the gods by all but the most rationalistic of physicians, and even they did not wholly deny the divine origin of dreams, as we will see in Chapter 5. What distinguished μάντεις from other types of interpreters was not their methods but the freelance nature of their activities, which made them more accessible to the public while also eliciting the disdain of many elites who felt threatened by their use of extra-institutional, "magical" power.[87]

Root-Cutters and Drug-Sellers

Root-cutters, or rhizotomists (from Greek ῥιζοτόμοι), were experts in the harvesting of plants for use in healing. They differ from the other practitioners in Gordon's list of "magical" healers in that they were not primarily concerned with giving direct treatment to sick people but rather procured the botanical materials that others used to treat them. Those who lived in or near cities sold their goods to drug-sellers (φαρμακοπῶλαι), who either re-sold them in raw form or combined them with other materials to create drug compounds.[88] Drug-sellers' shops could be found in the commercial agoras of Greek and Roman cities alongside other businesses, where

---

[85] Artemidorus's *Oneirocritica* describes one particular system that he has synthesized from numerous interviews and books, but it is still an idiosyncratic and inconsistent compilation, not a standard that others followed. Dillon notes two examples of interpreters using books to guide them (*Omens and Oracles*, 276–7).

[86] More will be said about medical uses of dream interpretation in Chapter 5.

[87] As we will see in Chapters 4 and 5, most members of the elite felt no hesitation about visiting a divine sanctuary or consulting a physician to receive or interpret divinatory dreams.

[88] The line between rhizotomists and drug-sellers was not sharply drawn; some drug-sellers may have cut their own plants, while some rhizotomists may have had shops where they sold to the general public. For more on this point (and on drug-sellers in general), see Laurence M. V. Totelin, "*Pharmakopōlai*: A Re-Evaluation of the Sources," in Harris, *Popular Medicine*, 65–85, and John Scarborough, "Drugs and Drug Lore in the Time of Theophrastus: Magic, Botany, Philosophy and the Rootcutters," *Acta Classica* 49 (2006): 1–29.

they served both practitioners and the general public.[89] In larger cities they sometimes congregated in specific neighborhoods.[90] Public opinion of them was equivocal—they supplied vital materials for health care, but they also had a reputation for dealing in poisons.[91] In rural areas where drug-sellers' shops were absent, rhizotomists probably sold their products directly to individuals.

From a social-systems standpoint, the work of rhizotomists and drug-sellers resembles a modern drug-supply chain. But the resemblance is purely formal; the substance of what rhizotomists did and their reasons for doing it differed radically from modern botanical medicine. Rhizotomists drew on the same stock of botanical knowledge that was used in traditional family-based cures, some of which has been shown by modern science to be clinically effective. But rhizotomists were not interested in plants that anyone could pick and use; they focused on plants that were thought to require special handling in order to activate or enhance their healing power. This included not only practical knowledge about when the plant should be harvested to maximize its potency and how it should be preserved after it was harvested but also esoteric knowledge regarding what rituals should be performed for each plant to bring its healing power under the harvester's control and protect the harvester from being harmed by suprahuman forces that gave the plant its effectiveness.

"The aim of rhizotomic knowledge-practices," observes Richard L. Gordon, "was . . . to locate φάρμακα/*medicamenta* as firmly as possible within a frame we can best describe as numinous."[92] To do this, rhizotomists surrounded the entire harvesting process with rituals while asserting that the power of the plant would remain dormant or even harm the user if their rituals were not followed. In some cases the rituals could be performed by ordinary people, while in others a specialist was required.

Examples of rhizotomists' harvesting rituals are abundant in both Greek and Roman literature. Theophrastus (371–287 BCE), the earliest botanical writer whose work has survived, acknowledges how much he has learned from them and repeats many of their prescriptions, thought he voices doubts about some of them. Here are a few examples from his *Inquiry into Plants*.[93]

> The peony, which some call *glykyside*, should be dug up at night, for, if a man does it in the day-time and is observed by a woodpecker while he is gathering the fruit, he risks the loss of his eyesight; and, if he is cutting the root at the time, he gets *prolapsus ani* [a prolapsed anus]. (9.8.6)

---

[89] Totelin, "Pharmakopōlai," 78–9; Scarborough, "Drugs and Drug Lore in the Time of Theophrastus," 12.
[90] Vivian Nutton, "The Drug Trade in Antiquity," *Journal of the Royal Society of Medicine* 78 (1985): 140–1.
[91] Totelin, "Pharmakopōlai," 68–70. The association was so strong that the common Greek word for a medicinal drug (φάρμακον) was also used to denote poison. The fact that ancient medicines were not regulated and might unintentionally produce poisonous effects added to the confusion.
[92] "From Substances to Texts: Three Materialities of Magic in the Roman Period," in *The Materiality of Magic*, ed. Jan N. Bremmer (Munich: Paderborn Fink, 2015), 144.
[93] All quotations are from taken the Loeb translation by Arthur Hort.

> As to cutting the kind of all-heal which is called that of Asklepios ... it is said that one should put in the ground in its place an offering made of all kinds of fruits and a cake; and that, when one is cutting gladwyn, one should put in its place to pay for it cakes of meal from spring-sown wheat, and that one should cut it with a two-edged sword, first making a circle round it three times, and that the piece first cut must be held up in the air while the rest is being cut. (9.8.7)
>
> One should also, it is said, draw a circle round the black hellebore and cut it standing towards the east and saying prayers, and one should look out for an eagle both on the right and on the left; for that there is danger to those that cut, if your eagle should come near, that they may die within the year. (9.8.8)

Several common features of rhizotomic practice can be seen in these examples: harvesting at night, using certain types of tools, drawing circles around the plant, facing in a particular direction, and making prayers and offerings while cutting the plant. Danger-narratives like the ones reported here are also common. When performed together, such rituals served to enhance public confidence in both the healing power of the plants and the value of the rhizotomists' skills.[94]

More plant-harvesting rituals are mentioned by other ancient authors, especially Pliny the Elder (23–79 CE) and the creators of the *Papyri Graecae Magicae* (*PGM*) (fourth century BCE to fifth century CE).[95] Some regulate the time when the plant should be harvested, including the season, the position of the stars, the time of day or night, and the weather conditions. Others involve preparations that the harvester must make before approaching the plant, such as fasting, ritual purification, wearing special clothing, removing garments, or gathering special tools to be used in harvesting. Still others prescribe what the harvester must do at the harvest site prior to cutting the plant, such as fumigating the site with a censer; presenting prayers and sacrifices to the plant or the gods who control it; naming aloud the illness for which the plant is being harvested and/or the person for whom it is being cut; chanting an incantation or spell; walking or dancing around the plant a certain number of times; drawing particular shapes on the ground in the vicinity of the plant; touching the plant with a specified object; and spitting in a prescribed manner. A related set of rules regulates how the plant is to be cut, including the type of tool to be used, which hand should be employed, whether one can look at the plant or not, and what part of the plant is to be removed. Still others explain what should be done after the plant is cut: holding it in the air with one or the other hand, laying it on the ground, wrapping it in a certain

---

[94] On the use of rituals to establish the authority of both the rhizotomists and their products, see Gordon, "The Healing Event in Graeco-Roman Medicine," 366–7. The durability and mobility of these traditions can be seen in the fact that the prescription for digging peonies is found nearly 400 years later in the writings of the Roman encyclopedist Pliny the Elder (*HN* 25.29), while the one for hellebore appears in both Pliny (*HN* 25.50) and his younger contemporary Dioscorides (*De mat. med.* 4.151).

[95] While there is a tendency in Roman circles for *magia* to be viewed as a dangerous foreign intrusion, rhizotomists were exempt from this negative classification. "Plant-picking traditions seem to have been normalized in Rome to the point that they were not considered a Greek or otherwise foreign import (which would likely condemn them to the category of *magia*), but rather an acceptable Italian practice" (Wallace, "Sorcerer's Pharmacy," 117).

kind of cloth, placing offerings in the hole from which the plant was dug, and even replanting the plant after it has served its purpose.[96]

Such a list seems bewilderingly complex to us, but it is no more complicated than the regimen that is followed in the modern harvesting of medicinal plants. The goal, too, is similar: to amplify the healing properties of the plant through proper handling. The worldview behind the rhizotomists' rituals, however, is radically different from modern science. It is fundamentally "magical," as evidenced by its presumption that the healing power of plants arises not from biological processes within the plant itself but from suprahuman forces inhabiting the plant that must be handled with care so that the harvester can gain mastery over them rather than being victimized by them. Rituals are the means by which this end is achieved. In such a system, "collecting herbs is an act of worship, and the herbalist understands that the powers contained in these plants emerge from the divinity within each part collected ... The plants' conversion into 'drugs' simply extends their powers for the kindly benefit of man."[97]

The system is also "magical" in the sense discussed earlier in this chapter: it involves the use of rituals by professional experts unaffiliated with the civic cultus to channel suprahuman powers to serve human needs. The methods of the rhizotomists were essentially a more developed and theorized version of methods that had been used by ordinary people from time immemorial but were now crystallized into a profession that would have required many years of training to master. Like most education in the ancient world, the bulk of it would have occurred within families whose members would have gained a reputation as having natural (god-given?) talents in this area. This in turn would have enhanced public confidence in the plant-based remedies that were sold by the local drug-seller or rhizotomist.

Whether the same can be said for the compounds created by the drug-sellers themselves is less clear from our scanty evidence. Both Pliny and the *PGM* speak of compounds involving materials that were rare, expensive, or both. Most were beyond the reach of the general public and must therefore have been created by drug-sellers, though this is never specified. Compounders probably used something like the recipes in Scribonius Largus's *Compositiones* (first century CE) to guide their work.[98] Some of these recipes are odd by modern standards, but few involve anything like "magical" practices.[99] Drug-sellers were secretive about many of their recipes, a behavior that is often associated with *mageia* in the ancient world, but secrecy was common in other settings as well.[100] Pliny and the *PGM* speak now and then of drug compounds that

---

[96] Excluded from this process are plants that are inherently "magical" and therefore do not require rituals to make them effective—see Pliny, *HN* 24.156–67, 26.18–20.
[97] Scarborough, "Pharmacology of Sacred Plants, Herbs, and Roots," 157–8. A wealth of information on harvesting practices can be found in Delatte, *Herbarius*, 39–200.
[98] For more on Scribonius's recipes, see Wallace, "Sorcerer's Pharmacy," 102–19; Harms, "Logic of Irrational Pharmacological Therapies in Aretaeus of Cappadocia," 43–177; and Ianto Jocks, "The Compositiones Medicamentorum of Scribonius Largus" (MRes thesis, University of Glasgow, 2013), available online at http://theses.gla.ac.uk/4892.
[99] Scribonius does mention a few quasi-magical cures here and there, but his skepticism is apparent. A different attitude can be seen when he speaks of using spells and rituals in the picking of medicinal plants, a practice that he generally approves. See Wallace, "Sorcerer's Pharmacy," 102–16.
[100] Nutton, "Drug Trade in Antiquity," 141–2; Dickie, *Magic and Magicians in the Greco-Roman World*, 27, 39–40; Delatte, *Herbarius*, 83–5.

involve what we might call "magical" preparation methods, but they say little about who was to prepare them. In the end, however, the question is probably moot, since few, if any, customers would have thought to distinguish products the produced by the drug-seller from those of the rhizotomists who supplied most of their materials.

Sorcerers

As with the word "magic," the use of the term "sorcerer" to designate a category of healers must be carefully delineated in order to avoid misunderstanding. In recent years it has become an increasingly common translation for the Greek noun γόης (pl. γόητες), which was previously rendered into English by such words as "charlatan" or "imposter" due to the negative connotations that it carries in the writings of many elite authors. The noun μάγοι, commonly translated as "magicians," is also used to describe these people, but μάγοι appears here and there as a term of self-ascription while γόης is invariably negative.[101] In Latin, the equivalent terms are *veneficus* and *magus*, both of which have negative associations in the writings of elite authors. In fact, the word *veneficus* is also used to denote a poisoner.

What is important for our purpose is to recognize that all of these terms belong to realm of elite discourse and do not reflect how such people thought of themselves or how they were viewed by people outside of elite circles. Many of those who were tarred with such labels were illiterate folk practitioners who likely never thought of their practices as belonging to any general category. As David Frankfurter has observed, literary descriptions of γόητες and μάγοι are in reality "learned construction[s] of danger, mysterious powers, and impure ceremonies" by elite authors which can only with caution be used as a "window into 'real' practices on the ground."[102]

With these caveats in mind, the term "sorcerer" will be used in this study as a shorthand label for ritual experts who specialized in the kinds of activities that elite authors associate with γόητες and μάγοι, but without the negative connotations that they give to these practices. More specifically, it will be used to describe healers who employed techniques like chants, spells, incantations, and amulets to channel suprahuman powers to relieve, remove, or protect people from illness or injury.[103] The discussion will include both the more visible (often semi-educated) practitioners

---

[101] Cf. Aune, "Magic," 262: "While γόης and ἀγύρτης are always used with a pejorative meaning and therefore no one every claimed to be a γόης or ἀγύρτης, μάγος typically has negative connotations, but is used very occasionally with a positive meaning (i.e., a priest or a wise man). ... Thus the γόης and ἀγύρτης are socially acceptable terms of abuse leveled against people who are thereby relegated to the margins of society and whose activities are judged to be deviant, antisocial or even illegal." This preference for μάγος over γόης is rather surprising as γόης is the older term, going back at least to sixth-century BCE Greece, while μάγος is associated with the hated Persians, as we saw earlier. For more on the meaning and connotations of these and related words, see Dickie, *Magic and Magicians in the Greco-Roman World*, 12–17; Graf, "Excluding the Charming," 30–7.

[102] Frankfurter, "Introduction," 30.

[103] This is not to say that such people did not also use their skills in less benign ways such as preparing curse tablets or deploying the "evil eye" to harm their clients' enemies. Such activities simply lie outside the scope of this study. This dual potentiality of "sorcery" has been recognized by anthropologists ever since the foundational research of E. E. Evans-Pritchard among the Azande people of northern Africa in the 1920s.

who plied their trade in the cities and thus came to the notice of elite authors and the (mostly illiterate) folk healers who labored in the shadows of history, serving poor clients in the villages and countryside of the Mediterranean world. The practices of the two groups may have differed in detail and level of sophistication—for instance, some of the *magi* whom Pliny criticizes recommend exotic remedies that would have been unavailable to rural healers—but their overall approach to healing was similar enough that we can treat them together without serious risk of distortion.

So where and how did sick people access "sorcerers" for treatment? In rural areas, the kinds of treatments associated with γόητες were part of the tradecraft employed by traditional folk healers whose services also included activities like supplying medicines and delivering babies. Such people were known to everyone since they were the primary health care providers outside of the family. Ancient authors do refer occasionally to wandering physicians in the countryside, and rural residents who lived close enough to a temple of Asklepios or another healing deity could always apply for help there if they wished.[104] But comparative studies and literary references suggest that illiterate folk healers were the first providers to be consulted when family-based treatments failed or when an illness was clearly beyond the skills of family members to treat.

In the cities, a similar role was played by γόητες or μάγοι who lived at a fixed abode and treated the people who lived around them. Physicians would have been more readily available in the cities, but poor people often could not afford their fees or their prescriptions. Many poor city-dwellers also hailed from the countryside and thus would have been more inclined to trust the ritual healers who had treated their ancestors than the unfamiliar city-based physicians. A sorcerer who recited an incantation or tied on an amulet to bring suprahuman powers to bear on an illness fit their view of the universe better than the naturalistic methods of the physician.

Literary sources also speak of wandering γόητες and μάγοι who moved from city to city offering their skills to people in need. Some combined healing skills with divination and dream interpretation and thus provided a broader range of options to those who were sick. Most probably traveled within a limited geographic area, but some moved permanently from the Roman East to the West in hopes of making their fortunes in a world open to new ideas.[105] Some brought their gods with them, and it was not uncommon for them to claim the power to do miracles, though it is clear today that most of their acts were little more than parlor tricks performed to impress the public and attract clients.[106] Vivian Nutton has such people in mind when he speaks about "the flashy charlatan [i.e., γόης] wandering the markets from city to city with garish clothes and appurtenances" who impressed people more than the stolid

---

[104] More will be said about these options in Chapters 4 and 5. The lines between the various types of practitioners were by no means clear—Peter Van Nuffelen notes that even the great physician Galen worried about being taken for a γόης as a result of his treatments ("Galen, Divination, and the Status of Medicine," 343).

[105] On magicians from the East who "exploited their exotic origins to win authority for themselves," see Dickie, *Magic and Magicians in the Greco-Roman World*, 106–12.

[106] This was definitely the case with the second century CE wonder-worker Alexander of Abonoteichos whose story is told by Lucian of Samosata, and likely true for some of the stories told about Apollonius of Tyana by Philostratus in the same era.

local physician.¹⁰⁷ "The public display," he explains later, "will have served to persuade spectators of the skill of the magician and encouraged them to approach him for help with their own problems."¹⁰⁸ Some were successful, but most plied a more humble trade, like the begging priests that Plato criticizes or the illiterate dream interpreters who shared their secrets with Artemidorus.

One other notable fact about ancient "sorcerers" that can be gleaned from the literary record is that many were women. Matthew Dickie points to evidence from the classical era onward that shows how in Greek circles, "women were brought in to heal the sick by applying amulets to them, over which they probably intoned an incantation."¹⁰⁹ Similar evidence is available from the Roman period. Dickie cites Plautus, Varro, Lucilius, and Porphyrion as referring to women using incantations to treat sickness, especially for other women.¹¹⁰ Two of the oldest surviving healing incantations, dated by scholars to the second century BCE, bear the names of women, one for curing inflammation and one for headache (*PGM* XX.4-19). The position of such women in Roman society was so well established that even after Roman authorities began passing legislation to punish harmful forms of magic, "the old women who performed incantations over the sick and who attached amulets to them were almost certainly left alone."¹¹¹

These and other references suggest that the most common ritual techniques used by γόητες for treating the sick were the recitation of oral formulae and the application of amulets. Other texts indicate that they were also active in prescribing medicines made from plants, animals, or minerals.¹¹² All three of these practices have deep roots in traditional Greek and Roman health care systems, as we saw in Chapter 2. The only clear difference is the level of artistry and complexity that appears in the more "professional" examples. Learning how and when to deploy these advanced healing techniques required many years of training at the feet of a skilled expert. This was true for "magicians" of all stripes: they learned their craft through apprenticeship with a master who instructed them both orally and experientially. Teachers and pupils alike guarded the secrets of their trade jealously from outside eyes both to protect the integrity of their discipline and to create an aura of mystery that enticed people to apply for their services.¹¹³ This emphasis on secrecy is especially apparent in the Greek magical papyri, where readers are repeatedly enjoined to keep their prescriptions secret.¹¹⁴

---

[107] *Ancient Medicine*, 155.
[108] *Magic and Magicians in the Greco-Roman World*, 231.
[109] Ibid., 85, 88, 91–3, 105, 129. Dickie also mentions women who performed incantations for other purposes such as purification or love-magic (96, 100–1, 104, 158–62, 181–4). It would be reasonable to suppose that at least some applied their skills to healing as well.
[110] Ibid., 128–9, 157.
[111] Ibid., 143.
[112] Both Pliny's descriptions of the *magi* and the *PGM* include such prescriptions. Leanne McNamara lists but does not discuss all three practices in her summary of the activities of the γόητες, noting their reliance on "a repertoire of amulets, spoken incantations and *pharmaka* [i.e., medicines] to treat illness" ("Conjurers, Purifiers, Vagabonds and Quacks'?," 15).
[113] On the secrecy of "magical" training, see Luck, *Arcana Mundi*, 15–16, 23; Dickie, *Magic and Magicians in the Greco-Roman World*, 39–40; Gordon, "The Healing Event in Graeco-Roman Medicine," 367.
[114] Noted by Jacco Dieleman, "The Greco-Egyptian Magical Papyri," in Frankfurter, *Guide to the Study of Ancient Magic*, 315.

(a) *Oral healing formulae* that can be attributed with some confidence to γόητες or μάγοι are known primarily from the Greek magical papyri (*PGM*). Many ancient authors refer to the use of spells and incantations in healing, but few were recorded apart from the *PGM*.[115] As with other materials found in Egypt, questions have been raised about the validity of using the *PGM* to speak about practices in other parts of the Mediterranean world prior to the high Roman Empire when most of the texts were written. Jacco Dieleman, an expert on the papyri, sees little danger in the practice because "similar materials circulated throughout the Roman Empire, as we know from ancient accounts as well as engraved gems and inscribed metal tablets that have been recovered from regions outside Egypt (some of which parallel texts in the papyri from Egypt)."[116] John Scarborough adds that the *PGM* mention rituals and substances that are found in literature written centuries earlier, a sign that they contain older material.[117] Whether the people described in these texts ever referred to themselves as *magi* (or μάγοι) is unclear, but the ideas and practices that appear in the *PGM* are consistent with what we know about the ritual experts who bore this name elsewhere.

Sickness is a common, though not dominant, concern in the *PGM*. The ailments that appear most often are fevers, shivering fits, epilepsy, headaches, eye diseases, scorpion stings, and various respiratory, urinary, gynecological, and dermatological problems.[118] Healing is offered through a variety of channels, including spells, amulets, exorcisms, and ingesting or applying medicines. Spells are less common than other forms of treatment, and some are so thoroughly Egyptian in language and ideas that they would not likely have been available to Paul and his audiences. But a few are general enough to serve as samples of what might have been prescribed by a "sorcerer" to members of Paul's congregations who were ill.[119]

> For migraine headache: Take oil in your hands and utter the spell, "Zeus sowed a grape seed; it parts the soil; he does not sow it; it does not sprout." (*PGM* VII.199-201)
>
> Another, for migraine headache: "OURBEDERAEIS OUROURBEDERAEIS OUROUROUBEDERAEIS EISTHES ABRASA ELECH BELLENOURE OUNOURE BAPHAMMECH, to you I speak, pounding headache: don't throb, don't rage, don't shake the teeth, don't produce mucus, don't produce a 'black-

---

[115] Gordon, "The Healing Event in Graeco-Roman Medicine," 365. Pliny quotes a few short incantations, but none of them are attributed to the *magi*. Georg Luck (*Arcana Mundi*, 36–7) and Matthew Dickie (*Magic and Magicians in the Greco-Roman World*, 208) point to their presence in the Gnostic and Hermetic literature, but the idiosyncratic nature of their contents renders them unreliable as a guide to practices elsewhere.

[116] Dieleman, "Greco-Egyptian Magical Papyri," 284.

[117] "Pharmacology of Sacred Plants, Herbs, and Roots," 157. A similar point is made by David Lincicum, who cites half a dozen texts from the PGM Supplement volume (52, 67, 70, 71, 72, and 73), dated by the editors to the first century CE or before, as evidence that "the types of spells found in the generally later Greek magical papyri had earlier currency and preserve earlier forms" ("Scripture and Apotropaism in the Second Temple Period," 73n58).

[118] Compiled from Dieleman, "Greco-Egyptian Magical Papyri," 303, and Magali de Haro Sanchez, "Between Magic and Medicine: The Iatromagical Formularies and Medical Receptaries on Papyri Compared," *ZPE* 195 (2015): 185.

[119] All translations except the last one are from Hans Dieter Betz, ed., *The Greek Magical Papyri in Translation, Including the Demotic Spells* (Chicago and London: University of Chicago Press, 1986).

out,' don't stir up convulsions. For if there is throbbing, raging, shaking of teeth, producings of mucus, producings of a 'black-out,' or stirrings of a convulsion." (*PGM* XCIV.45-60)

For swollen testicles: Take a cord from a coin bag and say with each knot "Kastor" once, "Thab" twice. (*PGM* VII.209-10)

Spell for all kinds of fever.
. . . housing-the-mists caught fire
at the top of the mountain caught fire
. . . sources, seven bears, seven lions;
and seven single dark-blue-eyed maids drew water
with dark-blue pitchers and extinguished the tireless fire. (*PGM* XX.6-11)[120]

(b) As we saw in Chapter 2, the wearing of *amulets* to treat or protect against illness or injury was ubiquitous in the Greco-Roman world, appealing to people of all social classes.[121] Dozens of recipes for making them can be found in the *PGM*, and scores of additional examples appear in Greek and Roman medicinal texts. But judging which ones were part of the traditional health care system and which were produced by "sorcerers" is a challenge. Pliny cites some sixty different substances that can be used as amulets to treat various conditions, but only fifteen of them are credited to *magi*. Those in the latter group must have come to him either from *magi* themselves or (more likely) from written sources where they were attributed to *magi*, since it is impossible to distinguish them from the others by their content. Pliny's approval or disapproval is also an unreliable guide in this case, since he cites without criticism many amulet recipes that sound as outlandish to modern ears as those that he attributes to the *magi*. A brief comparison will show how hard it is to distinguish the amulets that an elite male like Pliny accepted as valid remedies from those that he credits to the *magi*. If anything, the ones that he approves are more consistently "magical" by our standards than those that he rejects.

Pliny

For scrofulous sores, a person who is fasting should pick nine knots from a grass plant and roll them up in black wool with grease, then carry them to the house of the sick person and attach them to the body while saying three times, "Fasting I give a cure to a fasting patient," them repeat the same act for three days. (*HN* 24.180-81).

---

[120] Slightly modified from the translation offered by José L. Calvo Martínez in an unpublished paper titled "The 'Philinna Papyrus': A New Interpretation" (https://www.academia.edu/42592163/The_Philinna_Papyrus). He has made a compelling case for why the reconstruction and translation in Betz's edition of the *PGM* are wrong.

[121] Naomi Janowitz's definition of amulets cited in Chapter 2 is worth repeating here: "Amulets are any objects used to directly mediate between divine forces and a particular individual or place. They work by bringing some type of physical representation of the supernatural force into direct physical contact with the person/animal/place for which aid is sought" (*Magic in the Roman World*, 57).

To stop the chills of fever, remove the pith from a bugloss plant when it is withering while stating that it is being done to free a person from fever, then attach seven leaves from the plant to the sick person's body before a paroxysm begins. (*HN* 26.117).

To remove the pain of an aching tooth, place maggots grown on a *gallidraga* plant in a box with bread and tie it to the person's arm on the same side as the aching tooth. (*HN* 27.89).

To relieve attacks of gout, tie the hair from a child's first haircut (or any prepubescent child) around the affected part. (*HN* 28.41).

Magi

To eliminate groin pains, take a thread from a web and tie it with seven or nine knots, reciting the name of a widow as each knot is tied, and attach it to the groin. (*HN* 28.48).

To cure headache, tie a rope that was used to commit suicide around the temples. (*HN* 28.49).

To treat quartan fever, wear an amulet made of cat excrement and the claw of a horned owl, and do not remove it until the seventh periodic return of the fever. (*HN* 28.228).

To remove albugo of the eyes, gouge out the eyes of a frog when the moon is in conjunction, place them in an eggshell, and tie them around the neck. (*HN* 32.74).

None of these preparations, even the ones credited to the *magi*, necessarily required the services of a "sorcerer" to create or apply. But someone had to diagnose the condition and prescribe the proper amulet, including any rituals that were necessary to make the amulet effective. As Leanne McNamara notes, "An amulet's effectiveness did not lie wholly in the object, but also in the incantations, purification or other ritual acts which accompanied its production and wearing."[122] The most likely person to fill this role was the local healer whom the elite class denigrated as a *magus* or γόης.

Whether these local healers were familiar with the more elaborate amulets that we find in the *PGM* and the archaeological record is unclear. Literacy was required to carry out prescriptions that call for the writing or carving of words onto a piece of papyrus, a metal sheet, or a stone, but the actual work of writing or carving could have been performed by ordinary craftsmen such as metalworkers or gem-carvers under the supervision of a ritual expert who applied the appropriate chants and spells during the creation of the amulet or when it was applied to the body.[123] Some of the recipes

---

[122] "Conjurers, Purifiers, Vagabonds and Quacks'?," 8.
[123] Amulets to protect against or cure common ailments would have been mass-produced and available for purchase in a city market, but customized manufacture would have been required to treat more unusual problems or to create exotic items like gems or gold or silver scrolls. For a helpful survey of what the *PGM* say about how amulets are to be made, see Isabel Canzobre Martínez, "Magical Amulets User's Guide: Preparation, Utilization, and Knowledge Transmission in the PGM," in *Magikè téchne: formación y consideración social del mago en el Mundo Antiguo*, ed. Emilio Suárez

also require rare or expensive materials, especially the ones that were carved onto gemstones or sheets of gold or silver, so the healer who prescribed one of these amulets would have had to possess either the personal resources to acquire such materials or access to a wealthy patron who could afford them.[124]

Thus it seems that there were two classes of amulet-making sorcerers in the Greco-Roman world, one that served the general public (including Paul and his followers) and another, much smaller group that catered to the wealthier members of society. The latter class is the proximate source for the prescriptions that we see in the *PGM*, but we should be careful about drawing too sharp a line between the two groups as if lower-class sorcerers were incapable of using complex formulae like those in the *PGM*.

A few examples of amulet prescriptions from the *PGM* will highlight their distinctive character. The sample will inevitably be skewed since it is difficult to replicate here the multifarious signs, symbols, and shapes that were supposed to be written or carved onto many of the amulets, as evidenced also in the archaeological record. A simple version of this phenomenon can be seen in the last of the following examples.[125]

> Another amulet for the foot of the gouty man: You should write these names on a strip of silver or tin. You should put it on a deerskin and bind it to the foot of the gouty man named, on his two feet: "THEMBARATHEM OUREMBRENOUTIPE AIOXTHOU SEMMARATHEMMOU NAIOOU, let NN, whom NN bore, recover from every pain which is in his knees and two feet." You should do it when the moon is [in the constellation] Leo. (*PDM* XIV.1003-14)

> For discharge of the eyes: Write [this] on a piece of papyrus and attach it as an amulet: "ROURARBISAROURBBARIASPHREN." (*PGM* VII.197-8)

> A phylactery: "Great [god] in heaven revolving the world, the true god, IAO! Lord, ruler of all, ABLANATHANALBA, grant, grant me this favor, let me have the name of the great god in this phylactery, and protect, from every evil thing, me whom NN bore, [NN] begot." (*PGM* LXXI.1-8)

> *(In the following example, the triangular arrangement stands above the charm listed below it)*

---

de la Torre, Miriam Blanco Cesteros, Eleni Chronopoulou, and Isabel Canzobre (Madrid: Editorial Dykinson, S.L., 2017), 177–92.

[124] For more on the use of gemstones in amulets, including the archaeological evidence, see Véronique Dasen, "Healing Images: Gems and Medicine," *Oxford Journal of Archaeology* 33 (2014): 177–91, and Dasen and Nagy, "Gems," 416–55. The authors of the latter article observe that when gems were used as amulets, their "magical" quality was often known only to the user (422), a fact that might conceivably affect how Paul would assess them.

[125] All translations are taken from Betz, *Greek Magical Papyri*. This small sample contains all of the features that Henrik Versnel sees as typical of the spells and incantations in the *PGM*: the name of the affected person and their ailment; words believed to signify the secret names of mysterious deities invoked for assistance; and other words that appear to be a special divine language understood only by divinities ("The Poetics of the Magical Charm: An Essay in the Power of Words," in Mirecki and Meyer, *Ancient Magic and Ritual Power*, 112–17).

"Magical" Treatments 83

ABLANATHANABLANAMACHARAMARACHARAMARACH
BLANATHANABLANAMACHARAMARACHARAMARA
LANATHANABLANAMACHARAMARACHARAMAR
ANATHANABLANAMACHARAMARACHARAMA
NATHANABLANAMACHARAMARACHARAM
ATHANABLANAMACHARAMARACHARA
THANABLANAMACHARAMARACHAR
ANABLANAMACHARAMARACHA
NABLANAMACHARAMARACH
ABLANAMACHARAMARA
BLANAMACHARAMAR
LANAMACHARAMA
ANAMACHARAM
NAMACHARA
AMACHAR
MACHA
ACH
A

O Tireless one, KOK KOUK KOUL, save Tais whom [Taraus] bore from every shivering fit, whether tertian or quartan or quotidian fever, or an every-other-day fever, or [one] by night, or [even] a mild fever: because I am the ancestral, tireless god, KOK KOUK KOUL, immediately, immediately; quickly, quickly. (*PGM* XXXIII.1-25)

(c) The use of *medicinal substances* to treat illness has been covered already in Chapter 2 and in the present chapter when we examined the work of rhizotomists, so the discussion here can be brief. To judge from Pliny's critique, what sets the medicines of the *magi*/γόητες apart from those prescribed by other healers is the unusual nature of their contents or the atypical means by which they are applied.

On the content side, some of the recipes that Pliny disparages call for rare or expensive materials that were not available to traditional healers, while others use substances that were considered degrading or offensive by "civilized" men like Pliny. In the first category are medicines concocted from the body parts of exotic animals like hyenas, lions, camels, crocodiles, chameleons, hippopotamuses, basilisks, and "dragons," all of which produce multiple remedies (especially the hyena).[126] In the second category are prescriptions that involve human blood and body parts (especially

---

[126] Interestingly, Pliny has no problem with medicinal applications of similar body parts from more familiar animals. As elsewhere, it appears that the "foreignness" of a treatment renders it suspect. Pliny also describes a number of "magical" plants that he has heard of the *magi* using (*HN* 24.156–67), but these are left out of consideration here since most of them appear to be mythical.

those of dead criminals), the dung of various animals, and loathsome creatures like moles, ticks, and vultures.

As for cures involving atypical modes of application, two types of treatments can be identified here as well. In one type, medicinal materials are applied by some unusual technique; in the other, the application is accompanied by ritual words and actions that render it effective. Examples of the first type include varying the prescription according to the prevailing sign of the zodiac; setting an animal free after removing a portion for a cure; and prohibiting the patient from viewing the person who applied the cure for a certain number of days. In the second category the prescriptions are typically complex.[127] A few examples will illustrate the point.

To remove tertian, quartan, or quotidian fevers, take the parings of the patient's fingernails and toenails and mix them with wax while saying that a cure is sought for fever, then fasten them to the door of another man's house before sunrise. (*HN* 28.86). To cure a painful spleen, lay the fresh spleen of a sheep over the patient's spleen while stating the purpose of the application, then plaster the spleen into the wall of the patient's bedroom, "sealed with a ring thrice nine times," and state again the purpose of the cure. (*HN* 30.51). To treat quartan fever, tie a thread three times around a caterpillar in a linen cloth with three knots, stating with each knot the reason for tying it. (*HN* 30.101)

Like some of the other prescriptions that we have noted, there is nothing in these recipes that was in principle beyond the skill of an ordinary Greek or Roman. But knowing what remedy to use in a given situation and how exactly it should be applied to ensure its efficacy required an expert. That was the job of the healers that elite Greek authors called γόητες or μάγοι and Romans labeled as *venefici* and *magi*.

Conclusion

Identifying and analyzing "magical" modes of healing in the Greco-Roman world is a challenging task that requires careful attention to definitions and close sifting of both literary texts and archaeological data to avoid imposing modern categories and judgments onto ancient materials. The fact that so many elite authors held negative views of "magic" and its practitioners means that we often have to read against the grain of their writings in order to construct a nuanced understanding of the various types of healers whom they deride with this term. But it can be done, as this chapter has hopefully shown.

As used here, the term "magical healers" refers to men and women who worked in the cities and countryside as "freelance ritual experts" outside of the established

---

[127] Similarly complex applications can be seen in some of the treatments that Pliny approves. For example, to cure superficial abscesses, a poultice made from verbascum roots and leaves pounded and heated with wine should be applied to the sufferer's body by a virgin who is fasting and naked. As she applies it, she should touch him with the back of her hand and say three times, "Apollo tells us that a plague cannot grow more fiery in a patient if a naked maiden quench the fire." Then both parties must spit three times (*HN* 26.93).

civic or state cultus, using specialized (and often secret) skills and techniques to channel suprahuman powers to protect or cure individuals from illness or injury. At least three types of health care providers can be classed under this heading: diviners (including dream interpreters), root-cutters, and sorcerers. A certain amount of overlap can be seen in their ideas and practices, but they were different enough that literate observers (and presumably ordinary people as well) could tell them apart and use different labels to describe them, labels that in some cases were also used by the practitioners themselves. These distinctions were sustained over time by rigorous programs of apprenticeship and instruction by which novices were inducted into often secret rites that took years to master. Most would have specialized in a single system of practice, but we also hear of men and women who used a diverse set of skills to assist people with their problems, including issues unrelated to health care.

When Paul or a member of his congregations was suffering from a health problem, it would have been both natural and easy for them to consult any of the healing experts described in this chapter. But would they have done so? Or did Paul—whether as a Jew, a Christ-follower, or a member of the elite class—hold negative views of such people and teach his followers to avoid them? If so, why do we not hear about it in his letters?

To be more specific, would Paul have sought healing from a diviner who employed "magical" techniques to diagnose or treat an illness? Would it have mattered to him whether the person did or did not claim to receive revelations from Greek or Roman deities? What about a similar person who could interpret dreams? Would Paul have asked what gods the interpreter served or what interpretive methods they used? Or would he have judged them as anyone else would, by their records and results? Except when he was in the company of Jews or Christ-followers, all of Paul's daily social interactions would have been with people who honored non-Jewish deities, and it is hard to imagine him probing people's religious proclivities before paying them for fruits and vegetables in the agora or a massage at the baths. Would he have viewed the skills of a diviner any differently?

And what about buying medicines from a root-cutter or a drug-seller? Would he have asked what kinds of rituals had been performed when the plants were harvested, or whether any spells or incantations had been pronounced over them as they were being processed into medications? Would he have searched elsewhere if their preparations included prayers or offerings to Greek or Roman deities or other numinous forces? Did he differentiate as we might today between harvesting techniques that sounded "rational" and those that appeared bizarre or inexplicable? Or did he know or care enough to make such distinctions? If he chose not to ask about the methods used, would it have mattered to him if the seller voluntarily made a point of extolling the sacred rituals that had been used to ensure the potency of the medicine? Or did he accept this as an ordinary feature of life in a "pagan" city?

Finally, what would Paul have thought about that class of healers that elite authors derided as "sorcerers"? Would he have felt any reservations about consulting them? Why or why not? Would it have mattered to him what healing techniques they wished to use in his case? For example, might he have been willing to buy an amulet from them but not to have a spell or incantation recited over him? Would he have distinguished between healing chants that named a Greek or Roman god and those that used nonsense-sounding syllables? Would he have asked what rituals had been used in the creation of a particular amulet or medication, or would he simply buy whatever he was told would remedy his problem without probing further? Would he have purchased these items from some providers and not from others, depending on how they answered his questions? What advice would he have given to his followers about such matters, and how important was it to him that they follow his instruction?

These and similar questions will continue to dog us throughout this study, but they appear more acute when we turn from asking what kinds of healing techniques Paul might have accepted from friends and family (Chapter 2), most of whom were probably Judeans or Christ-followers, to what kinds of health care providers he might have consulted when these informal modes of care failed and how he would have advised others. The questions do not become easier as we turn to look at explicitly "religious" providers in Chapter 4 or medical providers in Chapter 5, nor do the answers become much clearer. But the more we know about the health care options that were available to Paul and his followers, the better we can frame the questions that we will eventually pose to Paul and his letters.

4

Religious Healing[1]

"Religion" and Healing

It has become popular in recent years to assert that Greeks and Romans did not share our modern concept of "religion." This claim is undoubtedly true if one means by it that they did not conceive of the suprahuman realm as distinct from the quotidian world of human society or delegate relations with that realm to a particular set of personnel and institutions who mediated its benefits to other individuals and the broader society. But the value of such judgments is limited, since similar statements could be made about many other societies both past and present. The definition of religion that is embedded in these assertions is deeply rooted in Western Christian experience, a system that is relatively anomalous in the history of religion. Certainly no modern anthropologist would accept it as a standard for judging the presence or absence of "religion" in a society. The fact that scholars of classics and biblical studies can accept such statements as meaningful reveals the continuing influence of Euro-American Christianity in both fields, where cross-cultural insights from anthropological and sociological studies of religion have been slow to gain acceptance.

This is not to say that anthropologists share a common understanding of religion that can be substituted for the one criticized above. The modern scholarly quest to formulate a universally valid definition of religion has failed to produce unanimity. But both Greek and Roman societies possessed all of the features commonly included in these definitions, particularly when we narrow the focus to beliefs and practices related to health and healing. Both Greeks and Romans credited at least some instances of illness and injury to deities or other numinous forces, and both made regular use of practices that they believed would motivate or manipulate these forces to heal sick or injured bodies. Such beliefs and practices would qualify as "religious" under any definition of the term, and they will be treated as such in this chapter without enclosing the word in quotation marks.[2]

---

[1] Some of the material in this chapter was published earlier in Christopher D. Stanley, "Paul and Asklepios: The Greco-Roman Quest for Healing and the Mission of Paul," *JSNT* 42 (2019): 1–31.

[2] The question of whether Greeks and Romans possessed a system of "religion" is different from the question of what Romans meant by the Latin word *religio*, which is used differently by different authors. Cicero defines it as "the pious cult of the gods" (*Nat. d.* 1.117), which implies both "a communal relationship with the gods" and "a system of obligations stemming from that relationship" (John Scheid, *An Introduction to Roman Religion*, trans. Janet Lloyd (Bloomington: University of Indiana Press, 2003), 22–3).

What Causes Sickness?

Diagnosing an illness in the ancient world meant something different than it does today. Even Hippocratic physicians had little reliable knowledge concerning the nature and causes of disease, so their diagnoses were not necessarily more accurate by modern medical standards than those of amateurs. Most interpreted physical symptoms through the lens of a theory that involved maintaining a balance among four bodily fluids called "humors" that kept the body in proper operation. Treatment meant using appropriate means to restore this balance when it was upset.[3]

A broadly similar approach lies behind ancient religious diagnosis and treatment: certain bodily symptoms were interpreted as evidence of an underlying problem that required a specific type of remedy. Where the religious approach differed from that of the physicians was in its understanding of what caused the illness and what should be done about it. Physicians blamed illness on malfunctions within the body, and treatment involved doing things to restore the body to proper functionality. Religious practitioners credited suprahuman forces outside the body, and treatment meant performing rituals to satisfy or repel the external forces afflicting the body.

Both Greeks and Romans believed that the physical universe was regulated by gods and spirits who lived in the same world as humans rather than intervening from outside. Unlike the gods, however, humans were subject to all of the vagaries and vicissitudes of mortality, including sickness, debilitation, and death. Some people were able to accept these developments as an inevitable consequence of being human, while others sought to identify more proximate causes for their suffering in order to make sense of their pain and perhaps find a way to remove it.

The most common explanation for specific cases of sickness and suffering was to credit them to gods or other numinous forces.[4] Various reasons could be cited as to why the gods might bring sickness and pain to humans. Sometimes they got caught in the middle of conflicts among the gods and suffered through no fault of their own. Sometimes they were in the wrong place at the wrong time, as when a god decided to oppose or punish a body of humans—a city, an army, a people—and innocent people were harmed along with the guilty. Still other sicknesses were caused by capricious deities or maleficent spirits who took pleasure in inflicting pain and suffering upon humans who fell into their grasp.

But there were also many cases in which it was thought that the actions (or inactions) of humans had brought them to the attention of deities or spirits who responded by imposing punishments. In some cases the offense was unintentional, as when an individual walked inadvertently over a hidden grave or trespassed unknowingly into a place that was sacred to or inhabited by a god or spirit. Such violations of purity and ritual standards are cited more often than we might expect as reasons for divine displeasure. Another common cause of judgment was negligence in performing one's

---

[3] More will be said on this subject in Chapter 5.
[4] Such beliefs were not limited to Greeks and Romans, as Dale Martin rightly observes: "The assumption that gods and other superhuman beings (such as daimons) may be vengeful or jealous or cause disease was shared by most people around the ancient Mediterranean throughout antiquity" (*Inventing Superstition*, 54).

duties to the gods, especially in cultic matters, such as failing to fulfill a vow or bringing a faulty animal to be sacrificed. Suffering could also result from mistreatment of others, especially those who were under the protection of a particular god or goddess such as Odysseus or Aeneas. Included under this heading are the dead, whose burial sites and memory had to be properly tended or else they would afflict the living. Worst of all was willful defiance of the gods such as profaning their cult, robbing their temples, or killing people to whom they had given protection. No ritual could remedy these faults or protect the violator from the effects of divine wrath.

Sickness was one of the afflictions that the gods could impose upon humans in response to any of these violations. Treating sickness under this scenario meant diagnosing the reason for the divine action (usually but not always some fault on the part of the sick person), prescribing the correct ritual to expiate or remove the offense, and performing or assisting in the performance of the ritual cure. In lesser cases the entire process could be carried out within the household, but more serious or persistent cases required the presence of a religious expert.

Several types of religious experts were available to give advice and treatment. For our purposes they can be divided into two broad categories: private and public. On the private side stood various types of freelance ritual experts who operated much like the practitioners that were discussed in Chapter 3. On the public side was the communal cult of the gods in its various expressions, including a series of regional healing centers. Both categories will be discussed in this chapter, but more attention will be given to the latter category since its societal influence was more dominant and pervasive.

Freelance Religious Healers

In the previous chapter we noted the presence of two types of freelance ritual experts whose approach to health care was more akin to religious than to "magical" modes of healing despite being often classed with the latter group. One was purifiers and the other was exorcists. Both are known only through the writings of elite authors. It is not entirely clear from their references whether certain people specialized in such skills or whether they were part of a broader repertoire of techniques used by different practitioners along with other healing methods. For the sake of our study it will be assumed that they were specialists since each method has its own view of the healing process that might have evoked different reactions from Paul and his followers than the public practices examined later in the chapter.[5]

Purifiers

As we noted earlier, both Greeks and Romans viewed ritual pollution as a possible cause of sickness, and both had similar systems for dealing with such pollutions, including

[5] For the sake of completeness, it should be noted that there were other types of freelance religious practitioners in the Greco-Roman world besides those treated here, such as the wandering priests of Cybele or the proponents of various "mystery religions." But it is not evident that any of them made health care a primary concern, so they are omitted from this study. Wandering Christ-followers like Paul could also be classed under this heading, as we will see in Chapter 10.

the time-honored ritual of sacrificing to various gods.⁶ But there also arose as early as the classical era in Greece a class of ritual purifiers who worked outside of the cultus to diagnose and treat illnesses and afflictions that they claimed were sent by the gods in response to various sorts of impurity. To remove such an illness, one had to pay for rituals of purification that they alone knew how to perform. From the literary record it appears that the techniques that they used were mostly similar or identical to those employed in the cultus, but they claimed to have specialized knowledge regarding what rituals should be applied in a given situation and how they should be performed. This includes sacrificial cleansing, which had to be performed by one of their number in order to produce the desired healing.

The limited evidence that is available suggests that purifiers shared their culture's understanding of the causes of ritual pollution while adding more to the list. When called in to diagnose an illness, they were likely to point to such arcane causes as an evil spell or curse from an enemy or the activities of dark deities like Hecate. Anxieties about such dangers are attested in many sources, but two examples from the late classical or early Hellenistic era can speak for the whole.

In a work titled "Characters," the philosopher Theophrastus (371–287 BCE) presents a scathing caricature of "the superstitious person" (ὁ δεισιδαίμων), someone whose life is dominated by fear of the gods and ritual pollution.

> He is apt, also, to purify his house frequently, alleging that Hecate has been brought into it by spells; and, if an owl is startled by him in his walk, he will exclaim "Glory be to Athene!" before he proceeds. He will not tread upon a tombstone, or come near a dead body or a woman defiled by childbirth, saying that it is expedient for him not to be polluted. . . . He would seem, too, to be of those who are scrupulous in sprinkling themselves with sea-water [a common purifier]; and, if ever he observes anyone feasting on the garlic at the cross-roads [where offerings were left for Hecate], he will go away, pour water over his head, and, summoning the priestesses, bid them carry a squill or a puppy around him [used in arcane cleansing rituals] for purification.⁷

Menander had a similar person in mind when crafting a scene in his *Phasma* in which a slave mocks his master's superstition regarding an illness (50–6). All of the treatments that he cites were common elements in the purifier's repertoire.

> If there had really been anything wrong with you, then you'd have to look for a real cure. But there isn't. Find an imaginary cure for your imaginary disease and persuade yourself that it's doing you some good. Get the women to wipe you round in a circle and fumigate you. Sprinkle yourself with water drawn from three springs, with salt and lentils added. ⁸

---

⁶ More will be said later about the role of cultic sacrifices as a channel for healing.
⁷ Excerpted from the 1870 translation by R. C. Jebb posted at https://www.eudaemonist.com/biblion/characters, section XVI. His rendering, though older, is much more readable than that of the 1929 Loeb translation.
⁸ Cited by Robert Parker, *Miasma: Pollution and Purification in Early Greek Religion* (Oxford: Clarendon, 1983), 207.

Caricature, of course, is not reality, but it has to bear some semblance to reality in order to strike its target, and there is ample evidence from more prosaic sources to indicate that such ideas and practices were common. Thus it appears that there was a ready market for the services of freelance ritual purifiers who claimed to be able to diagnose hidden impurities and remove them as a means of curing illness.

The range of methods employed by purifiers was broader than those mentioned in the texts just cited. Robert Parker explored the subject in his study of pollution and purification in early Greece, and his discussion has parallels in later Greek and Roman literature.[9] According to Parker's analysis, rites of expiation and purification were normally conducted facing east. The sick person usually sat in the middle of a circle as rituals were performed around them. Some of these rituals were drawn from the public cult, including sacrifices, lustrations, prayers, and incantations. Others resembled "magical" practices, such as spitting (a common practice for averting evil), laying a puppy on the sick person's abdomen to absorb the impurity, or burying the means of purification in the ground far from human habitation.

Various substances were used to purify the sick body and its environs from pollution based on the skills and judgment of the purifier.[10] As in religious rituals, water was the most frequent cleansing agent, though its collection and use were more narrowly delineated than in the cult. Salt water from the sea was considered most effective, followed by water that was drawn from several springs and mingled together. Pungent materials added to a fire—especially sulfur—could also have a purificatory effect. Certain plant materials were believed to possess the power to remove or avert impurities, including laurel boughs, olive branches, buckthorn, and squill. Numerous substances were used in rituals of transference to absorb the impurity from the sick person, including sacrificial animals, puppies, eggs, fleece, mud, and bran mash. The entire process was surrounded by incantations that made the rituals effective.

Many freelance purifiers were women. Among the many "mendicant holy women" that Matthew Dickie describes in his study of ancient magic are women who used purification rituals and incantations to cure illness. In later periods they appear in a more settled role in cities and towns. Most authors depict them as older women from the lower class of society, but Dickie offers evidence that some were younger and better situated. Limited evidence suggests that they sometimes worked in groups. Whether the same was true for male purifiers is unknown.[11]

Exorcists

Whereas purification rituals presume that the sick person is suffering justly due to some purity violation that incurred divine displeasure, the ritual of exorcism sees the sick person as an innocent victim of suprahuman beings who must be driven away

---

[9] A helpful investigation of Roman ideas about pollution that draws on Parker's work is Jack J. Lennon, *Pollution and Religion in Ancient Rome* (Cambridge: Cambridge University Press, 2014). Israel Israelowich observes rightly that "pollution and purification were inherent features of the Greco-Roman health-care system" (*Society, Medicine and Religion in the Sacred Tales of Aelius Aristides*, 46).

[10] The following summary is derived from Parker, *Miasma*, 226–32.

[11] *Magic and Magicians in the Greco-Roman World*, 88–90, 159, 182–4, 237–8, 298–9.

in order for the person to recover. To call these beings "demons" is misleading since ancient Greeks used the word δαίμονες to refer to beings who occupied a middle state between gods and humans and not to evil spirits who oppose God and attack humans.[12] But Greeks and Romans did believe that the suprahuman realm included malicious actors who sought to afflict the bodies of humans for their own ends. For the Greeks, it was the Nosoi and Keres; for the Romans, the *lemures* and *larvae* served as generic agents of harm, but most forms of sickness were caused by a particular deity or spirit who bore its name: Febris (fever), Macies (wasting), Tabes (corruption), Scabies (itching), and so on. Ideas such as these were rejected by more philosophically minded Greeks and Romans as unworthy of the divine, which they regarded as uniformly good and favorably disposed toward humans. But their views carried little influence with the masses, who stood firmly by their traditional beliefs.

Not all illnesses could be charged to harmful spirits. Their influence was seen most often in cases that seemed inexplicable by other means, such as epilepsy, insanity, and various forms of delirium where the person appeared to be "out of their mind."[13] The spirits that caused sickness were generally thought to attack the person from outside rather than invading and "possessing" their bodies as Jews and Christians believed.[14] The typical response to such attacks was to perform rituals to drive the spirits away. Simple apotropaic ("turning away") rituals like spitting on the ground or forming the hand into a "fig sign" with the thumb protruding from a closed fist were employed routinely by Greeks and Romans as a means of averting evil influences, but such acts were too weak to cure sicknesses caused by suprahuman beings. For this, one needed a specialist.

The common practice of labeling these specialists as "exorcists" is unfortunate since it evokes misleading images and ideas derived from Jewish and Christian history and modern popular culture. A term like "apotropaists" would be more suitable, but the rarity of this word in English renders it useless for most readers. The term "exorcists" will therefore be retained here with the understanding that (a) their aim was to drive away rather than cast out harmful spirits, and (b) these spirits were not evil beings allied with the devil as in Jewish and Christian usage.

Exorcistic healers appear only briefly and sporadically in Greek and Roman literature outside of the magical papyri, so it is difficult to paint a reliable picture of their activities.[15] As with other "magical" activities, the role is often associated with

---

[12] A helpful discussion of ancient Greek views of δαίμονες can be found in Martin, *Inventing Superstition*, 98–107.

[13] Luck, *Arcana Mundi*, 165.

[14] The earliest clear references to "possession" and exorcism outside of Jewish and Christian circles appear in the second century CE writings of Lucian and Plutarch and in Philostratus's account of Apollonius of Tyana. Roy Kotansky thinks that these later accounts reflect Jewish influence ("Greek Exorcistic Amulets," in *Ancient Magic and Ritual Power*, ed. Marvin Meyer and Paul Mirecki[Leiden and New York: Brill, 1995], 246).

[15] The oldest surviving reference to the use of rituals by experts to avert the influence of harmful spirits (here called δαίμονες) appears in the Derveni Papyrus (fifth century BCE), which mentions sacrifices, libations, bread offerings, and incantations. It is not included here because there is no clear reference to sickness in the text, but the rituals are nevertheless instructive. For a careful analysis of its contents, see Amir Ahmadi, "The 'Magoi' and 'Daimones' in Column VI of the Derveni Papyrus," *Numen* 61 (2014): 484–508.

older women who used a variety of rituals to protect or liberate people from harmful influences, whether caused by spirits, curses, or evil spells.[16] For the most part their practices seem to have resembled those used in the cultus for averting pernicious spirits from city or state: prayers, sacrifices, incantations, and purifications.[17] As with other practices disparaged by the elites, few details of their rituals have survived apart from what was included in the Greek magical papyri. Here we find many examples of charms and spells designed to drive away harmful spirits, along with instructions for creating amulets to avert or remove their influence. It is hard to judge how far these texts preserve the practices of earlier experts and what represents new developments, but it seems likely that they are at least broadly similar to methods employed in Greek circles for centuries. A few examples will show the types of incantations that exorcists might have used in Paul's day to repel spirits that caused sickness.

> A tested charm of Pibechis for those possessed by daimons: Take oil of unripe olives with the herb *mastigia* and the fruit pulp of the lotus, and boil them with colorless marjoram while saying, "IOEL OS SARTHIOMI EMORI THEOCHIPSOITH SITHEMEOCH SOTHE IOE MIMIPSOTHIOOPH PHERSOTHI AEEIOYO IOE EO CHARI PHTHA, come out from NN" (add the usual). *The phylactery:* On a tin lamella write, IAEO ABRAOTH IOCH PHTHA MESENPSIN IAO PHEOCH IAEO CHARSOK, and hang it on the patient. It is terrifying to every daimon, a thing he fears. (*PGM* IV.3007-19)[18]

> I, Abrasax, shall deliver. Abrasax am I! ABRASAX ABRASICHOOU, help little Sophia-Priskilla. Get hold of and do away with what comes to little Sophia-Priskilla, whether it is a shivering fit—get hold of it! Whether a phantom—get hold of it! Whether a daimon—get hold of it! I, Abrasax, shall deliver. Abrasax am I! BRASAX ABRASICHOOU. Get hold of, get hold of and do away with . . . what comes to little Sophia-Priskilla on this very day, whether it is a shivering fit—do away with it! Whether a daimon—do away with it! (*PGM* LXXXM. 1-27)

> [Protect] her, NN, o lord, [from all] evil acts [and from every] demonic visitation [and] . . . of Hekate and from . . . attack and [from every onslaught (?) in sleep . . . [from] mute daimons [and from every] epileptic fit [and from all] epilepsy and . . .and. (*PGM CXIV.* 1-14)

Carved gems were also used as exorcistic tools, though the extent of their availability in Paul's day is unclear.[19] Most depicted some sort of battle scene between a god and a

---

[16] Dickie, *Magic and Magicians in the Greco-Roman World*, 105–6.
[17] For a summary of these rituals, see Simboli, *Disease-Spirits*, 13–44. The use of purification rituals to avert suprahuman powers from epileptics is mentioned as early as the fifth century BCE by the author of *On the Sacred Disease*.
[18] The remainder of this particular charm shows Jewish and Christian influences, but the part cited here does not.
[19] According to Véronique Dasen and Árpád Nagy ("Gems," 433), the heyday of carved gems for healing was the second to third centuries CE, but examples are known from the late Hellenistic era. The material that follows is summarized from Dasen and Nagy, 435–8, and Dasen, "Healing Images," 178–83.

daimon who is blamed for the illness. Many included brief inscriptions invoking the *daimon* to leave the person alone. They could be set into rings, worn as pendants close to the ailment (neck, thigh, arm, back), or carried in a pouch on the body. Most were used to treat mysterious internal illnesses, especially those affecting the uterus and the stomach, as well as ailments that were hard to cure, such as gout or hemorrhage. Different materials were used to treat different conditions, and spells and incantations were recited during their creation to enhance their effectiveness. For the most part this preparatory activity would have been invisible to the wearer, who saw only the finished product, though spells might have been recited as it was applied.

Cultic Healing

Purifiers and exorcists had at best a mixed reputation in the Greco-Roman world as providers of religion-based health care. No such ambiguity attends the primary source of religious healing, the cultus of the gods. The term "temple healing" is sometimes used for this model, but this designation is overly narrow since religious healing could be sought in a variety of settings, including the home, rural shrines, temple buildings, and regional centers where the god Asklepios and his servants tended to the health needs of all who visited. Except for the home, which was discussed in Chapter 2, all of these sites were first and foremost venues for cultic veneration of the gods, whether Greek, Roman, or indigenous, and ritualized acts of worship played a vital role in their model of healing. The term "cultic healing" is thus a more fitting label for the services that they collectively provided.

The idea that gods can cure sick bodies was shared by virtually all Greeks and Romans apart from a few philosophers who saw the gods as being above such meddling in human affairs and a few more who flirted with atheism. The same was true for the various native cultures that came under Greek and Roman rule in the centuries before Christianity. Even Hippocratic physicians held this view, as we will see in Chapter 5. There was no sacred–secular divide in Greek or Roman culture by which religious ideas were excluded from "scientific" modes of health care.

Any deity could be petitioned for healing. Of the traditional Greek gods, literary sources mention Zeus, Pan, Hermes, Artemis, Herakles, Athena, Pluto, and the Nymphs, among others. Roman gods who were linked to healing include Salus, Valetudo, Castor and Pollux, Jupiter, Mars, Minerva, and Apollo. The Egyptian deities Isis and Serapis are also cited for their work in this area.[20] But the gods who were most renowned for their healing activity were Apollo, Asklepios (known to the Romans as Aesculapius), and the latter's daughter, Hygieia (conflated by the Romans with their health goddess Salus). Other sons and daughters of Asklepios also appear now and then with their father, but their popularity was minimal. A long list of indigenous deities also served as healers. In Asia Minor, where Paul spent much of this time, the primary indigenous

---

[20] Summarized from Georgia Petridou, "Healing Shrines," in *A Companion to Science, Technology, and Medicine in Ancient Greece and Rome*, ed. George L. Irby (New York: Wiley-Blackwell, 2016), 434–9; Nissen, *Entre Asclépios et Hippocrate*, 82–117; Penso, *La médicine romaine*, 1.28–35.

healers were the earth goddess Cybele and the Phrygian moon god Mên, both of whom were honored across the region.

Temples and shrines of healing deities were so numerous as to be accessible to virtually everyone in the Greco-Roman world. Every town or city had its temple of Asklepios where residents could present offerings and seek cures from the god, and similar petitions could be directed to other deities at their own temples. Historians have identified hundreds of healing centers dedicated to Asklepios and other gods around the Mediterranean world, placing them within reach of all but the most isolated residents.[21] Such data suggest that religious healing played a vital role in the health care system of the Greco-Roman world long after the rise of Hippocratic medicine. The two systems not only coexisted but actively borrowed from one another, as we will see in Chapter 6.

A proper analysis of the ancient cultic healing system would distinguish between rural shrines, civic temples, and regional healing centers. But evidence is scanty for the first two categories, and there are good reasons to think that similar practices prevailed in both settings for gods other than Asklepios, whose healing techniques were distinct enough to merit separate treatment. Our analysis will therefore begin with an overview of healing practices at the shrines of deities other than Asklepios and then shift to a more detailed examination of the Asklepian health care system.

Local Shrines (Non-Asklepian)

Because this study is concerned primarily with the health care options that were available to Paul and his followers, our investigation of non-Asklepian religious healing options will focus on Asia Minor. The regions from which enough material has survived to permit scholarly analysis are Lydia, Phrygia, and Caria in central and western Asia Minor. Before we review this material, however, it will be useful to summarize what is known more generally about the ways in which Greeks and Romans sought healing at local sanctuaries.

Giuseppe Penso describes a number of ritual techniques that were used at Roman temples by people seeking healing.[22] Some began with a formal procession to the temple, while others were more subdued. Sacrificial offerings were common in healing ceremonies, including animals, wine, wheat, and herbs. Divination was practiced on the bodies of sacrificial animals to discern the cause of the sickness or signs of the god's renewed favor. At the center of the ritual was supplication of the god in prayer by the sick person or the priest using language prescribed for the occasion. The entire system was founded on the principle of reciprocal exchange, with the sick person making offerings to the god either to expiate a past violation or to incite the god to provide a cure. Dedicatory inscriptions or sacrifices were used after healing was achieved to give thanks to the god.

Greek healing rites were broadly similar to those of the Romans since the latter adapted their own traditions to be more like the Greeks as part of their encounter

---

[21] More will be said about these centers later.
[22] *La médicine romaine*, 50–5.

with Greek culture. Prayers and sacrifices or offerings were vital to all forms of ancient Mediterranean religion, and similar ideas can be discerned regarding the role of the sacrificial ritual in relation to the petition for healing (as propitiation/expiation or inducement to divine action). Greeks were less fastidious than Romans about following prescribed forms of prayer, while divination played a larger role in Roman rituals. But the framework was the same.

Indigenous healing rituals were both similar to and different from those of Greeks and Romans, to judge from the evidence of Asia Minor. Angelos Chaniotis and Aslak Rostad have analyzed forty-five votive healing inscriptions that stood originally in rural shrines in northwestern Lydia and Phrygia.[23] The texts of these inscriptions reveal a strong link between sin and sickness. All were inscribed on steles that relate how the god punished the offerer with various physical ailments in response to some violation and how the god healed the person after the sin was acknowledged and requisite cultic acts were performed. A wide variety of violations is cited in the inscriptions, but most center on matters of ritual purity.[24] The erection of the stele in a public space was a vital element of the healing ritual, since it testifies to the god's righteous expectations of humans and elicits praise from viewers for the deity's mercy upon those who fulfill their obligations.[25] Some of the steles even give us a glimpse into the rituals that were involved in the reconciliation process. Stephen Mitchell describes two such specimens.

> A few of the inscriptions also carry a relief depicting the confession scene itself: a priest stands holding a wreath in one hand and the god's staff resting on a low base in the other; the confessor confronts him holding up his right hand as a pledge of honesty while he makes the confession; in a second case a woman confessor places an object on an altar while other figures, with right hands raised, look on, either as witnesses or to join in the praises of the god.[26]

Ailments that the inscriptions credit to the gods include eye problems (the largest number by far),[27] mental illness, gynecological diseases, and pains in the legs, arms, or genitals. Chaniotis finds no link between these ailments and specific gods: "Practically

---

[23] "Illness and Cures in the Greek Propitiatory Inscriptions and Dedications of Lydia and Phrygia," in van der Eijk et al., *Ancient Medicine*, 323–44; Aslak Rostad, *Human Transgression—Divine Retribution: A Study of Religious Transgressions and Punishments in Greek Cultic Regulation and Lydian-Phrygian Propitiatory Inscriptions ("Confession Inscriptions")* (Oxford: Archaeopress Publishing, 2020). A shorter, but still helpful, overview appears in Stephen Mitchell, *Anatolia: Land, Men, and God in Asia Minor*, 2 vols. (Oxford: Clarendon, 1995), 1.191–5.

[24] For evidence and analysis, see Rostad, *Human Transgression—Divine Retribution*, 121–44.

[25] Aslak Rostad notes (*Human Transgression—Divine Retribution*, 37–8) that the idea of reciprocity that is implied in these inscriptions and others from the region is identical to what we see in Greek and Roman religion, as are the rituals that are used. Their relevance is thus not limited to the region where they were found—as Rostad puts it, "There were no basic differences between religion here and other places in Anatolia" (39).

[26] Mitchell, *Anatolia*, 1.192.

[27] Chaniotis notes that eye problems are also the most common condition described in the healing tablets from the Asklepian center at Epidaurus in Greece as well as other sites. He attributes this to the debilitating consequences that blindness would have caused for a working man or woman in pre-modern societies ("Illness and Cures in the Greek Propitiatory Inscriptions," 327).

any local deity was believed to be competent to cause any kind of health problem."[28] Twenty-six different deities are named as causing suffering and healing, including both Olympian gods (eight localized variations of Zeus, three of Apollo, and Artemis) and indigenous deities (four variants of the moon god Mên, four of the earth goddess Meter, and assorted others).[29] In some cases the god is said to have taken the initiative in revealing the cause of the sickness by an oracle or a dream. Occasional references to physicians can be found in the inscriptions, but for the most part they lack the medical terminology and techniques that are found in many Asklepian accounts of healing, reflecting the local priests' ignorance of or disinterest in medical modes of healing. In their place we find references to sacrifices, purification rituals, prayers, and incantations.

A second batch of local inscriptions was studied by Cécile Nissen, who sought to identify all of the healing cults and physicians that are attested in the region of Caria in southwestern Asia Minor. Her multidisciplinary study, which draws on literary texts, epigraphy, archaeology, and numismatics, found evidence for thirty different healing sites and eighty physicians from the classical era to the late Roman Empire.[30] As in Lydia, the inscriptions name a variety of deities as healers, including Greek (Asklepios, Hygiea, Telesphorus, Apollo, Pluto and Kore, and the Nymphs), indigenous (Mên and two otherwise unknown figures, Hemithea and Arconessos), and Egyptian (Isis and Serapis) divinities.[31] Incubation (sleeping at a sacred site in hopes of receiving a dream from the god) is mentioned at one center, and confessions and dedicatory inscriptions of the type that Chaniotis found in Lydia and Phrygia are also attested.[32] Otherwise prayers and sacrifices seem to have been the most common modes of treatment. The only notable difference between the Lydian and Carian materials apart from the single reference to incubation is the increased presence of medical language in the latter, a pattern that reflects the presence of two major medical centers in the region and the resulting interaction between religious and medical healers in the management of sickness.

Taken together, the studies of Chaniotis and Nissen reveal the wide availability and diversity of healing centers in western Asia Minor, the site of several congregations of Christ-followers founded by Paul and his associates. Those who joined these groups would have been accustomed by a lifetime of experience to analyze and treat sickness in the manner described in these materials, interpreting suffering as a sign that they had offended one of the local deities and visiting local temples or shrines in hopes of

[28] Ibid., 330.
[29] Chaniotis includes two tables listing the names of all of the deities and the illnesses with which they are associated ("Illness and Cures in the Greek Propitiatory Inscriptions," 340–2). Rostad cites a broader study by de Hoz of religious inscriptions from the region that included the names of dozens of deities (*Human Transgression—Divine Retribution*, 26).
[30] *Entre Asclépios et Hippocrate*, 79.
[31] The Egyptian deities are unattested in the inscriptions that Chaniotis cites for Lydian and Phrygia; their presence here can be traced to the fact that Caria was periodically under Egyptian control. The inclusion of Pluto and Kore reflects a broader pattern of venerating the underworld deities in this region due to its unusual geothermal qualities, which include numerous hot springs, caves filled with noxious gasses, and periodic earthquakes. The springs also explain the presence of the Nymphs.
[32] Ibid., 114, 186–8, 257.

learning what they had done and how to remedy it. Here they would have followed the rituals prescribed by the temple personnel: offering sacrifices, reciting prescribed prayers, confessing their sins, engaging in purification rituals, and giving honor to the deity for anticipated or realized healing. Later they might have returned to erect a testimonial stele. This is the world that we must keep in mind when we turn in Chapters 8 and 9 to investigate how becoming Christ-followers might have affected the way in which Paul's converts treated physical ailments.

Asklepian Health Care

Of the many religious healing options that were available to Greeks and Romans in Paul's day, the most popular by far was the health care system that centered on the Greek healing deity Asklepios, whom the Romans adopted under the Latinized name of Aesculapius after he was brought to Rome in 293 BCE in response to a plague.[33] Historians and archaeologists have found evidence for up to 900 temples and shrines of Asklepios across the Greco-Roman world by the second century CE, and numerous literary references testify to the god's popularity.[34] Inscriptions and votive offerings in these temples testified to his healing power, and stories of his miraculous cures circulated orally throughout the Empire. Images of him as a kindly middle-aged man holding a wooden staff with a snake twined around it were sold in the agora for use at home. Stories and songs honored him as a compassionate and merciful savior who cared as much for the poor and lowly as the rich and connected, making him one of the few Greek gods who inspired deep personal devotion. Wherever healing was needed, Asklepios was there.

The idea of Asklepios as an accessible healer was reinforced by stories of how he became a deity. At least three different versions of the story are known, but all have certain common features.[35] Asklepios did not begin life as a god, but as a hero or demigod, the product of a divine father (Apollo) and a human mother (Coronis).

[33] According to Livy and Ovid, the Roman Senate consulted the Sibylline Oracles during a particularly virulent plague and was told that they must bring Asklepios to the capital. A delegation of elders was then sent to the god's healing center in Epidauros, Greece, to bring the god's cult image to Rome. Their efforts were forestalled when a large snake, an animal sacred of Asklepios, slithered onto their boat and settled onto the bow. Taking this as a sign of the god's presence, the delegation returned to Rome, where the snake slithered into the water and swam to a small island in the middle of the Tiber River. A temple to Asklepios (Latinized to Aesculapius) was soon built on the site and the plague ended. From then on, he became a Roman as well as a Greek deity.

[34] Information about the extent and availability of Asklepian temples in the Roman Empire is summarized by Hart, *Asclepius*, 165–82, who arrives at a total of 513 sites. Higher figures are given by Gary Ferngren, who counts 670 temples and shrines where Asklepios was worshipped alone or with other gods (*Medicine and Religion*, 67), and W. J. Riethmüller, who finds 177 Asklepeia in the Greek mainland and 732 outside of Greece (*Asklepios: Heiligtümer und Kulte*, 2 vols [Heidelberg: Verlag Archäologie und Geschichte], 2005). Primary sources for many of these centers are available in Edelstein and Edelstein, *Asclepius*, 1.370–452.

[35] The earliest literary account of the story comes from the fifth century BCE in Pindar's *Pythiae* II.1–58. Subsequent versions are given by Hesiod, Ovid, Diodorus, and Pseudo-Apollodorus (references in Hart, *Asclepius*, 6–11). Greek texts and translations of the extant materials about Asklepios and his divine descendants (including Hippocrates!) can be found in Edelstein and Edelstein, *Asclepius*, 1.1–107, followed by a series of additional texts that describe his deification and divine nature (1.108–82). The authors provide a thorough analysis and discussion of all of these texts in 2.1–138.

While pregnant by Apollo, Coronis took a human lover and incurred the god's wrath. In a fit of jealous rage, he (or his sister Artemis, in some versions) killed her. Apollo later regretted what he had done and rescued the baby Asklepios from his mother's body on the funeral pyre, then handed him over to the centaur Chiron to raise.

Chiron taught Asklepios the healing arts, and he was so adept that he soon surpassed both his master and his father in his skills. He was a kind and gracious man who cured all who came to him. In time, he healed so many people that Hades complained to Zeus that his kingdom was being deprived of subjects because Asklepios was preventing so many people from dying. In some versions of the story Asklepios even raised people from the dead; in others Zeus merely feared that this would happen.

Zeus, acknowledging the validity of his brother's concerns, struck Asklepios dead with a bolt of lightning. His father Apollo then killed the Cyclopes in retaliation for his death, but Zeus propitiated him by elevating Asklepios to the heavens as a constellation and a god. Humans soon began to build temples in his honor, and his cult spread as people came to these sites in search of healing and were visited by the god. Sometimes he was accompanied in these visits by one or more of his divine children, especially his daughter Hygieia (Greek for "health").[36]

This actual history of Asklepios's rise to prominence is more prosaic. He appears first in Greek literature in the *Iliad*, where his sons are named as healers who accompanied the Thracian contingent at the walls of Troy (ii. 729-33, iv. 192-219, xi. 504-20).[37] His reputation as a healer with close ties to the centaur Chiron is older than the *Iliad*, which mentions both points, but nothing more is said about him. When and where he first received honors as a god is unclear, but the oldest known healing complex to be erected in his name was at Epidauros in the northeastern Greek Peloponnese in the fifth century BCE. His cult spread rapidly from there as temples and healing centers were built across the Mediterranean world and beyond during the next few centuries.

Two major healing centers were constructed in Asia Minor in the fourth century BCE as direct extensions of the one at Epidauros. One was at Kos in southwestern Turkey and the other at Pergamon in northwest Turkey.[38] People came from all over Asia Minor, including the cities where Paul established congregations of Christ-followers, to be treated at these centers. Those who were too ill to travel on their own were carried by family or friends. Poor people would have found it difficult to afford the trip due to the rigors and costs of travel and the potential loss of several weeks of income, so their clientele consisted primarily of people who possessed at least a modicum of resources. Those at the upper end of society for whom time and expense were no barrier sometimes engaged in the kind of "medical tourism" that was popular

---

[36] For a helpful examination of the role of Hygieia as a healing partner with Asklepios, see Michael T. Compton, "The Association of Hygieia with Asklepios in Graeco-Roman Asklepieion Medicine," *Journal of the History of Medicine and Allied Sciences* 57 (2002): 312–29.

[37] The son whose work is acclaimed in the *Iliad* is Machaon, who along with the god's other children appears now and then alongside his father in later images but never attains prominence as a healing deity in his own right. Some scholars have traced the cult of Asklepios to Thrace on the basis of these passages and a later reference in Strabo (*Geog.* 14.39), but this is mere conjecture. No archaeological evidence supports such a claim.

[38] This same era marks the beginning of Hippocratic medicine, a commonality that will be discussed in Chapter 5.

with wealthy nineteenth-century Europeans, lingering for weeks to enjoy the spa-like facilities while receiving top-quality care for their bodies.[39] For these visitors, as Michael T. Compton observes, "The sanctuary had become a sanitarium."[40]

All of the major Asklepian health centers were laid out similarly and offered similar types of care. The entire compound was surrounded by walls that marked it as sacred, and temples of Asklepios and his family stood at their center. Sacrifices, offerings, and hymns were presented to the gods on a daily basis by a corps of priests, attendants, and slaves who managed all aspects of the temple's operation. A sacred well or spring stood near the temple where those who were seeking healing could cleanse their bodies and drink the healing waters before participating in the ceremonies.[41] Bath complexes and athletic facilities were available for those staying at the facility, accompanied in many cases by a theater that was used for musical and dramatic recitations and competitions. Covered stoas protected guests from the hot summer sun and provided a dry place for less privileged guests to sleep at night. Visitors of higher status slept in simple guesthouses on the premises or in the nearby town or city.

At the heart of the complex was the abaton, the sleeping chamber that distinguished Asklepian healing centers from all other types of health care.[42] Those who were sick slept on simple pallets on the floor in hopes of being visited by Asklepios in a dream.[43] Various rituals were required to prepare them for the divine encounter, including putting on a simple tunic, performing ritual washings, presenting a sacrifice at the altar, placing a small fee into a box, carrying torches around the sanctuary grounds, and contemplating the statue of the god and the inscriptions and votive offerings that testified to his healing power. Hymns and additional sacrifices and offerings by the temple personnel accompanied these rituals. All of these elements worked together to direct the sick person's mind toward the greatness of Asklepios and so intensify his or her faith in the god's power.[44]

---

[39] Israelowich, *Patients and Healers in the High Roman Empire*, 112.

[40] "The Union of Religion and Health in Ancient Asklepieia," *Journal of Religion and Health* 37 (1998): 304.

[41] Aelius Aristides composed an entire hymn in honor of this well—for Greek text and translation, see *In Praise of Asclepius: Aelius Aristides, Selected Prose Hymns*, ed. Donald A. Russell, Michael Trapp, and Heinz-Günther Nesselrath (Tübingen: Mohr Siebeck, 2016), 38–45. Some thirty sites associated with Asklepios also had hot springs, but there were none at the major healing centers. Other gods were also associated with these sites, suggesting that Asklepios was added later as his cult spread. For the evidence, see J. H. Croon, "Hot Springs and Healing Gods," *Mnemosyne*, 4th ser., 20 (1967): 225–46.

[42] The following description of the abaton ritual is based on a close reading of the literary and inscriptional evidence cited in Edelstein and Edelstein, *Asclepius*, 1.194–266, with support from summaries provided by various scholars. A detailed narrative of a fictional visit to the Asklepion at Pergamon that includes a description of the facilities and several accounts of visits to the abaton can be found in my historical novel, *A Rooster for Asklepios* (Buffalo: Amelia Books, 2020), 406–520.

[43] The idea that gods appeared to people in dreams was broadly accepted throughout the ancient world, and most people seem to have acknowledged a place for dreams in healing, even physicians (see Chapter 5). A discussion of divine dream appearances in literature going back to Homer can be found in William V. Harris, *Dreams and Experience in Classical Antiquity* (Cambridge, MA and London: Harvard University Press, 2009), 38–43.

[44] Olympia Panagiotidou offers an insightful argument from neuropsychology on how the placebo effect might have been activated by these rituals in "Religious Healing and the Asclepius Cult: A Case of Placebo Effects," *Open Theology* 2 (2016): 79–91. A fuller analysis can be found in Edelstein and Edelstein, *Asclepius*, 1.158–73.

Eventually everyone settled down to sleep in the abaton or the temple. Sometimes Asklepios or a member of his family would appear in a dream and effect a cure while the sick person slept, while at other times the god would prescribe a treatment regimen to be implemented by physicians who worked at the centers. Most of these divine prescriptions followed the standard methods of medical care: diet, exercise, purgation, baths, medications, blood-letting, and so on.[45] Some dreams included a visit by a sacred dog or snake who licked or bit the affected body part and immediately healed them. Dream interpreters were available afterward to help patients make sense of their dreams.

How many people actually received such dreams and how many went away cured is impossible to say, but archaeological and literary evidence suggests that the number was significant. Two types of archaeological material testify to their effectiveness. The first is votive images of body parts that had been healed during a visit. Thousands of these images representing virtually every part of the human anatomy have been excavated at both Asklepian healing centers and local temples. Most are made of unpainted terracotta, but stone and metal images are also known. Some were affixed to plaques giving the name of the person healed, but most are unmarked. Local craft workers created the images and the people who had been cured purchased them and presented them to temple personnel as thank-offerings. These offerings were hung on the walls of the temples and the abaton as material testimonies to future visitors of the healing power of the god.[46] So many of these offerings were donated over the centuries that they had to be cleared out periodically to make room for others.[47]

The second type of evidence for the effectiveness of Asklepian health care is epigraphic. Two large inscribed tablets from Epidauros (mostly fourth century BCE) tell brief stories of forty-three cures, most of them "miraculous" to a greater or lesser degree, and scattered examples have been found at other sites also.[48] Literary evidence suggests that such testimonial tablets and steles were common at Asklepian sanctuaries, where they were affixed to the walls or erected on stone bases. Most of them show Asklepios applying treatments similar to those used by physicians even when he is doing miracles, such as applying salves or performing surgery. Unlike human physicians, however, he shows no interest in diagnosing the cause of the illness;

---

[45] The overlap between medical and religious modes of treatment at the Asklepian healing centers will be discussed more fully in Chapter 6.
[46] The distribution of body parts is uneven; some temples have more of one body part and others another. Some interpreters have suggested that these differences reflect a degree of specialization among the various centers (e.g., Steven M. Oberhelman, "Anatomical Votive Reliefs as Evidence for Specialization at Healing Sanctuaries in the Ancient Mediterranean World," *Athens Journal of Health* 1 [2014]: 47–62), but this is difficult to prove since the differences might simply reflect the vagaries of what survived. Given the difficulties of ancient travel for most people, it seems more likely that every center would have treated whatever was afflicting people in their region.
[47] Oberhelman ("Anatomical Votive Reliefs," 49) notes that many of them were found piled together in pits or trenches within the temple grounds where they seem to have been ritually buried.
[48] Greek texts and translations of the Epidauran tablets can be viewed in Edelstein and Edelstein, *Asclepius*, 1.221–37 and 1.247–8, and online at https://topostext.org/work/648. Pausanius states that six such tablets remained at Epidauros in his day out of a larger collection (second century BCE) (2.27.3). These were probably compiled from earlier individual dedications. For inscriptions from other sites, see 1.238–40, 1.246–7, and 1.250–4.

the focus is exclusively on the cure. A few examples from the Epidauran tablets will indicate the types of healing that the god is said to have performed.[49]

> Euhippus had had for six years the point of a spear in his jaw. As he was sleeping in the sanctuary the god extracted the spearhead and gave it to him into his hands. When day came Euhippus departed cured, and he held the spearhead in his hands.

> A man with an abscess within his abdomen. When asleep in the sanctuary he saw a dream. It seemed to him that the god ordered the servants who accompanied him to grip him and hold him tightly so that he could cut open his abdomen. The man tried to get away, but they gripped him and bound him to a door knocker. Thereupon Asklepios cut his belly open, removed the abscess, and, after having stitched him up again, released him from his bonds. Whereupon he walked out sound, but the floor of the abaton was covered with blood.

> Hermodicus of Lampsacus was paralyzed in body. This one, when he slept in the sanctuary, the god healed and he ordered him upon coming out to bring to the sanctuary as large a stone as he could. The man brought the stone which now lies before the abaton.

Interestingly, faith in the god's healing power was not a prerequisite for healing.

> Ambrosia of Athens, blind of one eye. She came as a suppliant to the god. As she walked about in the sanctuary she laughed at some of the cures as incredible and impossible, that the lame and the blind should be healed by merely seeing a dream. In her sleep she had a vision. It seemed to her that the god stood by her and said that he would cure her, but that in payment he would ask her to dedicate to the sanctuary a silver pig as a memorial of her ignorance. After saying this, he cut the diseased eyeball and poured in some drug. When day came she walked out sound.

The third type of evidence for belief in the effectiveness of the Asklepian healing centers is literary.[50] Numerous ancient authors testify to their reputation as places where people were healed, and several relate cures that had occurred at these sites, including Aelian, Artemidorus, Philostratus, and the physician Galen (all second century CE). Others included fictional descriptions of visits to an Asklepian temple in their dramatic or poetic works, including Menander, Aristophanes, and Plautus. The fact that some of these texts are satirical and do not report a cure does not undermine their historical value, since the mockery works only if faith in the efficacy of such

---

[49] Bronwen Wickkeiser summarizes the cures that are claimed in these inscriptions: blindness, deafness, infertility, paralysis, ulcers and tumors, wounds, muteness, dropsy, baldness, φθίσις (an unidentified "wasting" condition), persistent headaches, a stone in the penis, gout, stomach disorders, pus, worms in the belly, lice, and epilepsy ("Appeal of Asklepios and the Politics of Healing in the Greco-Roman World," 107–8). See also Raphals, "Divination and Medicine in China and Greece," 93.

[50] Greek texts and translations of the authors cited here appear in Edelstein and Edelstein, *Asclepius*, 1.194–264.

visits was common. Even Christian authors admit that sick people were cured at the sanctuaries of Asklepios, though most attributed the healings to evil *daimones* rather than to the divine Asklepios.[51]

Our most valuable sources, however, are the writings of two second century CE authors who had spent time at Asklepian healing centers: Aelius Aristides and Pausanius. Both penned lengthy accounts of their visits, including multiple reports of divine epiphanies and cures that had occurred there.[52] Aristides's impressionistic description of his one of his dream-visits from Asklepios (*Oratio* 48.31–35) paints a vivid picture of what visitors might have experienced at the pinnacle of such a divine epiphany.

> For I seemed almost to touch him and to perceive that he himself was coming, and to be halfway between sleep and waking and to want to get the power of vision and to be anxious lest he should depart beforehand, and to have turned my ears to listen, sometimes as in a dream, sometimes as in a waking vision, and my hair was standing on end and tears of joy (came forth) and the weight of knowledge was no burden—what man could even set these things forth in words?

The regional healing centers were not the only places where sick people could pursue a healing encounter with Asklepios. Stories tell of Asklepios appearing to people who were sleeping at home, and the presence of votive body parts at local Asklepian temples proves that people were healed at these sites as well. Temples of Asklepios were generally rather small—even those in the major healing centers—but little space was needed for a sick person to sleep there, especially if they were coming in their hour of need and not as part of a major festival. Whether local temples used the same preparatory rituals as the regional healing centers is unknown, but the inner logic of the ceremonies was similar to that of the civic cult, so it seems likely that something along the same lines was done there. Similar questions can be raised about whether all local temples served as venues for sacred dreams or only those where the cultic staff possessed the requisite skills or training. The paucity of the records means that there is much that we will never know on the subject.

Finally, it is worth noting that Asklepios was not the only god who healed through dreams. Similar services were offered by other gods to those who slept in their temples, especially indigenous deities like Amphiaraus, Calchas, Podalirius, Isis, and Serapis.[53] But Asklepios was unmatched in the level of popularity that he attained as a healer and

---

[51] For the evidence, see Chapter 8.
[52] Aristides's *Sacred Tales* is a vital resource for anyone who wants to understand the daily workings of an Asklepian healing center in the second century CE, though like any firsthand report it reflects one person's biased perceptions. An excellent analysis of the place of medicine and religion in the *Sacred Tales* is Israelowich, *Society, Medicine and Religion in the Sacred Tales of Aelius Aristides*.
[53] See Israelowich, *Society, Medicine and Religion in the Sacred Tales of Aelius Aristides*, 72; John S. Hanson, "Dreams and Visions in the Graeco-Roman World and Early Christianity," *ANRW* 2.23.1397–8. According to Suetonius, Vespasian healed two men as the New Serapis after the god told them in a dream to visit his temple in Alexandria (Suet. *Vesp.* 7; cf. Tac. *Hist.* 4.81–2; Dio Cass. 65.8.1) (noted by Trevor S. Luke, "A Healing Touch for Empire: Vespasian's Wonders in Domitianic Rome," *Greece & Rome*, 2nd ser., 57 [2010]: 77).

the degree of personal devotion that he inspired. Some of this can be traced to the fact that he specialized in healing whereas other gods offered a broader range of services, but this cannot be the whole story. Just as important were his personality and the manner in which he carried out his practice. His images invariably show him wearing a kindly expression, while hymns and orations lauded him as the compassionate and merciful savior who was always open to the cries of those in need. He was not like other deities who sent weal one day and woe the next; he always did what was good. People felt confident that he cared for them and that he was inclined to help them. It is no wonder that the early church fathers felt threatened by his popularity and labored to present Jesus as a viable alternative, as we will see in Chapter 8.

Conclusion

The belief that gods and other suprahuman beings both caused and cured sickness was virtually universal in the Greco-Roman world. People in different regions had different ideas about the nature and identity of the gods and what led them to inflict pain and suffering upon humans, but most agreed that rituals played a vital role in alleviating their effects and producing healing. Differences can also be seen regarding what sorts of rituals should be performed to address various types of problems and who should perform them. But everyone seems to have agreed that more serious or persistent problems should be treated by someone with professional expertise.

Two broad classes of religious experts were available to treat sicknesses caused by divine beings and other forms of illness. The first class consisted of freelance purifiers and exorcists who offered their skills to individuals outside of the traditional cultic system. People who suspected that their illness might be a punishment for some sort of purity violation could call in a freelance purifier to diagnose and cleanse themselves, their possessions, and their family from the effects of ritual pollution. Those who feared that they were being attacked by harmful spirits might enlist an exorcist to drive the spirits away and prevent them from returning. How many people consulted either of these experts is impossible to say—they were broadly scorned by the literate elites, but they seem to have had a following among the populace.

The second class of ritual experts worked through the traditional cultus. Some were priests or attendants at local temples or rural shrines, while others served on the staff of one of the regional healing centers that were dedicated to the divine Asklepios. For the most part they prescribed traditional ritual cures: prayers, lustrations, sacrifices, offerings, divination, and so on. Some of the rural shrines also offered diagnostic services by which offenses against the gods could be ferreted out and remedied through the performance of rituals, while others—primarily, but not exclusively, those associated with Asklepios—provided venues where the sick could sleep overnight in the hope of receiving an immediate cure or a healing regimen from the god. All of these providers served people of every class and condition, but Asklepios was especially known for welcoming the poor and the desperate.

Given the importance of "religion" and cultic activity in the social and intellectual life of Greco-Roman antiquity and the ready availability of religion-based healers, we can presume that everyone who joined the early Christ-movement (apart from Judeans) had been nurtured from infancy in the systems of interpreting and treating sickness that have been discussed in this chapter. What is harder to assess is how their new affiliation affected their use of ritual healing experts. In view of the apostle Paul's declaration that "no idol in the world really exists" (1 Cor. 8:4) and his emphatic call for his followers to "flee from the worship of idols" (1 Cor. 10:14), we might suppose that they immediately ceased to consult religious healers for assistance with their ailments. But is this a valid inference? Paul himself acknowledges that the Corinthians continued to eat sacrificial meat "in the temple of an idol" (1 Cor. 8:10) and only cautions them against how it might be perceived; he does not tell them to stop doing it. He goes on to argue that because "idols" have no real existence, they are doing no wrong if they eat meat from animals slaughtered in the civic cult (1 Cor. 8:8-9, 10:25-26, 31). Would he have approved their continued reliance on ritual healers on similar grounds? Would he have approved some and not others? Or were their methods so deeply implicated in polytheistic beliefs about the identity and nature of the gods that they were beyond the pale for Christ-followers?

It is hard for us to imagine Christ-followers appealing to a ritual purifier or the priest of a rural shrine to find out what god they might have offended, and it is doubly difficult to envision them sleeping in an Asklepian temple in hopes of receiving a healing dream from the god. But that does not mean that it did not happen. If Paul thought that such practices posed a serious problem for the faith of his followers, we would have expected him to address the topic, perhaps by directing them to Jesus the compassionate healer as an alternative to Asklepios. Yet he says nothing on the subject, or at least not in the letters that we possess. Here as elsewhere his silence cries out for an explanation. These and other questions relating to Paul's beliefs and practices regarding sickness and health will be examined more closely in Chapter 9.

5

Medical Care

Hippocratic Medicine

Medical historians generally trace the beginnings of their discipline to the physician Hippocrates of Kos (460–370 BCE), whose name is associated with some sixty documents from antiquity that lay out various elements of what came to be known as a "scientific" approach to understanding and treating sickness and injury.[1] But this origin story veils as much as it reveals. Historians generally agree that Hippocrates was a real historical figure who systematized and developed certain trends in ancient Greek thought regarding the workings and care of the human body, but specifying his contributions more precisely is a challenge. The earliest biographical material comes from Soranus of Ephesus (second century CE), and many of the texts credited to him were in fact composed by followers in later centuries.[2] The problem is compounded by the positivistic and teleological orientation of many medical historians who have framed Hippocrates and his followers as the heroic and enlightened founders of a movement that struggled to overturn and supplant the ignorance and inefficacy of religious and magical modes of health care.

The reality is far different, as more recent historians have shown. Lisa Raphals summarizes the current consensus when she states that "Asclepian temple healing and Hippocratic naturalistic medicine were historically concurrent developments, and not an evolutionary process as represented by positivist historians of medicine."[3] Both movements arose and flourished in the same era (fifth to fourth centuries BCE) in the same geographic territories (southern Greece/western Turkey) as refinements of different aspects of traditional health care methods. The same is true for the "magical" treatments discussed in Chapter 3: all three systems have common roots

---

[1] For a good overview of the traditions about Hippocrates and the content of the various treatises, see Elizabeth Clark, "Hippocrates and Early Greek Medicine," in *The Oxford Handbook of Science and Medicine in the Classical World*, ed. Paul Keyser and John Scarborough (Oxford: Oxford University Press, 2018), 215–32.

[2] Even this statement oversimplifies the situation, as scholars have pointed to various discrepancies that suggest the Hippocratic treatises do not offer a consistent viewpoint but rather the diverse views of a living tradition. Jackson points to Alexandria as a possible site for their formation into the present corpus (*Doctors and Diseases in the Roman Empire*, 20–2). G. E. R. Lloyd agrees and posits a fourth century BCE date for the earliest collection (*In the Grip of Disease: Studies in the Greek Imagination* [Oxford: Oxford University Press, 2004], 41).

[3] "Divination and Medicine in China and Greece," 321–2.

and coexisted as alternate modes of healing throughout the Greek and Roman eras. Their practitioners spoke disparagingly of one another at times, but they also borrowed language, ideas, and practices from their competitors, as we will see in Chapter 6. The result was an overlapping web of treatment options from which sick people and their families could pick and choose as they wished. This was true even for the elites, who consulted religious and "magical" healers as often as Hippocratic physicians.

What then distinguished the medical approach from other modes of healing? At its base was an understanding of the human body that viewed sickness as a disruption of natural bodily processes rather than as something inflicted from outside, whether as a divine punishment or as an attack by evil spirits. The Hippocratic model did not entirely dismiss the divine from involvement in human health, but it insisted that the divine worked in and through the natural world, including the hands of the physician.[4] Miracles were possible and prayers could be useful alongside the remedies of the physician, but one should not ordinarily look to the gods for either causes or cures.

The medical view of sickness and health is rooted in classical Greek philosophy, from which it derived much of its theoretical framework regarding the nature of the human body and how it should be treated. Philosophical concepts that were incorporated into the Hippocratic model include the idea that the universe (including the human body) is composed of four basic elements (fire, air, water, and earth); the belief in universal flux and the importance of maintaining balance among the four elements; the vital role of "humors" and "pneuma" in the workings of the human body; and the idea that like attracts like.[5]

At the heart of the Hippocratic model was a belief that the body was energized and maintained by four essential "humors" (Greek χυμόι, literally "juices" or "fluids") that flowed through various channels within the body: blood, phlegm, yellow bile, and black bile.[6] Good health results when the four humors are properly balanced, while sickness indicates some sort of imbalance among them. The theory is well summarized in this pithy statement from section 4 of the treatise *On Human Nature*.

> The human body contains blood, phlegm, yellow bile and black bile. These are the things that make up its constitution and cause its pains and health. Health is primarily that state in which these constituent substances are in the correct proportion to each other, both in strength and quantity, and are well mixed. Pain

---

[4] This ambiguity of this view is expressed most clearly in *On the Sacred Disease*, where the author first says of epilepsy that "this disease is in my opinion no more divine than any other" (5.1–2), then goes on to observe that "there is no need to put the disease in a special class and to consider it more divine than the others; they are all divine and all human" (21.5–8) (Loeb translations).

[5] Jackson, *Doctors and Diseases in the Roman Empire*, 17–19; Nutton, "Healers in the Medical Marketplace," 22–4. The link between medicine and philosophy was never lost; the Roman physician and medical theorist Galen (second century CE) wrote an entire treatise (*That the Best Physician Is Also a Philosopher*) in which he argued that medicine is like philosophy in leading its practitioners to a better understanding of the universe and encouraging moral behavior (noted by Nutton, "Healers in the Medical Marketplace," 48).

[6] The idea of bodily humors actually predates Hippocrates, but he seems to have been the first to insist that there were precisely four of them and to frame a treatment regimen around this belief.

occurs when one of the substances presents either a deficiency or an excess, or is separated in the body and not mixed with others.[7]

Hippocratic physicians had no means of measuring the amount of each humor in the body, so they judged by the symptoms, which they determined by combining oral reports from the patient with rudimentary physical assessments. These included measuring the pulse and respiration, palpating the abdomen, peering into the ears and throat, and examining the color and quality of the patient's urine and excrement. If these investigations uncovered something that seemed out of the ordinary, the humoral theory gave them a framework for diagnosing the problem.

Hippocratic thought linked the four humors with the four fundamental qualities of the human body as defined by Greek philosophers: heat, coldness, moisture, and dryness. Blood was defined as hot and wet, phlegm as cold and wet, black bile as cold and dry, and yellow bile as hot and dry. The task of the physician was to use these associations to determine whether the sick person's body was experiencing too much or too little heat, coldness, moisture, or dryness (or some combination thereof), then to apply suitable treatments to increase or decrease the level of the affected humor until balance was restored. The modern recognition that different diseases can produce similar symptoms but require different modes of treatment was both unknown and unnecessary to Hippocratic physicians since their system credited all forms of illness to the same underlying causes and prescribed similar treatments for similar symptoms.[8]

This idea that sickness resulted from fluid imbalances in the body and not the actions of suprahuman forces led Hippocratic thinkers to speculate on why such imbalances occurred—what we today would call the underlying causes of sickness. Like modern physicians, they reasoned that changing or eliminating the conditions that caused these imbalances might enable them to ameliorate or even reverse the course of an illness. Their efforts were hampered, however, by their limited knowledge of the inner workings of the human body at a time when dissection of the human body was considered immoral and by their unfamiliarity with using measurement and experimentation to confirm or modify their theories. As a result, their ideas about causality were highly speculative and usually wrong. They did, however, draw some empirically valid inferences from observing their patients, including the modern-sounding observations that human health is affected by what people do with their bodies and the environments in which they live.

On the first point, Hippocratic physicians could identify correlations even when they could not properly explain the causal processes behind them. Physicians were taught to take detailed case histories that involved asking not only about the patient's physical symptoms but also about such lifestyle factors as diet, exercise, sleep, sexual

---

[7] Translation by J. Chadwick from Lloyd, *Hippocratic Writing*, 262.
[8] As odd as it sounds to us today, the Greek humoral theory formed the basis for Western medical treatment well into the nineteenth century until scientific discoveries led to the rise of germ theory. Something like germ theory also had its proponents in the ancient world, primarily the Roman poet Lucretius and the agricultural writer Varro.

activity, family history, and profession.⁹ Implicit in these questions was an awareness that some behaviors are more conducive to health and others to sickness. The answers given by the patient were then interpreted through a diagnostic model that analyzed the patient's symptoms and behaviors to determine which of the body's humors were out of balance, and treatments were prescribed to increase or diminish the relevant humors and so restore the proper balance. Sometimes the treatments involved medication, as in modern medicine, but often they involved changes in the patient's lifestyle.¹⁰

The second factor that Hippocratic theorists credited with having a causal influence on human health and sickness was the physical environment in which people lived. This idea is developed most fully in the treatise *On Airs, Waters, and Places*. The author begins by listing some of the environmental factors that medical theorists had identified as having an effect on human health, including the seasons, the types of wind, the qualities of water, the location and elevation of the site, and the nature of the soil. The remainder of the treatise is devoted to explaining how each of these factors influences human health, including their effects on the bodily humors. People who live in places with hot winds and ample water, for example, have heads that are moist and full of phlegm, with the result that "their digestive organs are frequently deranged from the phlegm that runs down into them from the head" (3.10-13). Building on this observation, the author lays out a long list of health problems that he says are endemic to such areas. Turning to those who live near marshy waters, the author observes that "their digestive organs, upper and lower, are very dry and very hot, so that they need more powerful drugs" (7.20-23). Such information, if it were valid, would certainly be useful to a practicing physician. The author also speaks at length about how various diseases rise and fall with the changing seasons and how environmental conditions affect men and women differently.

In both of these examples we see how the Hippocratic approach to health care, though built on a faulty theoretical foundation, was nevertheless prescient in the holism of its treatment regimen. It did not limit its focus to curing sick bodies; it also sought to preserve health. Several of the Hippocratic treatises include guidelines for healthy living, addressing such obvious topics as diet, exercise, and sleep along with less obvious influences like bathing, place of residence, and modes of transportation. Variations are provided for different ages, seasons, genders, and body types.

Much of the information in these treatises was written to guide physicians in their duties, but some sections read more like self-care manuals for the literate elites. Virtually all of their observations presuppose an upper-class audience that has a broad array of lifestyle choices and sufficient resources to purchase or do whatever the physician recommends. The limited options of the working poor are largely ignored, reflecting not only the usual upper-class bias of ancient literature but also the difficulty

---

⁹ Notable by their absence from this list are questions about sin, pollution, curses, and similar matters that presume divine causality.
¹⁰ Both Celsus (first century CE) and Galen (second century CE) have much to say about the daily regimen that should be followed to promote health, with special attention to diet and exercise. For an overview of their recommendations, see Jackson, *Doctors and Diseases in the Roman Empire*, 32–5.

that poor people faced in paying the fees demanded by private physicians. More will be said on this topic later.

Other Medical Theories

The Hippocratic model, while dominant in accounts of medical history, was in fact one of several systems of medical care that were available to treat sickness in the Greco-Roman world. Other schools of thought arose in the centuries after Hippocrates that shared the Hippocratic emphasis on empirical observation and treatment but rejected key elements of Hippocratic theory and practice. Physicians trained in these other systems competed for clients with the heirs of the Hippocratic tradition throughout much of the Roman world. It is thus misleading to speak of medical treatment as a monolithic alternative to "magical" and religious modes of health care in Greco-Roman antiquity. Ancient observers (including Paul and his followers) might have recognized a family resemblance among medical practitioners that distinguished them from the other forms of health care that we have examined thus far, but the beliefs of the various schools about the workings of the human body and their techniques for diagnosing and treating illness differed nearly as much as those employed by Chinese, Indian, and Western doctors today.[11]

By the time of Paul, the practice of medicine had coalesced into three main schools of thought with several offshoots.[12] The Hippocratic approach was carried on by the Dogmatic or Rationalist school, which used reason and experience (and the writings of their founder) to identify and repair the underlying bodily malfunctions that gave rise to each instance of sickness. The texts known today as the Hippocratic Corpus reveal the ongoing development of this school. On the whole it seems that they remained faithful to the theories and methods propounded by their founder, though diversity of thought can be observed on particular points.

The Empiricist school, which arose in the third century BCE in opposition to the Dogmatists, insisted that discerning the underlying causes of sickness was an unnecessary distraction because all such efforts were speculative and therefore unhelpful.[13] In their view, the physician should simply figure out by trial and error which treatments work best for each illness and apply them on a consistent basis. What

---

[11] As Molly Jones-Lewis rightly observes, "There was little agreement between groups of physicians about the basic principles on which the body functioned, let alone between individual physicians subscribing to the same schools of thought" ("Physicians and 'Schools,'" in Irby, *Companion*, 395).

[12] Extensive discussions of the various schools can be found in Prioreschi, *History of Medicine*, 3.76–173, and Flemming, *Medicine and the Making of Roman Women*, 81–124. The following summary draws on their descriptions along with other materials as noted. Lesser schools such as the Pneumatists and the Eclectics are not included here because they flourished either later than or geographically distant from the lands where Paul is known to have established congregations. The schools listed here all had historical connections to Asia Minor: Kos was the home of Hippocrates, ancestor of the Dogmatists; Carura housed a medical school that followed the semi-Empiricist path of Herophilos; and Bithynia was the home territory of the Methodist theorist Asklepiades.

[13] A good historical overview of the Empiricist school is Fabio Stok, "Medical Sects: Herophilus, Erasistratus, Empiricists," in *Oxford Handbook*, 359–80.

matters is not what causes a condition but what cures it. Their name, which comes from the Greek word ἐμπειρία ("experience"), reflects this pragmatic orientation.

Empiricists did not wholly ignore matters of causality, but their interest was limited to causes that could be observed, as when a person becomes nauseous after eating spoiled food or bleeds after being lacerated by a weapon. Over time their combined efforts produced a body of treatments that physicians could use to treat known patterns of symptoms even if they did not understand how the remedies worked. When faced with an illness not addressed in their training, they prescribed cures that had proved effective in treating similar conditions and made adjustments based on their results.

The third major school of medical thought and practice was the Methodists, whose name comes from their insistence on using the same basic method to treat all expressions of sickness.[14] Their founder, Asklepiades (first century BCE), rejected the teachings of both the Dogmatists, whose theories he viewed as overly complex, and the Empiricists, whose avoidance of theory left them with no ground for deciding what treatment should be applied to a given set of symptoms. According to his theory, all sickness can be traced to disruptions in the flow of miniscule particles that carry vital substances throughout the body via "pores" that are invisible to the human eye. Various factors can cause these pores to become constricted or dilated (or some combination of the two), leaving too many particles in some parts of the body and too few elsewhere. Constriction also makes the body excessively hot and dry, while dilation makes it overly cool and moist. The disruption of these invisible bodily processes creates the visible symptoms that we call sickness.

Since all sicknesses arise from the same bodily causes, all can be removed by the same basic method (hence the name of the school): relaxing what is constricted or tightening what is dilated. Special training is required to discern the nature of the malfunction behind a particular illness and to know what treatments should be applied to reverse it, but the system as a whole is so simple that Methodists boasted they could train a physician in six months rather than the many years that other schools required.

Literate members of all three schools criticized the theories and practices of their competitors, but it is hard to know how far these disagreements affected relations among individual practitioners or public perceptions of their discipline. It seems reasonable to suppose that their feuds created a degree of uncertainty in the minds of ordinary people regarding what kind of physician they should call in to treat particular episodes of sickness, but the evidence is slight.[15] They probably began by consulting people whom they knew or whom others had recommended and then moved on to other options if a cure was not forthcoming. All that matters for our purposes is the rich variety of diagnostic and treatment options that would have been available to Paul

---

[14] Helpful overviews of the theories and practices of the Methodists can be found in Ludwig Edelstein, "The Methodists," in Temkin, *Ancient Medicine*, 173–91; Nutton, *Ancient Medicine*, 187–201; and Michael Frede, "The Method of the So-Called Methodical School of Medicine," in *Science and Speculation: Studies in Hellenistic Theory and Practice*, ed. Jonathan Barnes et al. (Cambridge: Cambridge University Press; Paris: Editions de la Maison des Sciences de l'Homme, 1982), 1–23.

[15] Pliny, Galen, and Aelius Aristides all speak of physicians arguing around a patient's bed over what treatments to apply, but it is unclear whether these disagreements concerned the different theoretical perspectives of the various schools or the differing therapeutic judgments of individual physicians in the absence of a standardized treatment system.

and his followers if they wished to procure the services of a medical practitioner rather than (or in addition to) another type of healer.

The Social Location of Physicians

So what did it take to become a physician in the Greco-Roman world? Where and how did they ply their trade? Who consulted them, and why? What did people think of them by comparison with other types of healers? Greek and Roman sources supply at least cursory answers to many of these questions.

One of the key differences between ancient and modern forms of medicine is that there were no physical campuses where aspiring physicians were educated and no standard curriculum that they were expected to master. There was also no system of examinations or licensure to ensure that physicians had been properly trained and to certify that training to the public. A "school" of medicine in antiquity was only "a group of physicians who, having adopted the same or similar paradigms, taught medicine relying mostly on apprenticeship."[16] The three schools of medicine that we have examined in this chapter were systems of ideas and methods, not physical institutions. A school survived only as long as there were physicians who adhered to its teachings and applied its methods, and individual physicians had to heal people in the real world in order to gain clients. The bare fact that they had been trained in medical modes of treatment gave them no more claim to popular regard than any other health care provider.[17]

As with other trades in antiquity, medical expertise was passed on largely within families as a practicing physician (usually but not always the father) used oral instruction and hands-on experience to train children (usually sons, but occasionally daughters also) in the lore and skills of the medical system in which the practitioner had been educated. Some physicians also took on apprentices from outside the family who learned by the same means.[18] A smaller number received their training in a group setting at an Asklepian healing center where medical and religious modes of healing were commingled. Here, too, physicians learned only the perspectives and practices of a particular school—the Hippocratic model at Kos and Pergamon, the Empiricist approach at Carura in the Lycus Valley, and so on. No effort was made to expose students to other theories or methods since each school claimed that its approach was superior to the others. As a result, physicians who had been trained in one school of practice might offer a very different diagnosis and treatment regimen than another, making it difficult for a sick person to know whom to trust.

Another important difference between past and present medical care concerns the social status of physicians. While there were exceptions, medical doctors as a class were

---

[16] Prioreschi, *History of Medicine*, 2.644; Jackson, *Doctors and Diseases in the Roman Empire*, 58–9.

[17] According to William V. Harris, "Rationalistic Greek medicine was a marvelous structure and a major step forward from what came before it, but the fact is that, except in the face of moderate traumas, doctors' treatments generally did more harm than good" ("Popular Medicine in the Classical World," 7).

[18] On the normal modes of medical education, see Prioreschi, *History of Medicine*, 2.641–2, 645.

held in low esteem by the elites, who placed them on the same level as other craft workers who were paid for their services. The absence of any accepted criteria for determining who was and was not a qualified physician and the corresponding appropriation of the term by those whom Hippocratic physicians derided as "charlatans" also cast a pall of suspicion over the profession.[19] Their reputation was also affected by what Molly Jones-Lewis describes as their "unavoidable engagement with the body and the body's fluids, odors, and the unpredictability of disease and death" and the fact that many physicians were current or former slaves.[20] Popular prejudice against "wily Greeks" also played a role in Roman attitudes toward physicians, as medicine was widely considered a Greek import.[21] Here and there we hear of urbane physicians who were accepted in elite society, but they were the exception rather than the rule.

Little is known about how ordinary people perceived the social status of physicians, but it seems unlikely that they would have shared the negative judgments of the elites except toward those who were still enslaved, like the civic physicians that will be discussed later. But there is also no reason to think that they viewed physicians more highly than other types of healers or that the results produced by physicians justified such a view. Physicians were simply one of several types of health care providers to whom sick people could turn in times of need.

People who desired the services of a medical doctor would have found them readily available in the cities, where private physicians representing the various schools of medicine competed to serve those who could afford their fees.[22] Some maintained offices in the agora or elsewhere in the city, but much of their care was given in people's homes.[23] Civic physicians—slaves owned by the city for this purpose—treated those

---

[19] Noted by Prioreschi, *History of Medicine*, 2.667. Even Pliny, who exhibits a great deal of medical knowledge, devotes several pages of his *Natural History* to excoriating physicians (29.6-9). This confusion in the public mind is acknowledged in the Hippocratic treatise *Law*, where the author laments that "owing to the ignorance of those who practice it, and of those who, inconsiderately, form a judgment of them, [medicine] is at present far behind all the other arts." "Physicians are many in title," he concludes, "but very few in reality" (*Law*, 1).

[20] Jones-Lewis, "Physicians and 'Schools,'" 389. According to Rebecca Flemming, 80 percent of the physicians named in inscriptions in the Roman West in the first century CE were freedmen, slaves, or peregrines, unlike the Greek East where they are often mentioned in connection with elite families (*Medicine and the Making of Roman Women*, 51–2). For more on the subject, see John Scarborough, "Romans and Physicians," *The Classical Journal* 65 (1970): 298–300.

[21] Vivian Nutton estimates that more than 90 percent of Rome's doctors in the first century CE were Greek, compared with 75 percent in the second century and 65 percent in the third century ("The Perils of Patriotism: Pliny and Roman Medicine," in *From Democedes to Harvey: Studies in the History of Medicine* [London: Variorum Reprints, 1988], 37). On Roman views of Greek physicians, see Scarborough, *Roman Medicine*, 95–7, and María Ángeles Alonso, "Greek Physicians in the Eyes of Roman Elite (from the Republic to the 1st Century AD)," *Annales Universitatis Mariae Curie-Skłodowska* 73 (2018): 119–37.

[22] David Leith points to evidence from Galen and other Roman sources that shows how physicians from the major sects competed with one another in cities around the Empire ("How Popular Were the Medical Sects?" in Harris, *Popular Medicine*, 235–46). On the role of fees in limiting poor people's access to physicians, see Harris, "Popular Medicine in the Classical World," 45–6; Prioreschi, *History of Medicine*, 2.651–2; Flemming, *Medicine and the Making of Roman Women*, 53; and especially Norman Underwood, "Medicine, Money, and Christian Rhetoric: The Socio-Economic Dimensions of Healthcare in Late Antiquity," *Studies in Late Antiquity* 2 (2018): 342–84.

[23] Jackson, *Doctors and Diseases in the Roman Empire*, 65–7, 73–5; Patricia A. Baker, *The Archaeology of Medicine in the Greco-Roman World* (Cambridge: Cambridge University Press, 2013), 111. At

who could not afford private care. The quality of their skills is unknown, but it is unlikely that their expertise would have matched that of private physicians unless they had been trained prior to becoming enslaved.[24] Some members of the elite class also kept enslaved physicians to care for their families, but their numbers were small.

Physicians were less common in the countryside, where traditional remedies predominated. If the need was not urgent, people in smaller towns and villages could have consulted one of the many itinerant physicians who made the rounds of the rural areas.[25] Little is known about their training or activities, but the fact that they offered a type of care not ordinarily available in the local area might have given them a certain amount of prestige. If nothing else, they offered another option when traditional remedies failed.

Most physicians were men, but women also served as medical providers in the Greco-Roman world. Most worked as midwives (μαῖαι), though their expertise was not limited to managing labor and delivery. The physician Soranus of Ephesus (second century CE), whose treatise on gynecology was recognized as the authoritative guide on the subject for centuries, laid out a series of expectations for midwives that included not only physical and temperamental qualities but also intellectual and technical skills. "The best midwife," he says, should be literate (uncommon for women in his day) and possess a strong memory. She should be familiar with both the theory and practice of all branches of medicine so that she will be ready to treat any health problem that arises with her patients. She should know enough about diseases and their symptoms that she is not surprised by sudden changes in a patient's condition. In carrying out her duties, "she will be unperturbed, unafraid in danger, able to state clearly the reasons for her measures; she will bring reassurance to her patients, and be sympathetic."[26] In short, Soranus expects "the best midwife" to possess the same qualities that the Hippocratic Corpus lays out for good physicians.

How many practicing midwives measured up to this rather idealized portrait is hard to say, but the fact that Soranus can make such statements in all seriousness and follow them with an entire treatise of instructions for midwives about treating women's health problems suggests that his expectations were not beyond the reach of actual women and would not have been perceived as such by male doctors who consulted his treatise. Literary evidence suggests that most births were in fact managed by illiterate folk healers or family members, but Soranus's writings show that elite women and their husbands had as high expectations for their midwives as they did for physicians.

---

least eighteen buildings containing medical tools (i.e., offices or homes of physicians) have been found in Pompeii alone (Underwood, "Medicine, Money, and Christian Rhetoric," 358).

[24] On the training of slaves to be physicians, see Underwood, "Medicine, Money, and Christian Rhetoric," 361–2.

[25] Vivian Nutton speaks of "circuit doctors going through the countryside from a home base in a market town" who offered their services alongside those of local healers ("Healers in the Medical Marketplace," 53). Elsewhere he mentions "travelling doctors, wandering the roads of Greece or Judaea, touting their wares and their skills" (*Ancient Medicine*, 152). Cf. Harris, "Popular Medicine in the Classical World," 38–9.

[26] *Gyn.* 3–4. The quote is from Owsei Tomkin's translation published in 1991 by Johns Hopkins University Press.

The work of women as medical providers was not limited to being midwives; some also received formal training in medicine and practiced as physicians in the same manner as men. Holt Parker points to both literary (e.g., Plato, *Rep.* 454d2, 455e6-7; Mart. 11.71.7; Apul. *Met.* 5.10) and inscriptional evidence that attests to "more than sixty women who were recognized by their societies as medical practitioners, called by the normal word for physician with a feminine ending (Greek form, ἰατρίνη; Latin *medica*) or cited as authors of medical works or recipes."[27] Most, if not all, would have been trained at home by a sympathetic father, perhaps alongside their brothers. The available evidence suggests that they treated mostly women, but this is by no means certain. The fact that they were honored in inscriptions suggests that their services were valued by their communities.[28]

Treating Sickness

While there were deep and serious disagreements among the various schools of medicine on matters of theory, the methods that they used to treat illness and injury were broadly similar. Given their limited familiarity with the inner workings of the human body, it is surprising how many of their remedies have been validated by medical science. As in every society, people concerned with maintaining health were intelligent and practical enough to discover biologically effective treatments for sickness and to pass that knowledge on to others even if their ideas about why these remedies worked were faulty.

Viewed as a whole, the methods used by Greek and Roman physicians were surprisingly holistic. Medicines were available to treat most forms of sickness, but they were utilized in combination with other treatments such as diet, exercise, and hot springs that were designed to nurture the sick body and restore it to health. The same is true for acute injuries: medical remedies (ointments, bandages, splints, etc.) were accompanied by prescriptions for creating a post-treatment environment that was conducive to the natural healing of the body.

From Hippocrates on, ancient medical theorists tended to classify their treatment regimens under three headings: dietetics, pharmacology, and surgery. Practicing physicians used additional methods that do not fit readily into any of these categories. A broad survey of the most commonly used healing practices will help us to discern the kinds of treatments that Paul and his followers might have received if they had sought help from a physician.

(a) Managing the patient's *diet* was the first resort in virtually all forms of medical care. Foods were seen not merely as sources of nourishment but as vital contributors to the health or sickness of the body. Traditional Hippocratic medicine classified foods

---

[27] "Women and Medicine," in *A Companion to Women in the Ancient World*, ed. Sharon L. James and Sheila Dillon (New York: Blackwell, 2012), 122–3. Additional evidence can be found in Holt N. Parker, "Galen and the Girls: Sources for Roman Medical Writers Revisited," *Classical Quarterly* 62 (2012): 359–86, and Wainwright, *Women Healing/Healing Women*, 50–62.

[28] On inscriptions honoring female physicians, see Penso, *La Médecine Roman*, 107.

according to their effects on the bodily humors: some heated the body, some cooled it, some dried it out, and some increased its moisture. Digestion was the process by which these properties were released to form blood, phlegm, black bile, and yellow bile. Sickness occurred when the body possessed too much or too little of one of the humors. If the physician determined by a review of the patient's symptoms that the humors were out of balance, the patient might be told to eat more of certain foods to enhance the strength or distribution of humors that were low or to reduce or eliminate other foods to reduce the humors that were high. In cases of obesity, the physician might also recommend a weight-loss regimen. Little is said about why particular foods were linked to specific humors; physicians simply accepted the traditional associations and prescribed accordingly.[29]

Other schools of medicine also gave high priority to diet in their treatment of sickness, but the reasoning behind their prescriptions was different. For the Empiricists, dietary prescriptions were based on what was observed to work rather than any underlying theoretical perspective. Their advice to patients drew heavily on traditional dietary remedies as modified by their own experience. For the Methodists, the key dietary question was whether a particular food caused constriction or relaxation of the body's pore network, since they believed that all sickness arose from one or the other of these conditions. Foods were prescribed or prohibited to counteract whichever condition was causing a particular illness. The regimen might differ when different parts of the body were affected and could be modified if changes occurred in the symptoms or intensity of the illness.[30] As with the Hippocratics, the rationale for associating certain foods with one bodily effect and others with the opposite is only occasionally evident.

(b) When dietary changes failed to work or when the patient's symptoms appeared to demand stronger remedies, *medicines* were prescribed. Much has been said already about the use of medicinal substances in Greek and Roman healing, but a few comments are in order about how they were viewed and applied in medical circles. Most of the knowledge that the medical profession possessed regarding the effects of various plant, animal, and mineral substances on the human body came from traditional healers who had learned by trial and error. Medical theorists sifted this information through their own rationalistic intellectual framework to minimize the influence of "superstition" and supplemented it with the experience that physicians had gained from treating actual patients.[31] The result was a body (or more likely, diverse regional bodies) of pharmacological knowledge that could be transmitted orally to aspiring

---

[29] Sometimes the association is obvious, as with the ideas that wine warms the body and salt dries it out. But why bread should be described as warming and drying while vegetables produce the opposite effect is not immediately apparent to a modern reader. The same can be said for claims that various foods create high amounts of a certain humor, such as cabbage producing black bile or apples making phlegm.

[30] Edelstein, "Methodists," 183.

[31] This does not mean that the medicines were all "rational" in the modern sense. All of the ancient pharmacological compendia contain remedies and explanations that make no sense by modern medical standards. For example, many treatments were justified on the grounds of the so-called "doctrine of signatures" whereby a substance that bore a resemblance to either a body part or the cause of the illness or injury (e.g., worms or scorpions) was believed to be effective for curing that body part or condition. For more on the subject, see Harms, "Logic of Irrational Pharmacological Therapies in Aretaeus of Cappadocia," 195, 198–9, 309–15.

physicians and applied by those in practice to treat particular cases of sickness. Much of this knowledge was eventually compiled into written compendia by writers like Dioscorides, Scribonius, and Celsus, though how many physicians knew and could read their works is unclear.

These written collections provide valuable insights into the number and variety of medicinal remedies that were at least theoretically available to physicians and the varied ways in which they could be applied. The Hippocratic Corpus names at least 300 different substances that could be prescribed as medications for different conditions, while Dioscorides describes some 600 and Pliny over 900. Many were available locally through root-cutters or drug-sellers and were thus more likely to be included in a practicing physician's repertoire, while others involved expensive or exotic materials that would have been accessible only to those who served wealthy clients in the larger urban centers. The sheer breadth of these catalogs suggests that those involved in the medicine trade—traditional healers, root-cutters, drug-sellers, and practicing physicians—tested virtually every substance that they encountered to discover whether it might have healing properties. People were undoubtedly harmed or even died as a result of this uncontrolled testing, but it also produced many useful remedies. The side effects of some of these treatments would have been so unpleasant, however, as to make people wary of trusting the medicinal prescriptions of physicians.

As for how the medications were applied, the methods varied with the material. Some involved only a single substance while others required the mixing of different materials and special processing to bring out their medicinal qualities. For both types, the most common mode of application was ingestion, usually by mixing the substance with wine, water, or another liquid and drinking it. Some materials were processed into pills that could be carried around and taken orally as needed. Still others were injected directly into the rectum or vagina or inhaled after heating. Medicines that were designed to be absorbed into the body typically required multiple applications and the passing of time to produce effects. Those that were given to purge the body via vomiting or evacuation of the bowels—a very common mode of treatment—acted more quickly, producing effects that could be both violent and painful.

External application of medicinal substances was also quite common, especially in the case of injuries, where a variety of creams, salves, plasters, and similar dressings was available to treat wounds, lumps, or contusions prior to bandaging. Some of the manuals specify the precise substance to be applied to a particular type of injury and the mode of bandaging that should be used. Similar materials were used to treat rashes, abrasions, and various sorts of skin diseases. Numerous prescriptions are given for salves, ointments, liquids, and other materials that could be applied topically to the eyes, ears, nose, and mouth to treat localized ailments, with eye problems receiving the most attention. The latter would have been especially salient for Paul if he suffered from eye disease as many think he did.

Another mode of external application that was common among physicians in Paul's day was the use of amulets. Virtually all medical writers from antiquity accept the validity of amulets to treat at least some forms of sickness. Their mode of operation is rarely specified, perhaps because wearing them was so common as to place them beyond question. Some have suggested that their use by physicians is based on a belief that healing substances, like diseases, emit some type of particles that could affect body parts in the immediate area.[32] But the fact that they were used to treat internal as well as external ailments raises problems for this theory unless one posits that these particles could also penetrate the skin. Paul Jonathan Harms sees amulets as a specific application of a general theory regarding medicinal substances. He cites evidence from Aretaeus, Scribonius, and Dioscorides to demonstrate that in their way of thinking, "the material's medicinal power is conceived to be active independent of the manner of application. This means that to treat a particular condition a material could be applied as a plaster smeared on, a pill to be ingested or hung around the affected part."[33] Whatever the rationale behind them, there is ample evidence that amulets were an accepted mode of applying healing substances among Greek and Roman physicians.

(c) The practice of *surgery* was still in its infancy in Greco-Roman antiquity due to the absence of safe and reliable anesthetics and a general lack of knowledge about germs and antisepsis.[34] Anything that involved opening the chest or abdominal cavity was automatically rejected since death was certain in such cases.[35] Surgical techniques were applied often by military doctors to remove arrows, close wounds, set dislocations, relieve hemorrhages, and amputate limbs, and civilian physicians employed similar methods to treat analogous injuries. Less invasive surgery was practiced regularly to remove cysts, abscesses, skin lesions, and superficial tumors. Physicians also performed various forms of eye surgery (perhaps relevant to the apostle Paul), including cataract removal, along with minor surgery on the ears, nose, and mouth.[36] Cupping and bloodletting, both of which were commonly practiced, should also be mentioned here since they involved at least a minimal cutting of the skin.[37] More challenging procedures like trepanation (the removal of a small portion of the skull to reduce internal pressure) and the extraction of bladder stones were performed only by skilled experts.[38]

(d) Physicians of all schools held similar ideas about the importance of *physical regimen* to the treatment of sickness, even when they disagreed over why and how it worked. Rest and relaxation were prescribed for some conditions and exercise for

---

[32] This seems to be Galen's view, according to Caroline Petit, "Galen, Pharmacology and the Boundaries of Medicine: A Reassessment," in *Collecting Recipes: Byzantine and Jewish Pharmacology in Dialogue*, ed. Lennart Lehmhaus and Matteo Martelli (Berlin and Boston: De Gruyter, 2017), 63–6.

[33] "Logic of Irrational Pharmacological Therapies in Aretaeus of Cappadocia," 269. The idea is developed more fully in pp. 268–77.

[34] For a helpful overview of ancient surgical tools and techniques, see Jackson, *Doctors and Diseases in the Roman Empire*, 112–29.

[35] The lone exception is Caesarean birth, which in ancient times invariably resulted in or followed the mother's death.

[36] According to Vivian Nutton, "Galen expected any competent surgeon to be able to cure a wide range of eye conditions, including growths on the cornea and eyelid" (*Ancient Medicine*, 31). The first-century CE physician Celsus gives instructions for performing minor types of eye surgery in *De med.* 7.7, followed by discussions of surgery on the ear, nose, and mouth in 7.8–12. Fractures and dislocations are treated in book 8.

[37] For a description of common blood-letting practices, see Jackson, *Doctors and Diseases in the Roman Empire*, 70–3.

[38] Trepanation is discussed in the Hippocratic treatise *On Injuries of the Head*. The first-century CE physician Celsus describes the procedure for removing bladder stones in some detail in *De med.* 7.26.

others, depending on the type of illness and the ability of the patient.[39] Exercises mentioned in the literature include walking, marching, riding, running, wrestling, ball games, and riding in carriages or on horseback. Baths and hot springs also played an important role in heating, cooling, and massaging the sick body, though the manner in which they were used varied with the nature of the ailment and the school to which the physician belonged. Hot springs were categorized according to their mineral content, with different types of minerals being prescribed for different types of illness.[40] Other forms of heating and cooling were also employed in treatment, such as wrapping the body in blankets or swimming in ice-cold rivers. Yet another form of regimen was transferring the sick person from an unhealthy environment to a more salubrious setting. For the wealthy this might entail moving to a country residence, embarking upon a sea voyage, or taking a vacation in a dry climate. Remedies such as these were beyond the means of ordinary people.

(e) Another technique used by Greek and Roman physicians to diagnose and treat sickness was *divination*, specifically *dream interpretation* and *astrology*.[41] Several ancient medical writers talk about how dreams can provide information regarding the causes and cures of particular illnesses, though they disagree about the sources of these dreams and how they should be interpreted. The fourth book of the Hippocratic treatise *On Regimen* (fourth to fifth centuries BCE) speaks at length about the value of dream interpretation for the physician.[42] Without denying the possibility that the gods might communicate with humans through prophetic dreams, the author traces most dreams to the activity of the human soul, which uses the period of rest to convey symbolically what it has observed regarding the condition of the body. Dreams in which the body and the natural world follow their normal course denote bodily health, while those that involve some sort of struggle or a deviation from the natural order indicate a problem within the body. The treatise is filled with practical advice for physicians about how to interpret various types of dreams and what treatments to apply for each one. The popularity of this approach in Hippocratic circles is evident from the fact that it appears centuries later in the writings of the physicians Galen and Rufus of Ephesus (both second century CE).[43]

---

[39] In the Hippocratic treatise *On Regimen in Health* 3–4, physicians are encouraged to prescribe not only the amount of sleep a person should get but also the type of bed they should use and the kinds of clothing they should wear in the daytime, depending on the condition.

[40] For more on this topic, see Israelowich, *Patients and Healers in the Context of Culture*, 120–1; Dvorjetski, "Medicinal Hot Springs and Healing Spas in the Graeco-Roman World," 86–7. The latter article includes a long list of illnesses for which hot springs were thought to provide relief (84–5).

[41] A brief, but helpful, overview of the subject can be found in François P. Retief and Louise Cilliers, "Medical Dreams in Graeco-Roman Times," *South African Medical Journal* 95 (2005): 841–4.

[42] Dreams are also mentioned more briefly in other parts of the Hippocratic Corpus. For a review of these other texts, see Maithe A. A. Hulskamp, "The Value of Dream Diagnosis in the Medical Praxis of the Hippocratics and Galen," in *Dreams, Healing, and Medicine in Greece: From Antiquity to the Present*, ed. Stephen M. Oberhelman (Surrey and Burlington, VT: Ashgate, 2013), 34–54.

[43] The Galenic treatise *About Diagnosis from Dreams*, which is generally regarded as a collection of excerpts from Galen's writings, echoes the ideas and language of the Hippocratic *On Regimen*, while Galen himself says on more than one occasion that a remedy had been revealed to him in a dream. Rufus of Ephesus (late first to early second century CE) instructed physicians to ask patients about their dreams on the grounds that troublesome dreams might denote malfunctions in the bodily humors (*Medical Questions*, 5.33, cited by Harris, *Dreams and Experience in Classical Antiquity*,

Other medical writers held different views. Herophilos (fourth to third centuries BCE), an early forerunner of the Empiricist school, agreed that most dreams originate in the soul, but he regarded them as imaginative expressions of human desires and not as veiled commentaries on the body's health.[44] A different view prevailed among his successors, whose pragmatic, anti-theoretical orientation led them to embrace the possibility that dreams, like any other form of experience, could play a role in diagnosis and treatment. The third major school, the Methodists, rejected all medical uses of dreams as superstitious, if Galen's account of their ideas can be trusted (*On the Natural Faculties* 1.12).[45] If therefore Paul or one of his followers wished to know whether a particular dream might be relevant to the diagnosis or treatment of a health problem, they would have found more sympathy from a Hippocratic or Empiricist physician than one from the Methodist school.[46] For the same reason, it was likely that they would be asked about their dreams as part of the medical diagnostic process unless they happened to choose a Methodist physician.

Astrology played a similar role for at least some physicians. Ancient medicine has deep roots in Greek philosophy, where the nature of the heavens, the human body, and the influence of the former on the latter were common topics of speculation. Astrology grew out of these discussions. This common history explains why a significant number of Greek and Roman philosophers and medical writers link human sickness and health with the movement of the stars and planets, including Empedocles, Diocles, Theophrastus, Vettius Valens, Firmicus, and Democritus.[47] The Hippocratic treatise *On Airs, Waters, and Places* speaks several times about how the balance of the humors is affected by the movements of sun, moon, and stars.[48] The influence of astrology on medicine was particularly strong in the Hellenistic era. Marilynn Lawrence lists a number of astrological concepts that were taken up by medical theorists during this period: "(1) zodiacal and planetary melothesia (the association of astral phenomenon at birth with physical type), (2) iatromathematics (which included consideration of auspicious and inauspicious times), (3) sympathies and antipathies between healing

---

195). A helpful overview of the medical use of dreams in antiquity is Steven M. Oberhelman, "The Diagnostic Dream in Ancient Medical Theory and Practice," *Bulletin of the History of Medicine* 61 (1987), 47–60. For Galen's views on dreams, see Hulskamp, "Value of Dream Diagnosis in the Medical Praxis of the Hippocratics and Galen," 54–68.

[44] Retief and Cilliers, "Medical Dreams in Graeco-Roman Times," 843.

[45] Soranus (second century CE), writing from a Methodist perspective, sees attention to dreams as a female superstition (*Gyn.* 1.3). Cicero, while not a medical writer, expresses a similar view (*De div.* 2.148–9): "To believe that there is such a divine power behind them is a superstition that is at odds with genuine piety or religion" (noted by Hanson, "Dreams and Visions in the Graeco-Roman World and Early Christianity," 1400).

[46] Despite reports of success by such reputable physicians as Galen and Rufus, there is no reason to think that their medical interpretation of dreams yielded any better results than the "magical" interpretations described in Chapter 3. Cf. Oberhelman, "Diagnostic Dream in Ancient Medical Theory and Practice," 53.

[47] François P. Retief and Louise C. Cilliers, "Astrologie en geneeskunde in die oudheid en middeleeue," *Suid-Afrikaanse Tydskrif vir Natuurwetenskap en Tegnologie* 29 (2010): 5.

[48] The writings of Hippocrates and other ancient writers on the subject are examined in Dorian Gieseler Greenbaum, "Hellenistic Astronomy in Medicine," in *Hellenistic Astronomy: The Science in Its Contexts*, ed. Alan C. Bowen and Francesca Rochberg (Leiden and Boston: Brill, 2020), 350–80.

plants and celestial bodies, and (4) prognostication of the course of an illness, of life expectancy or recovery, based on the moment a person fell ill."[49]

At the practical level, astrological knowledge helped physicians to diagnose the causes behind specific cases of sickness (by crediting them to the influence of planets or stars) and to make decisions about proper treatment (by predicting the likely course of an extended illness like malaria). How many physicians actually knew and used astrology in Paul's day is hard to assess, though the popularity of the practice would have made such associations welcome to ancient audiences. This was true even among the elites, many of whom consulted astrologers for guidance when facing major decisions. In fact, Glen Cooper has argued that the discussions of planetary influences in Book 3 of Galen's *On the Critical Days* were included solely to make elite audiences more receptive to his scientific methods of diagnosis and treatment.[50] John Scarborough, by contrast, thinks that astrology played a more integral role in Galen's thought: "Galen deemed astrology as one of the great discoveries of the Egyptian astronomers, and believed that the moon's position in the good and evil planets had great power over the condition of his patients."[51] Whoever is correct, there is ample reason to suppose that Paul and his followers could have been exposed to physicians who consulted the movements of planets and stars when diagnosing and treating their illnesses or injuries.

(f) Various other treatments were offered by physicians on a less consistent basis. *Incantations*, disparaged by some medical writers and recommended by none, were nonetheless regularly employed as healing aids by both Greek and Roman physicians. Roman healers recited them from ancient times, and several sources mention their use by midwives to manage labor and delivery.[52] They also appear among the fruitless practices of those medical providers whom the Hippocratic authors deride as "charlatans."[53] In a later era, Galen criticizes a first-century CE physician named Xenocrates because his treatises were filled with incantations and other practices that Galen disapproved.[54] Medical historian Vivian Nutton summarizes the situation well: "Chants, charms, and so-called sympathetic or white magic all continued to be used, to a greater or lesser extent, within medicine."[55]

Closely related but less well known is the use of *music therapy* by ancient physicians. The belief that sounds have the power to move both body and soul was implicit in the use of incantations, and the effect of music in particular was broadly theorized by Greek philosophers, especially Pythagoras. Plato speaks of music as "an auxiliary

---

[49] "Hellenistic Astrology," *Internet Encyclopedia of Philosophy*, ISSN 2161-0002, https://iep.utm.edu/astr-hel/#SH2b.
[50] "Galen and Astrology: A Mésalliance?" *Early Science and Medicine* 16 (2011): 120–46. For a more nuanced analysis, see Vivian Nutton, "Greek Medical Astrology and the Boundaries of Medicine," in Anna Akasoy, Charles Burnett, and Ronit Yoeli-Tlalim, ed. *Astro-Medicine: Astrology and Medicine, East and West* (Firenze: SISMEL edizioni del Galluzzo, 2008), 17–31.
[51] *Roman Medicine*, 120. Retief and Cilliers claim that Empiricists and Methodists rejected the use of astrology in medicine, but they cite no sources for this assertion ("Astrologie en geneeskunde in die oudheid en middeleeue," 5).
[52] Zucconi, *Ancient Medicine*, 305; Wainwright, *Women Healing/Healing Women*, 39.
[53] Zucconi, *Ancient Medicine*, 211.
[54] Nutton, "Healers in the Medical Marketplace," 56.
[55] *Ancient Medicine*, 113.

to the inner revolution of the soul, when it has lost its harmony, to assist in restoring it to order and concord with itself" (*Tim.* 47D). Such views explain why physicians routinely prescribed music to treat patients plagued by mental disturbances.[56] Physical illness could also be treated with music; for example, the alternating music of flute and harp was prescribed as a treatment for gout.[57] Both the rousing hymns and the theatrical and musical performances that Aelius Aristides describes at the Asklepion at Pergamon were a vital part of the healing regimen, not merely a pastime to entertain wealthy clients. How often such therapies were prescribed by ordinary physicians is impossible to say, though we can guess that they were used more often with the wealthy who had ready access to musical performers.

Finally, a brief comment should be made about the role of *prayer* in the therapeutic regimen of physicians. As we will see in the next chapter, neither Greek nor Roman physicians drew any bright line between their own discipline and religious modes of healing. In fact, the same Hippocratic treatise that discusses the medical interpretation of dreams also tells which gods one should approach to cure various types of illness (*Regimen* 4.89-90). As Cécile Nissen observes, "Les prières font partie intégrante de sa thérapeutique, au même titre que les aliments, les boissons, lea bains et les exercises physiques."[58] A similar attitude can be seen in *On the Sacred Disease*, where the Hippocratic author, after disparaging the efficacy of purification rituals and incantations as mechanisms for treating epilepsy, proposes that people should instead supplicate the gods with sacrifices and prayers and bring gifts to their temples (4.40-42). The treatise *Decorum* specifically acknowledges the value of prayer as an aid to healing (87), and other texts commend it as well, especially in hopeless cases where the physician's skills had proved fruitless. In fact, "the inclusion of prayer in the Hippocratic corpus confirms that this was a mainstream method of prophylaxis, so common that even the Hippocratic author accepts it."[59] This is exactly what we should expect in a culture where virtually everyone (including physicians) regarded the gods as a vital force in human affairs.

This reference to hopeless cases raises a final point that should not be missed regarding ancient medical care. Despite their array of treatment methods, ancient physicians were very aware that not all sicknesses could be cured. As John Scarborough observes, "Once he has exhausted his stock of drugs, poultices, cupping glasses, theories of fluxes and their control through diet, the doctor simply says 'the patient cannot be cured.'"[60]

One of the vital skills of a successful physician was the ability to recognize such cases when they appeared and refuse to take them lest too many failures should diminish one's reputation with the public, leading to a loss of clients.[61] Few physicians

---

[56] Edelstein, "Greek Medicine in its Relation to Religion and Magic," 235–9.
[57] Christos F. Kleisiaris, Chrisanthos Sfakianakis, and Ioanna V. Papathanasiou, "Health Care Practices in Ancient Greece: The Hippocratic Ideal," *Journal of Medical Ethics and History of Medicine* 7 (2014): 6.
[58] *Entre Asclépios et Hippocrate*, 39.
[59] "'Conjurers, Purifiers, Vagabonds and Quacks'?" 9.
[60] *Roman Medicine*, 141.
[61] Molly Jones-Lewis sees a dual purpose behind the physicians' refusal to treat incurable conditions: it "protected patients from a doctor's unnecessary experimentation and intervention, and it also

even attempted to treat congenital abnormalities, and many avoided cases involving internal maladies that might turn out to be cancerous since they were considered incurable.[62] Some even refrained from treating the elderly for similar reasons. Opinion was divided over mental disorders, which ancient medical authors regarded as treatable through the use of diet, medicines, purging, blood-letting, exercise, and changes of environment. Practicing physicians would have avoided the more persistent cases, but some clearly made the effort since the literature speaks also about harsher remedies such as starvation, flogging, and, if all else failed, incarceration.[63]

Conclusion

Medicine was one of several modes of health care that were available to Greeks and Romans who needed help in dealing with an illness or injury. It differed from other systems primarily in its rationalist orientation that saw sickness as a disruption of natural bodily processes rather than as something inflicted from outside, whether as a divine punishment or an attack by evil spirits. It was not a wholly materialist system like modern medicine, as both theorists and practitioners left room for the divine to produce cures either through or independently of the hands of the physician. But medical care did not require divine activity, nor did its methods include any direct appeals to suprahuman powers. Its prescriptions aimed instead to repair or remove that which was disrupting the normal operation of the body so that it could resume its natural mode of operation. It also offered guidance regarding how to keep the body healthy and thus avoid such disruptive influences.

Greco-Roman medicine was not a unified system of thought or practice. Various schools arose over time with differing ideas about how the body works and what kinds of remedies should be applied both generally and in particular cases to restore it to health. As a rule, physicians learned the theory and methods of a single school through apprenticeship with a practitioner who had been trained in a similar manner. The result was a highly diverse medical landscape with followers of each school competing for patients in all of the major cities and many smaller communities across the Mediterranean world. People who needed health care might have found the diversity confusing, but most could have distinguished a physician from other types of healers.

As with other modes of health care, the remedies prescribed by physicians resembled those of the traditional health care system from which it was derived, but the medical cures were more developed and grounded in theory. Dietary

---

protected the physician from losing his reputation owing to too many deaths" ("Physicians and 'Schools,'" 388). A similar mentality can be seen at the Asklepian sanctuaries, where patients deemed to have a terminal illness were forced to leave lest they should die on the premises and pollute the sanctuary (not to mention harming the sanctuary's public image).

[62] The only congenital malformities that ancient physicians are known to have treated are clubfoot and hunchback, according to Garland, *Eye of the Beholder*, 123–8. On cancers, see Retief and Cilliers, "Tumours and Cancers in Graeco-Roman Times," 201–9.

[63] Garland, *Eye of the Beholder*, 137–9; Philip van de Eijk, "Cure and (In)curability of Mental Disorders in Ancient Medical and Philosophical Thought," in Harris, *Mental Disorders*, 307–38.

modifications, rest or exercise, medicinal substances, and even minor forms of surgery were employed in both systems to treat illnesses and injuries. Medical healers also absorbed practices from religious and "magical" modes of healing, including dream interpretation, incantations, amulets, astrology, and even prayer. The rationale for using these techniques was different in medical healing than in traditional health care, but methods alone would not have set physicians apart from other types of healers.

What then might Paul and his followers have thought about medical providers and their methods of treatment? Most modern readers probably assume that Christ-followers turned to physicians when they needed health care because that is what we do today. More astute observers might suppose that medical treatment was preferable because it was less entangled with the beliefs and practices of Greek, Roman, and indigenous religious systems. But there is no evidence to support these presumptions. Not only are there no references in the New Testament to Christ-followers consulting physicians, but as we will see in Chapter 8, Christians debated for centuries what types of health care were and were not permissible, with various church fathers condemning practices that the majority of Christians followed. In some cases the list of banned practices included reliance on "pagan" physicians. The same can be said for Judeans: their leaders, too, debated the propriety of various healing methods, with some arguing for a more conservative stance and others adopting a more liberal viewpoint. On the whole, it seems that Jewish leaders remained open to diverse modes of treatment long after Christians had narrowed their list of acceptable providers (Chapter 7).

Thus the fact that Paul was a Jew and a Christ-follower cannot be cited as a reason for supposing that he would have preferred or recommended medicine over other forms of treatment. Paul clearly had a need for health care in view of the many injuries and illnesses that he suffered, and his followers would have had similar needs by virtue of living in a world where health problems were ubiquitous. But there is nothing in Paul's letters to indicate whether he had any preference regarding what type of provider he or the members of his congregations should consult. Arguments from silence are invariably precarious, but Paul's silence on what would seem to be a significant point of theological and ethical concern is curious, especially in light of the attention that later Christians gave to the subject (Chapter 8). Whether we can retroject their concerns and arguments back into Paul's day will be examined in Chapter 9.

6

Overlapping Health Care Systems

A Web of Options

The last four chapters have highlighted the diversity and complexity of the health care network that would have been available to Paul and his followers wherever they lived or traveled. Unlike today, when much of the world regards Western medical science as superior to other forms of care, no system of treatment predominated in Greco-Roman society.[1] Rich and poor alike sought cures from a variety of "magical," religious, and medical experts who worked alongside traditional healers to treat the many illnesses and injuries that were a mundane element of life in the ancient world. This diversity produced "a 'medical market place' in which *authority* was in the hands of the health care providers but *power* remained in the hands of the sick, insofar as they chose which of the available treatment options to follow."[2] Relations among the different practitioners varied with time and place from cooperation to grudging acceptance to denigration to open hostility and efforts at repression. Making vital health decisions in the face of such varied treatment options would have been challenging to say the least.

Complicating matters further is the fact that the boundary lines between the various health care systems were fuzzy at best. Literary evidence suggests that the educated elites could tell them apart, guided perhaps by polemical texts in which proponents of the different systems commended their own methods and disparaged those of their competitors. But whether such distinctions were evident to the illiterate masses is doubtful. Since they were incapable of reading the polemics produced by proponents of the various schools, their judgments would have been based on their experience, where the language, ideas, and methods used in the different health care systems overlapped more than the polemical texts would suggest. Some of these overlaps can be traced to their common roots in traditional medicine while others reflect conscious borrowings from competing systems of care. A review of the nature and extent of these overlaps will help us to estimate how far it would have been possible for Paul and his followers to distinguish among the various systems so as to prefer or avoid one form of health care over others.

---

[1] The difference is less clear in practice, as ordinary people in much of the world actually prefer traditional forms of medicine. The health care system in countries like China or India where multiple forms of treatment coexist is quite similar to that of the Greco-Roman world.
[2] Israelowich, *Patients and Healers in the High Roman Empire*, 31 (emphasis his).

"Magical" Healing

The routine conflation of what later became "magical," religious, and medical modes of treatment in the traditional health care systems of Greece and Rome was described in Chapter 2 and need not be repeated here. The distillation of these traditional healing techniques into three distinctive systems—Hippocratic medicine, the cult of Asklepios, and "magical" healing—occurred in ancient Greece during the fifth and fourth centuries BCE as proponents of the first two systems labored to distance their treatments from the "magical" elements of traditional healing in order to attract clients. Suspicions of *mageia* were growing during this period because of its perceived foreignness, its independence from the local cult, and the fact that it could be used to harm as well as to help people. It is thus understandable that medical and religious healers would want to frame their own approaches as free from "magical" influence.

The effort was only partly successful, however, as the pragmatic syncretism of traditional health care resisted the efforts of religious and medical theorists and practitioners to establish methodologically coherent and distinct systems of thought and practice. All three of the health care systems examined in the last three chapters retained elements of traditional health care that were not wholly consistent with their theories, and all three continued to appropriate language, ideas, and practices from the other two systems throughout their history.

The fact that "magical" healing has much in common with religious healing is not surprising as suprahuman powers play an important role in both systems. Both presume that ill health can be caused by suprahuman forces, and both agree that appropriate rituals can influence these forces to put an end to human suffering. Many of their rituals were also similar, including purification rites, sacrifices, incense, libations, and prayers. Practitioners of *mageia* might have spoken more confidently about the power of their rituals to move suprahuman forces to do their bidding, especially those that were distinctive to them (incantations, charms, spells, ingestion of sacred substances, manipulation of objects, etc.), but this alone was not enough to differentiate them from traditional Greek and Roman religion where moving the gods to provide material benefits was a perennial concern.[3] The fact that their rites were performed by self-appointed experts to benefit individuals without reference to the civic cult aroused the suspicions of local leaders, as we saw in Chapter 3, but this individualized pattern of treatment was not materially different from what we see in the cult of Asklepios and other healing gods. The popularity of "magical" healing with the illiterate masses shows that they did not share the negative judgments of the elites concerning these practices. Instead, they seem to have viewed *mageia* as a particular application of commonly held beliefs about how humans should interact with the gods. For them, *mageia* was simply a form of popular religion.[4]

---

[3] As we saw in Chapter 3, certain philosophers objected to *mageia* on the grounds that it sought to manipulate the gods to do the will of humans, but the same objection could be raised against many forms of traditional religion. "Magical" healing did differ somewhat from traditional religion in attributing some illnesses to *daimones* whose power must be broken in order for healing to occur.

[4] As we saw in Chapter 3, most modern scholars have found no objective basis for distinguishing *mageia* from religion. As Georg Luck puts it, "One person's religion may be another person's magic"

Similarities between "magical" and medical modes of health care are less obvious since medical theorists typically denigrated "magical" healers as charlatans and frauds and the practitioners of *mageia* showed little interest in "medicalizing" their language and practices as was done in the cult of Asklepios.[5] From the perspective of those seeking to be healed, however, the distinction between the two systems was by no means sharp. Practitioners in both areas used similar treatment methods, including the ingestion or application of ritually prepared substances, the wearing of amulets, the interpretation of dreams, and the regulation of remedies by the movements of the heavens. These similarities, which mostly reflect their common roots in traditional health care rather than any direct borrowings or adaptations, may have been sufficient to blur the lines between the two systems in the eyes of the public. The presence in both Greek and Roman circles of healers who actively conflated the two approaches—those whom the elites derided as "charlatans"—also undermined the efforts of medical theorists to establish clear distinctions between medicine and "magic."

Religious Healing

As we saw in the previous section, most of the similarities between religious and "magical" healing can be traced to a shared worldview (including their belief in the importance of suprahuman forces) and their common roots in traditional modes of treatment, though the possibility of dialog and interchange between their practitioners cannot be ruled out. Clarifying whether and how far such mutual influence occurred is beyond the scope of this study, since our concern is with how the various health care systems would have been perceived by the public and not with how they developed. On this question the answer seems clear: "magical" and religious healing were regarded as points on a continuum and not as distinct systems of thought and practice.

With regard to medicine, there is ample evidence of ongoing interchange and influence between religious and medical systems of healing as Asklepian healing centers were increasingly "medicalized" over the centuries. Physicians were present to treat people who traveled to these centers seeking cures from the god, and the larger centers included all of the facilities that a physician might have needed to treat patients, including bath complexes and gymnastic facilities. Priests also provided medical care at some facilities, and some physicians served as priests. Both employed similar techniques of consultation and diagnosis (including dream interpretation) to assess the health of visitors, and both worked together to apply any treatments that were prescribed by the god in dreams.[6] Decrees honoring physicians were set up in the sanctuary at Kos, while the early collaboration between priests and physicians is

---

(*Arcana Mundi*, 135). Stephen Ricks speaks of a "religion-magic continuum" in which the dividing line between the two depends on the stance of the person speaking or writing ("The Magician as Outsider in the Hebrew Bible and the New Testament," in *Ancient Magic and Ritual Power*, ed. Marvin Meyer and Paul Mirecki [Leiden and New York: E. J. Brill, 1995], 143).

[5] More will be said on this topic later.

[6] Israelowich, *Patients and Healers in the High Roman Empire*, 65-6; Nissen, *Entre Asclépios et Hippocrate*, 227.

celebrated on coins from Epidauros (minted 323–240 BCE) depicting an altar on which a thymiaterion (incense burner) is flanked by two cupping vessels.[7]

Asklepios himself also took on an increasingly medical persona over time, being framed as "a divine healer who was trained in the art of medicine and continually followed the advances in medical practices."[8] Eventually he came to came to be regarded as the living embodiment of the art of medicine, one who possessed all of the skills, talents, and attributes of a good doctor.[9] The dream treatments that lay at the heart of Asklepian health care were also "medicalized" over time as the god increasingly relied on medical techniques (including otherwise impossible surgeries) to perform his miraculous cures or gave instructions for medical remedies (diet, exercise, baths, purging, ointments, etc.) to be applied to the sick person after they woke.[10] This pattern of clothing religious healing in medical garb led people to think of religious and medical healers more as partners than competitors: "Divine and human healing were thus complementary, and how and when each was to be used was a personal decision."[11]

Medical Healing

As we noted earlier, the presence of "magical" elements in medicine is due more to their common roots in traditional health care than any ongoing influence of the former on the latter. But we cannot wholly rule out the latter, especially among those practitioners whom elite authors deride as "charlatans." Clearly some of these people were presenting themselves as physicians or there would have been no cause for medical authors and their supporters to be concerned about them. Their presence and activities would have created ambiguity in the minds of the public about who was and was not a physician. The fact that their medical critics also included "magical" practices in their repertoire, as we saw in Chapter 5, would have muddied the waters still further. How many people were able to differentiate between medical and "magical" practitioners (or even cared to try) is hard to say, but it seems likely that most people would have viewed them as shades on a spectrum rather than as methodologically distinct systems of care.

---

[7] Hart, *Asclepius, the God of Medicine*, 136; photos of the coins can be found on p. 61. Translations of several inscriptions that were erected at temples of Asklepios from the third and second centuries BCE to honor particular physicians can be viewed online at http://www.attalus.org/docs/other/inscr_99.html.

[8] Panagiotidou, "Religious Healing and the Asclepius Cult," 83.

[9] Nutton, *Ancient Medicine*, 111–14. This dual role takes visible form in Aristophanes's play *Plutus*, where Asklepios appears dressed like a physician and uses medical tools to prepare a plaster for the eyes of a sick person (709–45).

[10] Israelowich, *Patients and Healers in the High Roman Empire*, 57–9; Helen King, "Comparative Perspectives on Medicine and Healing in the Ancient World," in *Religion, Health and Suffering*, ed. John R. Hinnells and Roy Porter (London and New York: Kegan Paul, 1999), 281. According to Aelius Aristides, physicians at the Asklepion in Pergamon sometimes had their prescriptions countermanded by the god in a dream, and they seem to have accepted the dream as a superior form of guidance (Lloyd, *In the Grip of Disease*, 55–6).

[11] Nutton, *Ancient Medicine*, 279.

Regarding medicine and religion, we have already seen how religious healers adopted some of the language and practices of medical providers, but the influence also moved in the opposite direction as Hippocratic physicians actively cultivated ties with religious healing. Physicians claimed Asklepios as the founder and patron of their discipline, and some even asserted physical descent from the god.[12] The original version of the Hippocratic Oath calls on Apollo, Asklepios, Hygieia, Panacea, and "all the gods and goddesses" to witness the physician's commitment to ethical service, while the *Law* of Hippocrates uses religious language to describe the transmission of medical knowledge.[13] Physicians worked on the staff of Asklepian sanctuaries, collaborating with the priests to interpret their patients' dreams and apply treatments prescribed by the god, and a few are known to have served as priests to Asklepios. Numerous inscriptions show them making benefactions to Asklepian temples and presenting sacrifices and votive offerings to Asklepios, his father Apollo, and his daughter Hygieia for themselves and those whom they had cured.[14] At Athens, physicians were required by law to offer sacrifices twice a year to Asklepios and to acknowledge him as the source of their healing power, and excavators have found medical instruments that physicians had dedicated to the god at his temple there.[15] Votive inscriptions show that people who were healed by physicians simultaneously credited the god for their cures.[16]

Similar ties can be seen in the area of ideology. Hippocratic authors insist that sickness is caused by natural physical and environmental forces, but that belief did not exclude divine causality. The treatise *On Airs, Waters, and Places* explains that all diseases are both divinely caused (because the forces within nature are divine) and divinely cured (because physicians use healing techniques and substances that were created and revealed by the gods, who also work through miracles).[17] Similar ideas can

---

[12] Prioreschi, *History of Medicine*, 2.645; Nissen, *Entre Asclépios et Hippocrate*, 262–4.

[13] The ancient version of the Hippocratic Oath begins with this asseveration (Loeb): "I swear by Apollo Healer, by Asclepius, by Hygieia, by Panacea, and by all the gods and goddesses, making them my witnesses, that I will carry out, according to my ability and judgment, this oath and this indenture." It also describes medical knowledge as "holy secrets" that should not be divulged except to fellow physicians. Similar language appears in *Law* 5: "Those things which are sacred, are to be imparted only to sacred persons; and it is not lawful to impart them to the profane until they have been initiated in the mysteries of the science."

[14] Nissen, *Entre Asclépios et Hippocrate*, 270–6; Wickkeiser, "Appeal of Asklepios and the Politics of Healing in the Greco-Roman World," 98–107. That this was not an external imposition upon a "secular" discipline is evident from numerous medical writings where Asklepios is honored. The celebrated Roman physician Galen (second century CE) describes Asklepios as his "paternal deity" and attributes his healing powers to the god of medicine (Christian Brockmann, "A God and Two Humans on Matters of Medicine: Asclepius, Galen and Aelius Aristides," in Russell et al., *In Praise of Asclepius*, 115–19).

[15] Nissen, *Entre Asclépios et Hippocrate*, 279–80; Nutton, *Ancient Medicine*, 111.

[16] Nissen, *Entre Asclépios et Hippocrate*, 279–80. Even the skeptical Cicero in one of his letters thanks Apollo and Asklepios (Latin "Aesculapius") along with his physicians for an act of healing (*Fam* 14.7.1, cited in ibid., 220).

[17] Cf. *Airs* 22: "To me it appears that such affections are just as much divine as all others are, and that no one disease is either more divine or more human than another, but that all are alike divine, for that each has its own nature, and that no one arises without a natural cause." The second century geographer Pausanius, who visited the Asklepion at Pergamon, expresses the duality more clearly: "Asclepius . . .is air, bringing health to mankind and to all animals likewise; Apollo is the sun, and most rightly is he named the father of Asclepius, because the sun, by adapting his course to

be found in *On the Sacred Disease*, which also affirms the value of sacrifices, prayers, and gifts to temples. Physicians often prescribed prayer in conjunction with other treatments, and patients whom they deemed incurable were commended to the will and power of the gods.[18] Those who could afford it were sent to Asklepian sanctuaries for treatment. Both medical and religious healers benefited from this relationship of mutual support: "The dedications of doctors increased the economic prosperity and architectural expansion of the Asklepieia, while the popularity of Asclepius enhanced the reputation of the physicians, increasing their authority and attracting new clients."[19]

Conclusion

It should be clear by now that the health care system that was available to Paul and his followers both before and after they joined the Christ-movement was varied and complex. Medical historian Vivian Nutton speaks of "the pluralism of Greek medicine" when describing this ancient cultural framework in which "magical," religious, and medical practitioners coexisted and borrowed from one another in an uneasy peace marked by critical judgments and periodic bouts of rancor.[20] Plinio Prioreschi's warning to modern interpreters is apt.

> We must not imagine . . . that there was a distinction between a more or less official medicine (i.e., the Hippocratic medicine) practiced by "doctors" and the healing activities of others similar to the distinction that we make today between "medicine," meaning by this term the officially recognized practice, and the so-called alternative medicine. . . . Besides the *iatroi* (physicians) and the priests of Aesculapius who practiced medicine in the shrines of the god, there were root-sellers (*rizotomoi*—root-cutters), drug-sellers (*pharmacopolai*), itinerant sellers of charms and purifications, midwives (*maiai*—whose activities may not have been confined to what we call midwifery), lithotomists (as mentioned in the *Oath*), gymnastic trainers, and, finally, magicians and other charlatans. How distinct in the mind of everybody were the *iatroi* from the others is not clear.[21]

---

the seasons, imparts to the air its healthfulness. . . .It is the course of the sun that brings health to mankind" (*Achaia*, 23.7). For more on physicians and divine causality, see Israelowich, *Patients and Healers in the High Roman Empire*, 34; Lloyd, *In the Grip of Disease*, 46–50; Edelstein, "Greek Medicine in its Relation to Religion and Magic," 208–17, 226–32. By contrast, medical authors had little room for causation by demons, which they linked to the quackery of magic (Edelstein, "Greek Medicine in its Relation to Religion and Magic," 219).

[18] Edelstein, "Greek Medicine in its Relation to Religion and Magic," 239–44; Michael T. Compton, "The Union of Religion and Health in Ancient Asklepieia," *Journal of Religion and Health* 37 (1998): 207–8; Martin, *Inventing Superstition*, 47.

[19] Olympia Panagitidou, "Asclepius: A Divine Doctor, A Popular Healer," in *Popular Medicine in Graeco-Roman Antiquity: Explorations*, ed. William V. Harris (Leiden and Boston: Brill, 2016), 97. Several modern investigators have remarked on the total absence from the medical literature of any attacks on religious healing or Asklepian healing centers—see Lloyd, *In the Grip of Disease*, 52; Wickkeiser, "Appeal of Asklepios and the Politics of Healing in the Greco-Roman World," 49; Edelstein and Edelstein, *Asclepius*, 139.

[20] Nutton, "Medicine in the Greek World, 800-50 BC," 16.

[21] Prioreschi, *History of Medicine*, 2.639–40.

To suppose that Paul or anyone else in the ancient world could have chosen to rely exclusively on one system of healing (e.g., some form of "secular" medicine) while avoiding all others (e.g., healers who adhered to "pagan" religious beliefs or practices) is to replace historical analysis with Western intellectual prejudice. No "secular" healing institutions existed in Greco-Roman antiquity, and the ancient health care system was too complex and messy for such distinctions to be practicable. Helen King's pithy comment is apt: "As post-Enlightenment beings, we separate medicine from both magic and religion, and call this liberation, or progress; the Greeks did not."[22]

Such presumptions also stifle historical inquiry insofar as they impose limits on Paul's practice without justification. As we will see in Chapters 7 and 8, there is a wealth of evidence that Judeans and Christian used the services of Greek and Roman healers in the first few centuries of the Common Era, including those who offered "magical" and religious remedies. We cannot therefore infer from Paul's Jewish or Christian identities that he would have rejected or even been troubled by the use of "pagan" healing practices. Only by carefully sifting the historical evidence can we determine what counts as a reasonable presumption regarding Paul's ideas and practices in this area.

---

[22] "Comparative Perspectives on Medicine and Healing in the Ancient World," 281.

Part II

Judean and Christian Health Care Systems

7

Judean Approaches to Health Care

Introduction

In the previous chapters we examined the health care options that were available to ordinary people in the Greco-Roman world where Paul and his followers carried on their lives both before and after they became Christ-followers. In the remaining chapters we will focus more narrowly on what can be known about the health care beliefs and practices of people who shared Paul's distinctive social and religious views, that is, Judeans[1] and Christians.

All of our ancient sources testify to the unease that Judeans and Christians felt regarding any sort of interaction with gods or spirits other than the God of Israel, so it is natural to ask whether that unease extended to the Greco-Roman health care system, where all forms of treatment presupposed polytheistic beliefs about suprahuman powers. Paul's letters tell us nothing specific about his views on the subject, but we have ample testimony regarding what other Judeans and Christians thought and did to treat health problems in the centuries before and after Paul. A careful examination of this evidence will enable us to develop an informed opinion regarding what Paul might or might not have found acceptable in this area. It will also give us material by which to test modern assumptions regarding the limits of ancient Jewish and Christian (including Pauline) monotheism.

Our study will begin with Judaism, since Paul's beliefs and practices in all areas of life would have been heavily influenced by his Jewish upbringing. Though he believed that God had commissioned him to bring the message of Jesus to polytheistic gentiles who were ignorant of the God of Israel, Paul's negative opinion of non-Jewish religious beliefs and practices is apparent throughout his letters (Rom. 1:21-25, 1 Cor. 8:4-7, 10:20-21, 2 Cor. 6:16-18, Gal. 2:15, 1 Thess. 2:9, etc.). Such opinions were not unique to Paul; similar statements can be found in many other Judean writings from the era. We might therefore anticipate that Paul and other Judeans who shared his devotion to his ancestral traditions would have avoided most, if not all, of the "pagan" healing practices described in Chapters 2–5. Whether the evidence supports this presumption is the subject of the present chapter.

---

[1] As I explained in the Introduction (note 54), I have chosen in this book to translate words derived from the *Ioudai-* root differently depending on context: traditional renderings ("Jewish," "Judaism," etc.) are used when discussing matters of ideology and praxis, while "Judeans" is used when referring to the people who held those views.

Our review of Judean healing practices will begin with a survey of what can be gleaned from the Hebrew Bible about how sickness and healing were viewed by the Yahwistic editors of the canonical text. No effort will be made to distinguish between real-world practices and the ideology of the editors, since our concern is not with what was actually done in ancient Israel but with how the contents of the sacred text influenced the views and practices of Judeans in Paul's day. The remainder of the chapter is devoted to a careful investigation of what ancient sources tell us about how Judeans in the centuries around the turn of the era viewed and used (or avoided) the three systems of Greco-Roman health care described in the previous chapters: "magical," religious, and medical. Attention will also be given to whether and how far Judeans might have developed their own versions of these practices that were more consistent with their religious ideology. The chapter will conclude with some reflections on what these inquiries might suggest regarding how the apostle Paul handled matters of sickness and healing insofar as he remained faithful to his Judean roots.

According to Scripture

The claim that Judean beliefs and practice in Paul's day were heavily shaped by the content of the Jewish Scriptures requires no justification since everyone agrees that the sacred text was central to Jewish life. The amount of scriptural knowledge that particular individuals possessed would have varied with their literacy levels and social class, but even the illiterate masses would have absorbed the central stories and tenets of the Scriptures in oral form from early childhood.[2] Whether this instruction would have included biblical ideas about sickness and healing is unclear since the subject is not often addressed in the Jewish Scriptures, as we will see later. Most probably heard little on the subject and were thus ill-equipped for assessing the compatibility of Greek and Roman healing practices with their sacred text. This observation should be kept in mind when we encounter evidence of Judeans engaging in healing practices that seem to us inconsistent with the content of the Jewish Scriptures.

So what do the Scriptures say about sickness and healing? On the causes of sickness, reflection is sparse. Most texts treat it simply as an unpleasant occurrence that needs to be remedied. When a cause is given, it is almost always the mighty hand of Yahweh, who uses bodily suffering to discipline or punish his people.[3] The Scriptures are clear that Yahweh created and directs all of the forces of nature, including the human body, so any pain or suffering that comes to humans through the natural world must be rooted directly or indirectly in the divine will. Nature itself is not divine as Greek and

---

[2] Even in Israel, less than 10 percent of the population would have been able to read simple texts and sign their names during the imperial era, according to the careful research of Catherine Hezser, *Jewish Literacy in Roman Palestine* (Tübingen: Mohr Siebeck, 2001).

[3] Masculine pronouns and adjectives are used in this chapter when referring to the deity as our concern is with how God is presented in the Hebrew Bible and not with contemporary theology or praxis. Feminine imagery is used here and there to describe Yahweh, but the vast majority of references depict the deity in male terms and all of them use exclusively masculine pronouns and adjectives.

Roman medical writers would have it, but everything in the visible world owes its existence to Yahweh and operates according to his will. Demonic causation, which plays a notable role in later Jewish thought, is absent from the Jewish Scriptures, even from the book of Job, where the "Satan" who afflicts Job with bodily sores is not a devil or demon but one of the "sons of God" who present themselves before Yahweh in heaven (Job 1:6-8, 2:1-2). As such, he acts against Job only after receiving permission from Yahweh.

As for what humans should do when faced with illness, the answers vary from text to text, but all three modes of treatment examined in the previous chapters are represented. For the sake of consistency, the material will be analyzed under these same headings. Because the Hebrew Bible is fundamentally a religious text, however, we will alter our previous order and discuss religious modes of treatment first, followed by "magical" and then medical healing.

Religious Healing in the Hebrew Bible

In cases where sickness is sent directly by Yahweh as a form of discipline or punishment, the only cure is repentance. This view is expressed clearly in texts where sickness is inflicted upon the people as a whole (Lev. 26:14-18, 1 Kgs 8:37-40, 2 Chron. 7:13-14, Amos 4:10, etc.), but it also appears in stories about individuals (2 Sam. 24:1-17, Job 42:1-17, Dan. 7:24-37).[4] Similar ideas can be seen in several psalms where the petitioner confesses sin as part of an appeal for healing (32, 28, 41, etc.). None of these texts say anything about using ordinary methods to cure illness—where religious violations are involved, religious treatments alone can suffice.

Even in cases where no sin is involved, prayer to Yahweh is presumed to be the most effective remedy for sickness. Numerous texts describe Yahweh as a god who heals (Exod. 15:26, Deut. 32:39, Job 5:18, Ps. 41:3, etc.), and several stories show him healing people who are sick in response to prayers (Gen. 20:17, 1 Kgs 17:17-23, 2 Kgs 20:2-7). Healing is explicitly linked with prayer in 2 Chron. 6:28-30, and the psalms are filled with the laments of sick people praying to Yahweh to relieve them of sickness. Insofar as the psalms provided a template for prayers at the Jerusalem temple, many others besides the authors would have used them to give shape to their own appeals for healing.

In the vast majority of texts involving religious healing, Yahweh acts directly and miraculously. No reference is made to anything like the Asklepian treatment centers that were so common in the Greek and Roman worlds.[5] The only human agent who

---

[4] Sin is not explicitly cited as the cause of sickness in 1 Kgs 8:37-40, but Yahweh is called to forgive the people in v. 39 and all of the other forms of suffering in the chapter are blamed on sin, so it is likely that the same cause should be inferred here. In Job, the sickness is not inflicted because of sin but as part of a divine wager, yet by the end of the story Job is repenting of a sin that might best be described as presumption (42:1-6). The text never says that Job was cured, but it is clearly implied in his reversal of fortune.

[5] Hector Avalos (*Health Care and the Rise of Christianity*, 43) suggests that the sanctuary at Shiloh might have been a place where people went for healing based on 1 Samuel 1, but there is nothing in this passage to suggest that Elkanah went there seeking a cure for Hannah's infertility. He also mentions the site of the bronze snake Nehushtan in 2 Kgs 18:4 as a possible healing shrine (Num.

is shown healing sickness is the prophet. Most of the relevant examples are associated with Elijah or Elisha, but we also read of Isaiah healing king Hezekiah in 2 Kgs 20:2-8. For the first two prophets, the cure is almost always instantaneous and miraculous, while for Isaiah it involves a treatment that might be labeled as medical (applying a poultice to a boil, 2 Kgs 8:7).[6] Prophets also engage in prognosis, announcing in advance the outcome of a disease (2 Kgs 1:3-4, 8:7-13, 14:1-18, 20:1-6; cf. 1 Sam. 1:12-17). But these stories are exceptions; there is no evidence in the Hebrew Bible that healing was a regular part of the duties of a prophet.

Certain forms of sickness are said to impart ritual impurity. These conditions were treated by isolation from the community for the duration of the illness. Examples include the skin lesions that the priests are called to inspect in Leviticus 13-14 and the "leprosy" that appears in the stories of Miriam in Num. 12:10-15, Naaman in 2 Kgs 51-14, and Uzziah in 2 Chron. 26:20-21. The laws about bodily discharges (including menstruation) in Leviticus 15 might also be included here insofar as they pertain to conditions that were considered abnormal and thus disordered from a male standpoint. Nothing in these texts suggests that isolation itself effected healing; its sole purpose was to protect the community from contagion. The same is true for the purification rituals that are mandated in some instances—they were done to mark the person publicly as cured, not to aid the healing process. In fact, only one of these texts—Elisha's order for Naaman to bathe in the Jordan River (2 Kings 5)—says anything at all about treatment. For the most part these purification texts seem to presume that healing, if it occurs at all, happens naturally with the passage of time, not as a result of ritual action.

In summary, the Hebrew Bible offers no clear instruction for performing religious healing other than repentance and prayer. Allowance is also made for miraculous healings, but the only ones described in the Scriptures take place at the hands of prophets. Whether such healings could still be expected in an era devoid of prophets was an open question in the time of Paul.

"Magical" Healing in the Hebrew Bible

The Hebrew Bible contains many texts in which activities that might be called "magical" are condemned, including some that call for the death penalty (Exod. 22:18, Lev. 20:6, 20:27, Deut. 18:9-14, 2 Chron. 33:1-6, Jer. 27:9-10, Ezek. 13:17-23, Mic. 5:12-15, etc.). Several different Hebrew words are used to describe these activities; in English they

---

21:4-9), but the text says only that people were offering incense to the image, not that they were using it for healing. The only passages where the sanctuary of Yahweh plays any role in healing are 1 Kgs 8:37-40, where Solomon asks Yahweh to heal those who pray toward his temple, and Lev. 14:1-32, where people healed of skin disease are required to go through a cleansing ritual at the sanctuary (noted by Hector Avalos, *Illness and Health Care in the Ancient Near East: The Role of the Temple in Greece, Mesopotamia, and Israel* (Atlanta: Scholars Press, 1995), 358–9). The latter passage is only indirectly relevant, however, since the ritual is performed after the healing has occurred, not as a form of treatment, and the priest serves only a ritual function, not as a healer.

[6] The lone exception to the instantaneous cures of Elijah and Elisha is 2 Kgs 5:8-14, where Elisha tells Naaman to wash himself seven times in the Jordan River to be healed. Even here we read that Naaman was disappointed that Elisha did not heal him immediately (v. 11), an observation that reaffirms the norm.

are commonly rendered by terms like "sorcery," "witchcraft," and "divination," while those who practice them are designated as "sorcerers," "witches," "wizards," "spiritists," "mediums," "soothsayers," "augurs," and the like. Many texts associate these practices with foreigners and people who serve deities other than Yahweh (Exod. 7:10-12, 8:6-7, 1 Sam. 6:1-2, Isa. 2:6-9, etc.), but whether these texts reflect historical reality or slander is hard to say. As we saw in Chapter 3, similar charges of foreignness were used in ancient Greece to vilify religious practitioners (often women) who offered needy individuals access to the divine without regard to the civic cult and its officials. The same concern can be seen in the Bible, where criticism centers on the legitimacy of the practitioners (as judged by the religious ideology of the Yahwistic elites) rather than the efficacy of their practices.[7] Even the necromancy of 1 Samuel 28 is depicted as effective despite official censure. Such freelance practitioners were viewed as threatening by those who managed and benefited from the official cult, and it was in their circles that the books we know as the Jewish Scriptures were written and edited.

Many interpreters have assumed that these biblical prohibitions against "sorcery" would have precluded the use of magical healing techniques by Judeans who took their Scriptures seriously, but there is nothing in these texts to warrant such a conclusion. None of the relevant verses mention sickness or healing, and the Hebrew Bible contains a number of stories in which cures are effected by methods that most would describe as "magical." Examples include using mandrake plants as a treatment for infertility (Gen. 30:14-18); gazing on an otherwise idolatrous bronze statue of a snake to be healed from snakebite (Num. 21:4-9); and offering golden images of tumors to Yahweh along with sacrifices to end an outbreak of tumors (2 Sam. 6:4-18). Also relevant are several texts in which religious officials manipulate sacred objects to access divine power, including the *sotah* ritual in Num. 5:11-31; the transference of sins to a goat in Lev. 16:7-22; the divinatory use of the Urim and Thummim in Num. 27:18-23 and 1 Sam. 14:41 LXX (cf. 1 Sam. 28:6); and the casting of lots in Lev. 16:6-10, Josh. 18:3-10, 1 Chron. 24:31, 26:12-16, and Neh. 10:34.[8]

Notably absent from all of these passages is any divine or human criticism of acts that in other contexts might be judged as violations of biblical prohibitions. In fact, their positive outcomes could be taken to imply that Yahweh approves (or at least condones) such practices. Texts like these led Gideon Bohak, one of the leading experts on Jewish magic, to the conclusion that "there is no clear-cut biblical prohibition of magic or divination" in the Bible. What is prohibited, he says, is consorting with foreign practitioners.[9] Subsequent history shows that these and similar texts provided

---

[7] Gideon Bohak lays particular stress on this point ("The Use of Engraved Gems and Rings in Ancient Jewish Magic," in *Magical Gems in their Contexts*, ed. Kata Endreffy, Árpád M. Nagy, and Jeffrey Spier (Budapest: L'Erma di Bretschneider, 2019), 10–19, *Ancient Jewish Magic*, 13–27). Similar views can be seen in Yuval Harari, "Ancient Israel and Early Judaism," in *Guide to the Study of Ancient Magic*, ed. David Frankfurter (Leiden and Boston: Brill, 2019), 142–50, who notes also the absence of specific information about what the condemned people were doing.

[8] All but the last of these examples come from Gideon Bohak, *Ancient Jewish Magic*, 28–34. Bohak also notes the stories of the Israelites carrying the ark into battle in 1 Sam. 4:1-11 and Samson's hair in Judg. 16 (cf. 15:2-5), but these stories actually undermine his point since the purported cult magic fails in both cases.

[9] Ibid., 18.

"an extremely useful set of paradigms for postbiblical Jewish practitioners to choose from."[10]

In short, Judeans like Paul who looked to the Scriptures for guidance regarding the acceptability of using "magical" healing techniques would have found ambivalent views on the subject. As long as the practice did not involve direct appeals to foreign gods, there was no explicit prohibition on their use and several verses that could be cited in their favor. This observation will prove useful later in the chapter when we look at what Judeans actually did in this area.

Medical Healing in the Hebrew Bible

Medical healers are rarely mentioned in the Hebrew Bible, and virtually nothing is said about the home-based treatment regimens that form the first line of treatment in every society. These omissions can be credited to the nature of the text, which focuses on "religion" to the exclusion of many other aspects of daily life in ancient Israel. Gary Ferngren is surely correct when he observes that "it is inconceivable that at any time the Israelites lacked knowledge of the rudimentary treatment of wounds and uses of herbs for various ailments in which natural causality was evident" while also observing that "we have no evidence that any systematized therapeutics existed in early Israel."[11]

The few references to what we might call medical healing in the Hebrew Bible paint a mixed picture of its practitioners.[12] On the positive side, the work of two Hebrew midwives is commended in Exod. 1:15-21, as is that of the Egyptian physicians who embalmed Jacob in Gen. 50:2. The lament in Jer. 8:22 over the absence of a physician who could (metaphorically) heal Judah implies a positive view of physicians, as does the presumption that "balm of Gilead" is an effective remedy (cf. 46:11, 51:8). The efficacy of some type of healer also seems to be implied in 2 Kgs 8:29 and 9:15, where the king of Israel is said to have returned home for his wounds to be treated. On the negative side, Asa's use of physicians in 2 Chron. 16:11-12 is framed as a rejection of Yahweh as healer. The unreliability of medical treatment is presupposed in Job 13:4, where Job disparages his friends as "worthless physicians," while the limits of medicine are similarly acknowledged in Jer. 30:12-13 where a wound is described as "incurable."

Here and there the Hebrew Bible gives a few details about the activities of physicians. Where a venue for treatment is cited, it is invariably the home; nothing is said about any type of medical office or treatment center (1 Sam. 16:14-23, 19:11-16, 2 Sam. 12:15-20, 13:5-9, 2 Kgs 4:18-37, 20:1-7).[13] The use of unspecified medicines is mentioned in Prov. 17:22, Jer. 30:13 and Jer. 46:11, while Ezek. 47:12 refers specifically to healing leaves. Isa. 1:6 speaks metaphorically about treating wounds and sores by cleaning them and applying oil and bandages, and Ezek. 30:21 refers to binding and wrapping

---

[10] Ibid., 26. As we will see later, later Jewish debates centered on whether certain practices are too foreign, not whether they involve manipulation of suprahuman forces.
[11] *Medicine and Religion*, 29.
[12] The Hebrew word *raphaim*, generally translated as "physicians," comes from the Hebrew word meaning "to heal" and might therefore better be translated as "healers" in order to avoid importing modern ideas of a formal medical system into ancient Israel.
[13] Noted by Avalos, *Illness and Health Care in the Ancient Near East*, 251-2.

a broken arm. None of these texts says anything about who applies the treatment; all are simple enough to have been done by a family member as well as a physician. The only passages in which specialized skills are presupposed are 1 Sam. 16:14-23, where music is used to treat a chronic mental disturbance, and Leviticus 13-14, where priests are commissioned to diagnose skin diseases. Even here the remedies are not explicitly medical—the former treatment is done by someone who is not identified as a healer, while in the latter, the skill is limited to diagnosis; no cure is offered other than segregation from the community.[14]

In sum, the Hebrew Bible offers at best a vague and ambivalent endorsement of medical healing when it is provided by fellow Yahwists. Nothing is said about the acceptability of consulting providers from outside the community, nor is there any clear recognition of a class of medical experts whose cures are to be valued above those provided within the family. Judeans in Paul's day who were weighing the legitimacy of seeking treatment from a Greek or Roman physician would have found little guidance on the subject from their Scriptures.

Judeans and Religious Healing

By the turn of the era, Judeans in both the land of Israel and the Diaspora had been engaged for centuries in negotiating how much of polytheistic Greek and Roman culture they could accept and what should be avoided. Virtually every point on the ideological spectrum had its supporters, from conservatives who rejected all but those elements necessary for daily living to liberals and "apostates" who fully immersed themselves in Greek life and thought. Discerning a coherent view on any subject amid such diversity is a fool's errand, so the best that we can hope to do here is sketch the range of ideas and practices regarding sickness and healing that can be discerned in our sources.

Virtually all Jewish writings from the Second Temple era and beyond take for granted biblical teachings about the divine causation of at least some illnesses, the power of God to heal, and the value of prayer as a channel for obtaining healing. Opinion was more divided on matters of purity and impurity, so it is hard to assess how far people might have followed the biblical mandates of isolation for certain types of health problems, especially in the Diaspora.[15] Similar disagreements can be observed regarding the propriety of religious healing on the Sabbath, a question that is debated not only in the Gospels but also in the Mishnah and Talmud.[16] Variety is also evident in

---

[14] The author known as Pseudo-Philo expands on the biblical story by depicting David as an exorcist who sings an exorcistic psalm (for which the author supplies lyrics) to drive the evil spirit away from Saul (60.1-3).

[15] Several of the healing stories in the New Testament show people whom the Torah would have placed under this mandate (various lepers, the woman with the bloody discharge) approaching Jesus along with the crowds. As for Judeans in the Diaspora, it is hard to imagine how such isolation would have worked in a Greek or Roman city or who would have enforced it.

[16] Later Jewish texts portray the synagogue as a site where health care services are provided, a practice that would have made them look rather like Asklepian healing centers in the eyes of outsiders.

Jewish beliefs regarding the possibility of miraculous healings, with some seeing them as a viable possibility and others (perhaps the majority) relegating them to the past.[17]

In general, however, Judeans seem to have hewed fairly closely to biblical teachings on the value of religious healing during the Second Temple era. But the hegemony of religious approaches was facing increasing challenges from the growing popularity of magical and medical modes of healing. The tension is apparent in a text like Sir. 38:1-15, which affirms the utility of physicians (as long as they are faithful Jews, v. 14) as channels of God's healing power while insisting that prayer, confession, and sacrifice should be the first line of treatment.

> [9] My child, when you are ill, do not delay,
>   but pray to the Lord, and he will heal you.
> [10] Give up your faults and direct your hands rightly,
>   and cleanse your heart from all sin.
> [11] Offer a sweet-smelling sacrifice, and a memorial portion of choice flour,
>   and pour oil on your offering, as much as you can afford.
> [12] Then give the physician his place, for the Lord created him;
>   do not let him leave you, for you need him.
> [13] There may come a time when recovery lies in the hands of physicians,
> [14] for they too pray to the Lord
> that he grant them success in diagnosis
>   and in healing, for the sake of preserving life.

Similar preferences for religious healing can be seen in other Judean texts. According to *Ep. Arist.* 232-3, "freedom from sorrow" and protection from "death, disease, pain, and suchlike" come from prayer and righteous behavior.[18] In *T. Job* 38:7-8, when Job's friends offer to bring their physicians to treat his ailments, he rebuffs them with the assertion, "My healing and my treatment are from the Lord, who also created the physicians." According to *1 En.* 40:9, God has given the angel Raphael authority "over all disease and every wound." Nothing is said about how humans can avail themselves of this healing power, but the depiction of Raphael as one of four angels who are incessantly "interceding and praying on behalf of those who dwell upon the earth" and "expelling the demons and forbidding them from coming to the Lord" suggests that healing is an act of divine mercy that lies beyond human control. This reading is reinforced by the author's claim in *1 En.* 7:2 and 8:3 that medical and magical forms of healing were revealed to humans by fallen angels (to be discussed later). It is hard to imagine a stronger endorsement of religious healing over competing practices.[19]

But whether that was true in Paul's day (or in the Diaspora) is unclear. For references, see Bohak, *Ancient Jewish Magic*, 314–15; Twelftree, *Paul and the Miraculous*, 52–3.

[17] On the latter point, see Twelftree, *Paul and the Miraculous*, 35–60.

[18] Translation by J. H. Schutt in *The Old Testament Pseudepigrapha*, ed. James H. Charlesworth (2 vols; Garden City, NJ: Doubleday, 1983–85).

[19] A different picture of Raphael can be seen in Tobit, where the angel reveals to Tobit's son, Tobias, a substance that can be applied to Tobit's eyes to heal his blindness. In this case Raphael is sent by God in response to human petitions (3:16-17), not as a free act of mercy, and the cure is effected through a normal human healing technique, albeit under the guidance of the angel.

One question that is not often raised in discussions of religious healing is whether Judeans in Paul's day might have used healing practices that were directly or indirectly associated with non-Judean deities. Such activities would appear to be precluded by the frequent injunctions in the Jewish Scriptures against worshipping other gods and the judgments that Yahweh is said to have inflicted upon the people of Israel when they ignored these prohibitions. But there is ample evidence in the historical record that Judeans disagreed about the meaning and implication of these strictures, and some (those whom their traditionalist peers classed as "apostates") actively ignored them.

Examples abound. According to 1 Macc. 1:43, during the time of Antiochus IV, "many Israelites delighted in his [the king's] religion; they sacrificed to idols and profaned the sabbath." The author seems to have in mind here a group of Judeans who voluntarily chose to participate in the cult of Greek gods as opposed to those who submitted in order to save their lives. Josephus's account of this era ascribes such behaviors specifically to Menelaus and the sons of Tobias, whom he says "wanted to leave behind their ancestral laws and polity and follow those of the king and the Greeks" (*Ant.* 12.240). To this end, they surgically hid their circumcision and "abandoned all of the other ancestral customs and imitated the practices of the other nations" (*Ant.* 12:241). The accuracy of this characterization can be challenged: did these people indeed renounce their ancestral traditions and identity as Josephus suggests, or did they incorporate elements of Greek practice into their lives while remaining devoted to Israel's god in their own minds? However we answer the question, it is hard to imagine how anyone who embraced Greek customs could have avoided visiting Greek temples and participating at least passively in the cultic worship of Greek gods.

From a later era, we know that Herod the Great paid for the construction of several temples for Greek and Roman gods (including the divinized Augustus) both in Israel and in other lands, and he surely would have been present when the ones in Israel were formally dedicated with prayers and sacrifices to the resident deity. Whether he participated in the rituals or simply watched is unknown. But it is hard to see how he could have served Roman interests in Caesarea, his usual place of residence, without visiting the temple of Roma and Augustus during public rituals, especially when Roman officials from other parts of the Empire were in town. Herod's sons and family would have faced similar pressures to compromise, a fact that lends credence to Josephus's claim in *Ant.* 18.141 that a branch of his descendants "abandoned the observances of their Judean homeland and aligned themselves with the customs of the Greeks." Yet another Judean whose duties would have required him to be present for Roman rites was Philo's nephew Tiberius Julius Alexander, who served as procurator of Judea from 44 to 46 CE and as prefect of Egypt from 66 to 69 CE. According to Josephus, he "did not continue in the ancestral customs" in the same manner as his father (*Ant.* 20.100). The meaning of this statement is disputed, but there is nothing to indicate that he abandoned Judaism altogether as is often supposed.[20]

---

[20] For more on these and others who engaged in "high assimilation" to Greek and Roman culture, see John M. G. Barclay, *Jews in the Mediterranean Diaspora from Alexander to Trajan (323 BCE-117CE)* (Berkeley: University of California Press, 1996), 103–12.

All of these examples (with the partial exception of the last one) come from the land of Israel, where Greek and Roman cultic activities were limited, and involve members of the elite class, who were likely the only Judeans in that region who would have felt pressured to participate in "pagan" rituals. In the Diaspora, by contrast, every Judean faced such challenges on a daily basis. The only way to avoid being present at cultic activities honoring the patron deities of a Greek or Roman city was to avoid all public gatherings and entertainments since prayers and sacrifices were offered routinely at such events. Some Judeans did just that, giving rise to charges that their people were misanthropic.[21] But many others did not: inscriptional evidence shows that they attended theater performances so regularly that seats were reserved for them, and literary evidence indicates that they were present at other public gatherings where cultic worship took place. Paula Fredriksen describes the situation well: "Every time we encounter a Jewish ephebe, a Jewish town councilor, a Jewish soldier or a Jewish actor or a Jewish athlete, we find a Jew identified as a Jew who obviously spent part of his working day demonstrating courtesy to gods not his."[22]

But was their participation only passive? Or did some go farther and seek treatment from healers who were associated with Greek or Roman deities? Might they, for instance, have visited an Asklepian healing center for treatment or consulted a Greek "magician" for ritual purification or exorcism? If they did, would they have participated in cultic rituals as part of their cure, or did they accept only "secular" remedies? We might suppose that only Judeans who had renounced their ancestral traditions and become "apostates" would resort to such methods, but the record shows otherwise. As we will see later, there is ample evidence that Judeans who were loyal to their religion employed "magical" healing techniques that originated in polytheistic religion, and it is only a short step from there to seeking treatment from a Greek or Roman religious healer, especially if one was convinced that it was the god of Israel and not a Greek or Roman deity who made the cures effective.[23] One need not believe in the divinity of Asklepios to benefit from the treatments that were available at an Asklepian healing center, including medical interpretations of dreams.

A few tantalizing pieces of evidence suggest that at least some Judeans did in fact visit Greek or Roman temples and engage with the resident deity despite the apparent conflict between such behaviors and the injunctions of the Jewish Scriptures. Most

---

[21] Numerous examples of such charges from both Greek and Roman authors can be found in Menachem Stern, ed., *Greek and Latin Authors on Jews and Judaism*, 3 vols (Jerusalem: Israel Academy of Sciences and Humanities, 1974–1984), and Louis H. Feldman, *Jew and Gentile in the Ancient World: Attitudes and Interactions from Alexander to Justinian* (Princeton: Princeton University Press, 1993).

[22] "How Later Contexts Affect Pauline Content, or: Retrospect Is the Mother of Anachronism," in *Jews and Christians in the First and Second Centuries: How to Write Their History*, ed. Peter J. Tomson and Joshua Schwartz (Leiden: Brill, 2014), 21.

[23] In the Babylonian Talmud ('Abod. Zar. 55a), a sage named Zunin approaches R. Akiva seeking an explanation for the apparently well-known fact that people would enter a pagan shrine (of Asklepios?) crippled and come out cured. Akiva does not deny the reality of the healings, but rather answers with a parable that essentially credits the healings to Israel's god—the person just happened to go to an idol's temple at the moment when God had preordained that the sickness would end. The question of whether a Judean might legitimately visit such a temple for healing does not come up, but the implicit point of the parable is to deny any efficacy to such visits.

interesting is a third century BCE inscription from a temple in Greece that was commissioned by "Moschos, son of Moschion the Jew [or 'Judean'] at the command of the god Amphiaraos and the goddess Health [i.e., Hygieia], having seen a dream in which Amphiaraos and Health commanded him to write it on stone and set it up by the altar."[24] Amphiaraos was a Greek hero who was associated with healing, while Hygieia was Asklepios's daughter. Here we have a clear example of a Judean not only erecting a votive stele in a Greek temple but doing so at the behest of two Greek healing deities, most likely after sleeping at the temple.

From around the same time we have three graffiti inscribed by self-identified Judeans in the precincts of an Egyptian sanctuary at El-Kanaïs that was dedicated jointly to the Greek god Pan and his Egyptian counterpart Min.[25] In two of the three, either "God" or "the god" is "blessed" or "praised." All three were carved into a stone facing intermingled with other graffiti honoring Pan or Min, so it would be natural to conclude that these Judeans were honoring the local god just as other travelers did in the ancient world. We cannot be certain of their intent, but the graffiti do show us Judeans who felt comfortable both visiting and carving inscriptions in the vicinity of a pagan temple. One of them even mentions that it was his third visit.

Equally interesting is a second century BCE inscription from Iasos in southwestern Asia Minor that honors a man named Niketas of Jerusalem, son of Jason, for donating 100 drachmas to support a local festival for Dionysus.[26] The reference to Jerusalem is proof of his Judean origins, while the designation of him as a metic (μέτοικος) signifies that he was a local resident and not a visitor. The inscription does not prove that he took part in the festival or its cult, but it does show that his support was conscious and not merely accidental.[27] Less clear are two Jewish epitaphs from the second and third centuries CE that include the standard pagan abbreviation "D.M.," ("dis manibus"), which refers to the Manes, Roman spirits of the dead.[28] The expression is formulaic, but it is still noteworthy that these two families saw no problem with using Roman religious formulae on the tombstone of a Judean.

Two final examples relate to the manumission of slaves. One, an inscription from Delphi that dates to the second or first century BCE, shows a person named Ioudaios freeing a slave at the temple of Apollo using the common fiction of selling the slave

---

[24] The inscription, published in 1952, was first highlighted in 1955 by D. M. Lewis in his article "The First Greek Jew," *Journal of Semitic Studies* 2 (1957): 264–6. The inscription appears on a stele erected to commemorate Moschos's liberation of a slave, so it does not relate directly to healing.

[25] The graffiti are analyzed by Karen Stern in her recent book, *Writing on the Wall: Graffiti and the Forgotten Jews of Antiquity* (Princeton and Oxford: Princeton University Press, 2018), 60–6.

[26] I owe this reference to Paula Fredriksen, "Judaizing the Nations," *NTS* 26 (2010): 237, n. 11. The text of the inscription can be found online at http://www.attalus.org/docs/other/inscr_136.html.

[27] The decision by a Judean to honor Dionysus might not be a as strange as it looks. Irina Levinskaya, observing that Plutarch identified the Jewish god with Dionysus in *Quaest. conv.* 4.6.1-2 and Tacitus refuted the association in *Hist.* 5.5.5, suggests that the identification of the two might have been widespread (*Book of Acts*, 100, n. 103). If this is true, Niketas might have justified his donation to a festival for Dionysus as a veiled way of honoring the god of Israel.

[28] Noted by Erich S. Gruen, "Diaspora and the 'Assimilated' Jew," in *Early Judaism: New Insights and Scholarship*, ed. Frederick E. Greenspahn (New York: New York University Press, 2018), 63.

to the deity.²⁹ The fact that the manumission takes place in a Greek temple under the auspices of a Greek god is remarkable. The second example is a first-century CE manumission inscription from the Bosporus region of Asia Minor that begins by acclaiming "the Most High God, Almighty, blessed," and ends with the phrase, "under Zeus, Ge, Helios."³⁰ The fact that the freed slave is dedicated to "the prayer house" suggests that the dedicator, Pothos, was a member of the local Judean community, though he could also have been a God-fearer. On its face, the inscription recognizes the authority of the Greek gods Zeus, Ge, and Helios as protectors of the freed slave, though it has been suggested that the author was following a standard formula used in Greek manumissions.³¹ Its absence from other Judean manumission texts from the region, however, casts doubt on this explanation.

None of this proves that Judeans in the Diaspora made a practice of approaching Greek or Roman gods for healing, but it does suggest that we should not summarily omit this possibility from a discussion of ancient Jewish approaches to healing. Contrary to modern opinion, Jewish monotheism in Paul's day did not invariably preclude the existence or power of other gods. Paula Fredriksen lists a number of ways in which Judeans around the turn of the era (including Paul) integrated the gods of other nations into their belief system while reserving supremacy for the god of their ancestors.³² Philo's commentary on Genesis (7:27) depicts them as celestial bodies operating under the authority of the God of Israel, while some of the LXX translators refer to them as *daimones*, by which they mean divine beings inferior to the God of Israel. The book of Jubilees describes them as evil spirits who lead the nations astray, while apocalyptic authors paint them as dark enemies of the almighty God and his followers who at the proper time will be overcome and compelled to bow their knees to the God of Israel.

In short, foreign deities had power, but it was nothing compared with the might of the creator of the universe. They were capable of helping or (more often) harming humans, but it was futile to placate them with prayers and offerings since human affairs lay under the ultimate control of the sovereign deity. To worship such beings was to dishonor the one divine being who deserved to be reverenced and thus to court divine wrath.

The apostle Paul's ambivalence in 1 Corinthians 8 and 10 about the nature and existence of other gods—are there many of them (8:5) or none (8:4), or are they *daimones* and not true gods (10:20)?—would have been entirely at home in this Judean ideological environment. In fact, he had probably heard all of these arguments from other Judeans prior to becoming a Christ-follower. What matters for our purposes is that a Judean who wished to consult a Greek or Roman religious healer or visit an

---

²⁹ Ibid., "Diaspora and the 'Assimilated' Jew," 63–4. Gruen cites the location of the inscription as *Inscriptiones Judaicae Orientis* I, Ach 44.
³⁰ To view the Greek text and English translation, see Irina Levinskaya, *The Book of Acts in Its Diaspora Setting* (Grand Rapids, MI: Eerdmans, 1996), 239–40. The inscription is discussed in pp. 105–16.
³¹ Ibid., 240; E. Leigh Gibson, *The Jewish Manumission Inscriptions of the Bosporus Kingdom* (Tübingen: Mohr Siebeck, 1999), 109–23.
³² Summarized from "How Later Contexts," 21–2, 25–6; "Judaizing the Nations," 240–1; and "How Jewish Is God? Divine Ethnicity in Paul's Theology," *JBL* 137 (2018): 196, 200–3.

Asklepian treatment center could have found Judeans who would approve or at least condone such actions even if others condemned them. Where the dividing line should be drawn between appropriate and inappropriate engagement with the cults of non-Judean deities was a matter for debate in the time of Paul.

Judeans and "Magical" Healing

References to Judeans practicing μαγεία appear relatively often in Greek and Roman literature.[33] The earliest reference comes from the Syrian polymath Posidonius (second century BCE), who describes Judeans as "addicted to magic" and reports that they used incantations to make the asphalt of the Dead Sea coalesce for cutting.[34] Several decades later, Strabo tells his readers that Moses, whom he describes as an Egyptian priest, promoted the practice of temple incubation: "Those who made fortunate dreams were to be permitted to sleep in the temple, where they might dream both for themselves and others" in hopes of receiving "some gift or sign from the God" (*Geog.* 16.2.35). Pliny the Elder (first century CE), as part of his history of magic, claims that Judeans possessed their own magical traditions distinct from those of the Magi. The reference is brief and cryptic, stating only that there is "another branch of magic [*magicē*], derived from Moses, Jannes, Lotapes, and the Jews" (*HN* 30.11).[35]

The idea of Judeans as experts in μαγεία is also found in later writers. According to Origen, the philosopher Celsus (second century CE) claimed that all Judeans, not just one branch, were descended from "magicians and deceivers" (γοήτων καὶ πλάνων). Origen's response, which he apparently intended as a denial, actually strengthens the force of Celsus's charge as he relates how Judeans use the names of Abraham, Isaac, and Jacob in conjunction with that of their God to perform exorcisms, incantations, and magical rites (*Cels.* 4.33).[36] The satirist Lucian of Samosata, writing around the same time as Celsus, paints a similar picture, listing "the spells of Jews" as one of several deceptive remedies that people suffering from gout might pursue in their desperation to be cured (*Pod.* 173). He also relates in some detail the story of a "Syrian from Palestine" (most likely a Judean) restoring a man to health by casting out the demon that was causing his sickness (*Philops.* 16). Even John Chrysostom (third century CE), a rabid opponent of Judaism, grudgingly admits the efficacy of Judean magic as he struggles to convince his Christian audience to stop consulting Judean healers who use incantations, amulets, charms, and spells to cure the sick (*Adv. Jud.* 8.5.6; cf. 8.6.11).

---

[33] The following references are taken from Dickie, *Magic and Magicians in the Greco-Roman World*, 223–5; Janowitz, *Magic in the Roman World*, 25; and Graf, *Magic in the Ancient World*, 6–8.

[34] Posidonius's views are known only from references by other authors; this report comes from the first-century BCE geographer Strabo (*Geog.* 16.2.43).

[35] Fritz Graf points also to Acts 7:22 ("Moses was educated in all the wisdom of the Egyptians and was powerful in speech and action") as a possible allusion to ancient views of Moses as a magician (*Magic in the Ancient World*, 6–7).

[36] Whether Origen intended to include Judeans among those who used these names to perform magic is not entirely clear since he mentions also that "treatises on magic in many countries" acknowledge the power of these names.

The intensity of his rhetoric suggests that these healers were popular in Christian circles.

The idea that ancient Judeans would gain a reputation as "magical" healers is surprising on its face since the Hebrew Bible prohibits "sorcery" and similar activities. But as we saw earlier, none of these prohibitions speaks explicitly about sickness or healing, and the Bible contains a number of stories in which people use healing practices that could be described as "magical" and receive no criticism from either the narrator or the deity. Whether these stories were ever cited in Paul's day to justify questionable healing techniques is unclear, but later sources show rabbis debating the permissibility of various healing techniques and quoting Scripture in support of their arguments.

Both Second Temple and rabbinic literature offer conflicting opinions about "magical" activities in general and magical healing in particular. As in ancient Greece and Rome, elite authors are generally more critical than the masses, where practices that might be classified as μαγεία were deeply embedded in traditional modes of healing. Opinion also changed over time among the elites, with negative views being more common in earlier texts and critical acceptance dominating later texts. The change coincides with shifting attitudes toward Greek and Roman culture more generally: earlier authors tend to amalgamate "magic" with other foreign practices that should be rejected as threats to the social and ideological power of the Judean elites while later texts reflect the elites' acquiescence in all but the most offensive Greek and Roman practices. The starkness of the shift can be seen in texts like b. Sanh. 17a and b. Menaḥ. 65a, which claim that Rabbi Yoḥanan required all candidates for membership in the Sanhedrin to be "masters of sorcery" (בעלי כשפים).[37]

The fact that elite authors were debating the propriety of Judeans engaging in "magical" practices implies that at least some Judeans in Greco-Roman antiquity were using "magic" in their daily lives since otherwise there would have been no cause for debate. Evidence for the use of such practices runs wide and deep in Judean literature. Our review of this material will begin with an overview of texts from the Second Temple period that reveal the competing elite attitudes on the subject, then turn to material that shows what Judeans were actually doing.

Second Temple Sources[38]

Perhaps the earliest literary example of magical healing appears in the book of Tobit, where an angel reveals to the hero, a Torah-observant Judean, a miraculous cure for cataract blindness that involves catching a giant fish that leaps from the water to eat him,

---

[37] Noted by Gideon Bohak, "Prolegomena to the Study of the Jewish Magical Tradition," *CurBR* 9 (2009): 120, who observes that such knowledge was needed "not only in order to detect and deter magicians, but also in order to beat them at their own game, and to gain the upper hand against other offenders as well." The Hebrew word translated here as "sorcery" is the same one that appears in Exod. 22:18 and Deut. 18:10 where the practice is condemned.

[38] Not all of the materials treated in this section were actually written in the pre-70 era, but they are included here because their contents are more like those of the earlier period than the rabbinic materials.

cutting it open, and applying bile from its gall bladder to the eyes of his afflicted father. The application of a healing substance to the eyes is a common medical treatment, but the strange account of what caused the cataracts (sparrow droppings falling into Tobit's eyes) and the note in 4:10 that physicians had been unable to cure Tobit weigh against a medical reading of the text, while the presence of a death-dealing demon in another part of the narrative situates the story squarely in a "magical" milieu. The successful cure is prescribed by an angel, so it clearly has the divine imprimatur. The setting of the story among ordinary people could be taken as a sign that the elite author is aware that "magical" ideas and practices were common among the masses.

The book of Jubilees traces human knowledge of the healing arts to the days before the Flood, when one of the "angels of the presence" taught them to Noah so that he and his descendants could use them to counteract the deceptions and diseases by which evil demons would seek to turn them away from God (10:10-12).[39] The author seems to imply a personal familiarity with written collections of exorcistic healing formulae when he states that "Noah wrote down in a book everything (just) as we had taught him regarding all the kinds of medicine, and the evil spirits were precluded from pursuing Noah's children" (10:13). Later we read how prince Mastema, the leader of the demons, empowers Pharaoh's magicians to imitate Moses's miracles but is unable to give them the ability to heal (48:9-11). Implicit in this story is a claim that all successful healing comes from God, regardless of the method used, since demons can only inflict illness, not cure it. The references to demons in both stories situate the author's understanding of sickness and healing squarely within the "magical" realm.[40]

Writing some two centuries later, the author of book 1 of the Sibylline Oracles credits the first generation of humans after the Flood with discovering the arts of bird-divination, drug-cures (φαρμακίη), and magic (μαγικὴ), which the author classes together with other useful skills like plowing, carpentry, sailing, and astronomy (1:85-93). The description of the discoverers as "the most righteous of the ones who were left" (1:88) underlines the positive regard with which the author viewed these arts.

Josephus also paints a generally positive picture of μαγεία, especially in his account of Solomon, which stands in a long tradition of depicting the king as an expert in esoteric practices.[41] Most relevant for our purposes are his claims that Solomon composed incantations for alleviating sickness and that he knew and transmitted to others the art of expelling demons to cure diseases (*Ant.* 8.2.45). The use of incantations is explicitly forbidden in the LXX renderings of several Torah texts (Lev. 19:31, 20:6, 20:27, Deut. 18:11), but as Phillip Jewell has observed, Josephus conveniently omits any mention of these or any other texts relating to "sorcery" when summarizing the Jewish laws in *Antiquities*.[42] The fact that he credits such actions to Solomon suggests that the

---

[39] The angels described here are clearly good ("all the angels of the presence and all the angels of holiness," 2:18), not the fallen angels of 1 Enoch 7 that will be discussed later. This and the following translation are taken from James C. VanderKam, *The Book of Jubilees* (Louvain: Peeters, 1989).

[40] As we saw in Chapter 3, the idea of demonic causation plays virtually no role in Greek or Roman medical texts.

[41] For a brief summary of this tradition, see Dennis C. Duling, "The Eleazar Miracle and Solomon's Magical Wisdom in Flavius Josephus's 'Antiquitates Judaicae' 8.42–9," *HTR* 78 (1985): 14–17.

[42] "Flavius Josephus' Terminology of Magic: Accommodating Jewish Magic to a Roman Audience," *Journal for the Academic Study of Magic* 5 (2009): 28.

omission of these laws is not accidental but reflects Josephus's own discomfort with blanket condemnations of "magical" practices.

Even more surprising are Josephus's positive comments about the "witch of Endor," whom he cites as an example for others to follow in *Ant.* 6.14.4. Following a summary of 1 Samuel 28 in which he hews fairly closely to the biblical story line, Josephus offers the following encomium on the woman's behavior.

> It is right to commend the woman for her generosity, for though the king had forbidden the use of the art which had bettered her situation and though she had never seen him before, she did not hold it against him to have condemned her sort of skill or refuse him as a stranger with whom she was not acquainted, but gave him sympathy and comfort and urged him to do what he felt disinclined to and despite her poverty readily and kindly offered him the one thing she had, with no prospect of being rewarded for her kindness or seeking anything from him in the future, as his life was ending.... It is well to imitate her example and to do good to all who are in want and to regard nothing as better than this, or more beneficial to mankind, for it renders God favorable and ready to grant us good things.[43]

While it is surprising to see a Judean commending as a model of righteous conduct the female practitioner of a magical art that the Bible explicitly condemns as "defiling" (Lev. 19:31, Deut. 18:11), it is even more remarkable to note the sympathetic language that Josephus uses to describe her profession ("the art which had bettered her situation"). Rather than condemning her, he appears to view the woman as the innocent victim of an unjust edict that prevented her from earning her living.[44]

A different picture emerges from several texts that voice negative opinions of "magic" in general and magical healing in particular. According to 1 Enoch, it was a group of fallen angels, not "angels of the presence," who taught humans the use of "magical medicine, incantations, the cutting of roots, and ... plants" (7:1).[45] These same angels are credited a few verses later with disseminating knowledge about incantations and astrology, both of which the author associates with deception (8:3). These and similar

---

[43] Translation by Patrick Rogers (2010–16) from the interlinear Greek-English text of Josephus's works posted online at http://www.biblical.ie/page.php?fl=josephus/Greek%20Texts. Josephus's positive view of the woman is highlighted by Jewell, "Flavius Josephus' Terminology of Magic," 29–30.

[44] Josephus's attitude toward "magic" is not entirely positive. In his account of Moses in the court of Pharaoh, he shows Moses drawing a sharp distinction between his own miracle-working power, which he credits to God, and the "magic arts and tricks" employed by Pharoah's priests (*Ant.* 2.13.3). He is also aware that μάγοι can be frauds, as in his account of how a Judean named Atomos pretended to be a μάγος at the instigation of the Roman procurator Felix in an effort to dupe Agrippa's sister Drusilla into leaving her husband and marrying Felix (*Ant.* 20.7.2; cf. 20.8.6). Elsewhere he speaks negatively about women who use their herbal skills to create love-potions and deadly poisons (*War* 1.29.2, 1.30.1, *Ant.* 15.4.1, 15.7.4, 17.4.1), echoing a fear that was common among both Greeks and Romans. But these scattered references, none of which involves healing, do not undermine the broadly positive view that we see elsewhere in Josephus's writings.

[45] Translated from Ethiopic by Ephraim Isaac in Charlesworth, *Old Testament Pseudepigrapha*, 1:5–89.

skills are described as "eternal secrets" that humans should never have possessed (9:6). Their revelation by the fallen angels is what eventually led God to send the Flood.

A negative view is also apparent in Ps.-Phoc. 149, which advises its readers to "make no potions, keep away from magical books."[46] The Greek word rendered here as "potions" (φάρμακα) can refer to either "medicines" or "poisons," but the call to avoid them suggests that the negative meaning is in view here.[47] More subtle is the decision by LXX translators to render the general biblical injunctions against "sorcery" and similar activities with terms referring to magical practices that were common across the Greek world (necromancy, divination, bird-augury, incantations, *pharmaka*, etc.).[48] Similar updating of the biblical text can be seen in 2 Baruch's account of the accession of Josiah, where the author tells how the king "destroyed and removed the magicians, enchanters, and diviners from the land" (66:2). Magical practices are mentioned in both the Hebrew and Greek accounts of king Manasseh's reign (2 Kgs 21:6/2 Chron. 33:6), but they are absent from the biblical story of Josiah's reform. Their insertion by the author of Baruch reflects a distinctly negative view of "magic."

A more nuanced example of negative opinion can be seen in Philo. Not all forms of magic are bad, in his view—there is a good type (ἀληθῆ μαγικήν), developed by the Persian Magi and studied by both kings and ordinary people, "by which the facts of nature are presented in a clearer light," and a bad type, "pursued by charlatan mendicants and parasites and the basest of the women and slave population," that involves purifications, enchantments, charms, and incantations (*Spec. Laws* 3.101).[49] The latter type is a counterfeit and perversion of the first type. Philo does not speak specifically about magical healing, but all of the practices that he categorizes as bad were used to treat sickness. Elsewhere he claims that Moses condemned all forms of divination ("haruspices, purificators, augurs, interpreters of prodigies, incantators, and those who put their faith in sounds and voices") because they rely on ambiguous and impious means of knowing the future rather than listening to and obeying God's prophets (*Spec. Laws* 1.59-65). These practices are less directly related to healing, but the passage reveals an even broader condemnation of popular magic than we might have gleaned from the previous text.[50]

In summary, elite Judean authors from the Second Temple era were divided over the propriety of engaging in "magic" and magical healing. The very existence of these divisions shows that at least some Judeans were using the practices under debate since

---

[46] Translation by P. W. van der Horst in Charlesworth, *Old Testament Pseudepigrapha*.
[47] Fear of poisons is one of the most cited reasons for avoiding "magic" in the Greco-Roman world. This is clearly what lies behind the injunction in the Hippocratic Oath against physicians giving their patients a φάρμακον.
[48] Noted by Bohak, *Ancient Jewish Magic*, 77.
[49] Noted by Harari, "Ancient Israel and Early Judaism," 155. Philo's comments on the biblical injunction against sorcery, by contrast, make no reference to magical practices but associate it only with mystic initiation rites (1.319-23) and poisoners (3.93-9). A fuller exposition of his favorable view of the Persian Magi can be found in *Prob.* 74, where he says that they "silently make research into the facts of nature to gain knowledge of the truth and through visions clearer than speech, give and receive the revelations of divine excellency."
[50] Philo's condemnations are not just theoretical interpretations of Torah texts but concrete applications of Mosaic principles. They imply that "magical" practices, including healing, were common enough in the Judean community to warrant censure and a warning to keep away from them.

otherwise there would have been no reason to speak of them. More direct evidence can be found in a range of texts that describe what Judeans were actually doing during this period.

A surprising amount of evidence regarding Judean practices can be found in the New Testament. A Judean μάγος named "bar Jesus" or "Elymas" appears briefly in Acts 13:6-12 as an opponent of Paul during his visit to Cyprus. Paul encounters him in the court of the Roman proconsul Sergius Paulus, but no reason is given for his presence there; he could have been a regular adviser to the ruler or a wandering μάγος who happened to be present when Paul arrived. The nature of his skills is also left unexplained, though Luke's vilification of him as a "false prophet" might suggest that he specialized in divination, a topic of special interest to Roman elites like the proconsul.[51]

Better known is the story of the μάγος Simon in Acts 8:9-25. Whether he should be classified as a Judean depends on what we mean by the term. In v. 9, Luke states that he was using unspecified acts of μαγεία to astonish the "ἔθνος of Samaria," a term that could refer to either the ancient Israelite capital (re-founded by Herod the Great in 30 BCE as a Roman city named Sebaste) or the region in which it appears. But Luke consistently uses "Samaria" to refer to a geographic territory (Acts 1:8, 8:1, 8:5, 8:9, 8:14, 9:31, 15:3), not a city, so the "ἔθνος of Samaria" must be Luke's designation for the people known elsewhere as "Samaritans." Samaritans were not actually "Judeans" in either the geographic or the religious sense, but they were similar enough to make Simon the μάγος appear as a broadly "Jewish" character and not as a "pagan."

A final example from Acts that might be useful here is Luke's story of a group of itinerant Judean exorcists (including the "seven sons of Sceva") in Acts 19:13-20. Luke does not describe their activities as μαγεία, but exorcism was a common form of magical healing, and their use of the "name" of Jesus in v. 14 recalls later magical texts in which divine names are recited in an effort to channel esoteric powers to serve the user's interests, including removing sickness. The story is preceded by an account of people being healed (linked explicitly here with the expulsion of demons) by the seemingly "magical" technique of laying cloths that had touched Paul's skin on the bodies of the sick (19:11-12) and followed by a report of people in Ephesus burning what appear to be "magical" books (19:19). This broader context suggests that the Judean exorcisms in 19:13-16 should also be viewed as "magical" acts.

Another reference to a Judean exorcist appears in Mk 9:38-40, where Jesus's disciples report to their master how they had silenced a Judean who was using his name to cast out demons. Their statement that he is "not one of us" and their efforts to stop him imply that he was not a Christ-follower, since Jesus had previously authorized his disciples to cast our demons (6:6-13). In his reply, Jesus confounds them by approving of Judeans who are not his followers engaging in exorcism. The opposite view can be seen in Mt. 7:22, where Jesus refuses to allow into his kingdom those who do "works of power" in his name, including prophesying and casting out demons, but do not obey him. In the Matthean literary context, these are clearly Judeans.

---

[51] The fact that he was cursed with blindness in v. 11 could be taken as an ironic judgment on either a healer or a "seer."

In neither of these stories does Jesus contest the ability of Judeans to perform such acts of power. Instead, he acknowledges their validity while insisting that such skills do not automatically mark one as a citizen of God's kingdom. This approach parallels the way the Gospel Pharisees view Jesus: they admit the efficacy of his healings and exorcisms but refuse to recognize them as evidence that he has been sent by God (Mt. 9:34, 12:24). Together these texts suggest that methods of drawing on suprahuman powers to cure sickness and expel demons were known and practiced by at least some Judeans in the first century CE even as their meaning was contested.

Similar activities are described in Judean texts from the era. Josephus relates how he witnessed the magical power of Solomon at work when a Judean named Eleazar drew out a demon through a man's nostrils by holding below his nose an amuletic ring containing a special root prescribed by Solomon and commanding the demon to leave in the name of Solomon while reciting incantations that Solomon had composed (*Ant.* 8.2.46-47). The attribution of a specific root-cure to Solomon suggests that Eleazar was familiar with a book of "Solomonic" magical cures that was known and used by at least some Judeans around the time of Paul.[52] Josephus clearly accepts the validity of Eleazar's action since he cites it as a proof of Solomon's greatness (8.2.49).

Another mode of exorcistic healing appears in Josephus's account in *War* 7.6.3 of a desert plant called *baaras* that drives away illness-causing demons when brought into their presence. No rituals are needed to make it effective; the healing power resides in the plant. In fact, the plant is so powerful that it resists being dug unless it is first doused with the urine or menstrual blood of a woman or else someone digs a trench around it and ties a dog to it so that the animal can pull it out, at which point the dog dies.[53] Expelling demons as a method of curing sickness was also practiced in the Dead Sea community, where several fragmentary psalms appear to have been written for that purpose.[54] Prayer also played a role in exorcistic healing, as we see in the story from the Genesis Apocryphon (col. 20) where Abraham prays to God to drive out the "pestilential spirit" that had afflicted the Egyptian Pharaoh and his household when Abraham asked God to protect Sarah from being violated by him.

A broader approach to magical healing can be seen in Josephus's description of the Essenes in *War.* 2.8.7, where the "magical" quality of their studies is routinely toned down in English translations. A more culturally sensitive rendering would describe the Essenes as being "extraordinarily devoted to the treatises of the ancients, selecting especially those sections that benefit soul and body, to which end they investigate how to cure sufferings by means of roots, apotropaic substances [amulets?], and the

---

[52] Josephus claims that the event was witnessed by Vespasian and his soldiers while they were engaged in putting down the Jewish revolt, which would place it in the late 60s CE.

[53] The fact that the latter prescription has parallels in Greek pharmacological texts does not take away from the fact that it is approved here as a Judean cure.

[54] The phenomenon is discussed in two articles in *Demons and Illness from Antiquity to the Early-Modern Period*, ed. Siam Bhayro and Catherine Rider (Leiden: Brill, 2017). The first is by Ida Fröhlich, "Demons and Illness in Second Temple Judaism: Theory and Practice" (81–96); the second is by David Hamidović, "Illness and Healing through Spell and Incantation in the Dead Sea Scrolls" (97–110).

properties of stones." In short, Josephus claims that the Essenes studied ancient books in order to learn and develop recipes for magical healing.[55]

The reference to "apotropaic substances" in the passage just cited highlights the importance of amulets as a means of curing or warding off sickness and demons in the Second Temple era. In fact, the wearing of amulets goes back much earlier in Judean history, as evidenced by the discovery in 1979 of two silver amulets from the sixth-century BCE containing a version of the priestly benediction in Num. 6:24-26. The next oldest samples come from the early Roman era.[56] The archaeological evidence for written Judean amulets is extensive for the post-70 era, with most consisting of narrow strips of metal inscribed on one side and rolled up or folded so that they could be attached with a cord to the affected body part.[57] But these are only the tip of the proverbial iceberg since, as we saw in Chapter 3, non-textual amulets were far more common than written ones in all parts of the Greco-Roman world. Identifying such items in the archaeological record, however, is difficult because of their unmarked status and their often perishable nature.

Discerning which amulets were used by Judeans is even more challenging. Only in rare cases have scholars been able to positively identify an unmarked amulet as Judean, as in the case of a child's shirt found in the Cave of Letters in the Judean wilderness that contained pouches filled with items like shells, seeds, salt crystals, and other unidentified materials.[58] Amuletic jewelry (rings, pendants, etc.) sometimes contains carved images or other markings that reveal their "magical" function, but their use was limited primarily to the wealthy. Even the presence of Judean words (including divine names) and images on amulets is no sure marker of Judean provenance since magic in the Roman imperial era was highly cosmopolitan and non-Judeans often used materials derived from Judaism due to their perceived power.[59] Material evidence alone is therefore an uncertain indicator of the use of amulets by Judeans in the Roman world.[60]

The literary evidence is also rather sparse for the Second Temple period. According to 2 Macc. 12:40, some of the Judean soldiers who fell in one of the early battles against

---

[55] What Josephus meant by "treatises of the ancients" is never explained, but the presence of magical terminology in the passage suggests that he might have had in mind something like the written compendia of magical recipes that are mentioned by other ancient authors.

[56] See the discussion in Roy Kotansky, "Textual Amulets and Writing Traditions in the Ancient World," in Frankfurter, *Guide to the Study of Ancient Magic*, 535–6.

[57] Described in Martínez, "Magical Amulets User's Guide," 179–80. Martínez notes the similarity of these exemplars to amulets described in the *PGM*, where even non-Judean amulets are commonly called φυλακτήριον. See also Hanan Eshel and Rivka Leiman, "Jewish Amulets Written on Metal Scrolls," *JAncJud* 1 (2010): 189–99.

[58] Described by Gideon Bohak, "Jewish Exorcism Before and After the Destruction of the Second Temple," in *Was 70 CE a Watershed in Jewish History? On Jews and Judaism before and after the Destruction of the Second Temple*, ed. Daniel R. Schwartz and Zeev Weiss (Leiden: Brill, 2012), 282.

[59] The Greek magical papyri contain many examples of "pagan" amulets and incantations that include divine names and symbols derived from Judaism. The difficulty of determining which ones might have been produced or used by Judeans makes them unreliable as sources for "Jewish magic." That fact and their generally late date (third to fourth centuries CE) explain why they are not cited as evidence in this chapter.

[60] Gideon Bohak has been especially assiduous in developing criteria for identifying Judean amulets and assessing particular exemplars: see *Ancient Jewish Magic*, 115–22.

the Greeks were wearing "sacred tokens (ἱερώματα) of the idols of Jamnia, which the law forbids the Jews to wear."[61] While the author attributes the men's deaths to this forbidden practice, the text reveals that at least some Judeans in second century BCE Palestine trusted in "pagan" amulets to protect them from harm. The Testament of Job, written around the turn of the era, tells how God gave Job three multicolored cords to tie around his waist, at which point "the worms disappeared from my body and the plagues, too" (47:4-8). The story goes on to relate how Job at the end of his life gave one of these cords to each of his three daughters so that by wearing them "it may go well with you all the days of your life" (46:9). The Greek word used in 47:11 to describe these cords (φυλακτήριον) shows that the author meant for them to be understood as amulets of healing and protection provided by God.[62]

While it is possible to read the limited Second Temple material as a sign that amulets gained currency among Judeans only in the post-70 era, most scholars view such a conclusion as erroneous in view of the difficulty of identifying amulets in the archaeological record and the limited nature of pre-70 Judean writings. The fact that the Mishnah treats the wearing of amulets as a common and unremarkable practice also suggests that their use in Palestine goes back much farther than the rabbinic era.[63] This is even more likely for the Diaspora: the absence of criticisms or warnings against such a universal practice suggests that Judeans outside of Palestine saw no difficulty with the use of amulets. It is possible that they drew the line at wearing amulets containing images of pagan deities, but even here clear evidence is lacking.[64]

Rabbinic Sources

By the rabbinic era (third to sixth centuries CE), the evidence for Judeans engaging in "magical" practices is abundant for both Palestine and the Diaspora. "Sorcery" continues to evoke condemnation from the rabbis (m. Sanh. 7:4, 7:7, 7:11, 10:1, m. Šhab. 6:10, etc.), but most of the practices over which Judeans had been divided in earlier times were now broadly accepted even by scholars. The list of "mighty acts" that rabbis are said to have performed is extensive and thoroughly "magical":

> Rabbis are presented in rabbinic literature as able to cause harm through a curse, slay by words or by a look, send a snake for whose bite there is no cure, make rain or adjust its strength, control the sea, fill a field with cucumbers and gather them through speech, fill a valley with dinars of gold by means of words, kill a snake by merely touching it, raise up dead bodies from the ground, revive the dead, cope with demons, overcome practitioners of *keshafim*, and a great deal more.[65]

---

[61] Discussed in Bohak, *Ancient Jewish Magic*, 119–20.
[62] Φυλακτήριον is a common word for amulets in Greek literature. There is nothing in the passage to suggest that these cords were "phylacteries" such as Judeans used when praying.
[63] More will be said on this subject later.
[64] The story cited earlier from 2 Macc. 12:40 suggests that this was the view in Judea, but we cannot presume from this text that the same was true in the Diaspora.
[65] Harari, "Ancient Israel and Early Judaism," 158–9; sources cited in 159, n. 50.

Even so, questions continued to be raised about certain practices that appeared overly foreign, particularly those that resembled the worship of pagan deities. The rabbinic term for these practices is "Ways of the Amorites," a reference to texts such as Exod. 34:10-16 and Deut. 7:1-6 where God warns the Israelites against engaging too closely with the Canaanites or their gods. The question of what acts qualified for inclusion under this heading was an ongoing (though not overly frequent) topic of debate.[66]

Several criteria are cited by different rabbis for distinguishing between permissible and forbidden types of magic. The most important for our purposes relates to the purpose of the act, as several rabbinic texts cite healing as an acceptable reason for performing otherwise questionable rituals. The prevailing view is summarized in b. Šab. 67a: "Whatever is used as a remedy [רְפוּאָה] is not forbidden on account of the ways of the Amorite."[67] The Mishnaic lemma for this comment (m. Šab 6:10) is an opinion by Rabbi Meir that reads, "One may go out [on the Sabbath] with the egg of a locust or with the tooth of a fox or with a nail from a stake as means of a cure." This rather cryptic ruling was initially rejected by "the Sages" out of a concern to guard the sanctity of the Sabbath, but it was eventually endorsed in the Talmud on the grounds that all of these items are useful as amulets to ward off or cure various ailments (earache, sleep problems, and inflammation, respectively). The same remedies are mentioned by Pliny the Elder, so they clearly originated as "pagan" customs.[68] The change of opinion is remarkable: a set of pagan healing practices has become so essential that they are permitted as exceptions to the prohibition against working on the Sabbath.

This is far from the only reference to amulets in the rabbinic corpus—in fact, their use was so common as to be unremarkable. As Gideon Bohak puts it, "Contrary to our own instinctive assumption that amulets are a magical implement, the rabbis saw amulets as a standard constituent of a person's daily garments."[69] Judeans who were experts at crafting amulets were held in high regard, as evidenced by the comment in m. Šab 6:2 that one may only wear an amulet (קָמֵעַ) on the Sabbath if it was produced by an expert (הַמֻּמְחֶה). Building on this opinion, the Talmudic authorities discuss such questions as whether the effectiveness of an amulet affects its legal status, what makes an amulet effective, and whether an amulet that contains

---

[66] For a list of practices that the rabbis did and did not include under this heading, see b. Šab. 67b. Giuseppe Veltri identifies a number of similarities between the rabbis' category of exclusion, "Ways of the Amorites," and Pliny's depiction of the "deceitful Magi" in his *Natural History*—see "The Rabbis and Pliny the Elder: Jewish and Greco-Roman Attitudes toward Magic and Empirical Knowledge," *Poetics Today* 19 (1998): 63–89.

[67] Translation from the Soncino Talmud, available online at https://halakhah.com/shabbath/shabbath_67.html. The more recent online translation by Rabbi Adin Even-Israel Steinsaltz will also be used at times in the quotations that follow. Most of the texts cited in this section are taken from the Babylonian Talmud rather than the Mishnah or Palestinian Talmud since references to "magical" practices (including demons) are much more frequent in the former than in the latter. The ideological background for Babylonian magic is Akkadian rather than Greek, but the pattern of influence is similar to that of Greek culture (including "magical" ideas and practices) on Diaspora Jews like Paul. On points of contact between Talmudic and Akkadian magic, see M. J. Geller, "Akkadian Healing Therapies in the Babylonian Talmud," Max-Planck-Institut für Wissenschafsgeschichte Preprint 259, available online at http://www.mpiwg-berlin.mpg.de/Preprints/P259.PDF.

[68] Veltri, "The Rabbis and Pliny the Elder," 69–70.

[69] *Ancient Jewish Magic*, 370.

the divine name should be treated as holy (b. Šhab. 61a-b). Surprisingly, the rabbis voice no discomfort with the idea that the name of Israel's god might be written on an amulet, a practice that both literary and archaeological evidence shows was common at the time. Such discussions reveal both a keen desire by the rabbis to provide guidance for their followers regarding the use of amulets and a total lack of concern about their "magical" quality.

The rabbis also approved and even recommended a variety of healing practices that recall the "magical" techniques described in Chapter 3. A few examples will suffice for the whole.[70]

> To cure a migraine, slaughter a wild rooster using a silver dinar and let the blood run over the side of the head that is hurting, being careful to avoid getting it in the eyes, then hang the body on the doorpost and rub it upon entering or leaving the house. (b. Gitt. 68b).
>
> To heal a daily fever, take a newly-minted dinar to the salt pools and collect its weight in salt, then bind the salt to the neckline of the person's garment with a thread made of hair. (b. Shab. 66b).
>
> To relieve a tertian fever, procure seven thorns from seven palm trees, seven slivers from seven wooden beams, seven pegs from seven bridges, seven types of ashes from seven ovens, seven types of dust from seven door sockets, seven types of tar from seven boats, seven cumin seeds, and seven hairs from the beard of an old dog, then bind them to the neckline of the person's garment with a thread made of hair. (b. Shab. 67a).

A similar attitude can be observed regarding healing charms and incantations. According to the Mishnah, Rabbi Akiva sought to exclude from the world to come anyone who "whispers over a wound" (m. Sanh. 10:1),[71] but the rabbinic corpus as a whole rejects his view. In fact, the Talmud contains scores of verses that explicitly or implicitly approve the use of healing incantations, with many even specifying the wording to be used. The following examples are typical.[72]

> While waiting for a remedy to be delivered to counteract the effects of a poison, recite the sentence, "Poison, poison, I remember you, and your seven daughters, and your eight daughters-in-law." (b. Pesaḥ 116a).

---

[70] Some of the cures are much longer and more complicated—for examples, see b. Gitt. 69a-70a. Three equally complex healing rituals are described in the third- to fourth century CE magical text known as *Sefer Ha-Razim*, where angels play a vital role in effecting the will of the magician. The rituals are described at 1.29-34, 2.95-103, and 2.183-5. The text also gives instructions for preparing a special oil that "has great healing power" in addition to its primary role as part of a ritual to reveal the month of one's death (5.19-42).

[71] The meaning of this text has been debated: did he mean to exclude all "whispering" of incantations, or only this particular application, which includes a recitation of Exod. 15:26? The relevant passage in the Talmud gives three other limiting interpretations (b. Shab. 101a).

[72] These are actually some of the shorter ones—longer examples can be viewed in b. Shab. 66a and 67a.

To heal a wound, say over it, "A drawn sword and a readied sling, its name shall not be ache, sickness, and pains." (b. Shab. 67a).

To stop a nosebleed, bring a priest named Levi to the sufferer and have him write his name backward, or else have any man write, "I Papi Shila bar Sumki" backwards, or alternately, "Ta'am deli kesaf, ta'am deli be-me pegum." (Gitt. 69a).

Exorcism as a form of "magical" healing also continued into the rabbinic era, though the rabbis say little about how it was done. References to demons and the trouble that they cause appear often in the Babylonian Talmud (less so in the Jerusalem version), and demonic causation is presupposed in many of its instructions regarding healing. But only one account of exorcism is actually described, and it does not involve sickness.[73] Exorcistic healing formulae that use Judean divine names and symbols are common in the Greek magical papyri, but it is hard to know which of these formulae have Judean origins and which represent foreign appropriations of Judean language. Their value for our purposes is therefore limited.[74]

Christian sources from the early rabbinic era supply a bit more information on the topic. Ireneaus (*Haer.* 2.6) states that Judeans adjure demons to depart in the name of God, while Origen (*Cels.* 4.33) and Justin (*2 Apol* 85) give the more specific phrase, "the God of Abraham, and the God of Isaac, and the God of Jacob." Justin adds that they use purifications and fumigations as part of the process. Archaeological excavations in Egypt, Palestine, and Iraq also offer a window onto Judean practice with the discovery of dozens of exorcistic amulets, ostraca, *lamellae*, and incantation bowls inscribed in Hebrew and Aramaic dating from the third to the seventh centuries CE.[75] The language, methods, and imagery used in these materials are broadly similar to those found in earlier exorcistic sources, so there is ample reason to suppose that such materials were also used among the rabbis.

In summary, the available materials suggest that the rabbis were comfortable with virtually all forms of "magical" healing, including the ritualized application of healing substances, the wearing of amulets, the recitation of incantations, and the performance of exorcisms. Objections were raised only over practices that were seen as veering too close to idolatry, and even here the boundary was fuzzy.[76] The ambiguity is evident in m. Sanh. 7:6, which follows the biblical text in calling for the stoning of idolaters while allowing some surprising exceptions. Cultic acts such as bowing, making offerings, and professing devotion to another god are clearly beyond

---

[73] For a survey of the material, see Ronald H. Isaacs, *Ascending Jacob's Ladder: Jewish Views of Angels, Demons, and Evil Spirits* (Rowman & Littlefield, 1997). The exorcism story appears in b. Me'il. 17a-b. This story and two others from later sources are discussed by Meir bar-Ilan in "Exorcism by Rabbis," an online English translation of an article originally published in Hebrew (available at https://www.scribd.com/document/58278471/Exorcism-by-Rabbis).

[74] Two spells that have a firmer claim to have originated with Judeans are discussed by Emma Abate in "Contrôler les démons: formules magiques et rituelles dans la tradition juive entre les sources qumrâniennes et la Gueniza," *RHR* 230 (2013): 273–95. An online English translation is available at https://www.cairn-int.info/article-E_RHR_2302_0273--controlling-demons.htm.

[75] For overviews of the material, see Abate, "Contrôler les démons"; Eshel and Leiman, "Jewish Amulets"; and Michael Swartz, "Jewish Magic in Later Antiquity," in *The Cambridge History of Judaism* (Cambridge: Cambridge University Press, 2006), 699–720.

[76] The entirety of the Mishnaic tractate 'Abodah Zarah is devoted to clarifying what constitutes overly close association with idolatry, but none of its provisions relate specifically to healing.

the pale, but hugging, kissing, washing, oiling, and dressing a deity's statue are not deemed capital offenses, though they do count as violations of the law.[77] The same is true for making oaths in the name of a non-Judean deity. Leniency is also apparent in the handling of necromancers and sorcerers: those who practice such arts are condemned to death, but not those who seek their services (7:7). A further limit is applied later to the execution of sorcerers: only those who perform genuine works of magical power, like harvesting cucumbers from a field without picking them, are condemned, while those who merely give the illusion of doing so (probably the vast majority of practitioners) are exempt (7:11).[78] In all three cases the rulings serve to narrow the definition of prohibited practices so that it applies only to the most egregious violations. As with other cases where the rabbis sought to limit the negative consequences of biblical laws, it seems unlikely that many people ever met these qualifications. If this was the case in late antique Palestine, it is even more likely to be true for the Diaspora of Paul's day where no self-appointed body of rabbis was seeking to shape the consciences and behaviors of the resident Judean community.

Judeans and Medical Healing

As we saw earlier, some Judeans in the Second Temple era preferred to rely solely on God to treat their health problems. But medical healing was also well respected among the elites, and some of their care was undoubtedly provided by Judean physicians. Even so, there is little evidence in the surviving Judean literature that any class of Judeans preferred medical care over religious or "magical" forms of treatment.

The earliest reference to medical healers in Judean literature appears in Sir. 38:1-15, a portion of which was quoted earlier (vv. 9-15). In the section that was not cited (vv. 1-8), the sage tells his followers to "honor the physician (רופא/ἰατρὸς) before he is needed" and claims that "his wisdom comes from God" (vv. 1-2; cf. v.6). Medicine, too, is a divine gift: "The Lord created medicines (תרופות/ φάρμακα) out of the earth, and the sensible will not despise them" (v. 4). Applying God-given skills and praying to God for assistance, the drug-maker (רוקח/μυρεψὸς) formulates medicines from the fruits of the earth and the doctor applies them to assuage pain (vv. 7, 13-14). Through their labors, health is preserved and God is glorified (vv. 6, 8). Only sinners refuse their care; kings and nobles honor them and reward their labors (vv. 2-3, 15).

The author clearly holds medical healers in high esteem, but they are still secondary to the hand of God in the healing process. There is a time to call in a physician (v. 13), but prayer and repentance should be the first line of defense (vv. 9-11).[79] Even the

---

[77] The Mishnah specifies no punishment in this case; the Talmud fills the lacuna by ordering flogging (b. Sanh. 63a). It is worth noting that unless this discussion is entirely theoretical, it offers further evidence of Judeans visiting the temples of pagan deities and participating in their rites.

[78] According to b. Sanh. 67b, a similar exemption applies to rabbis who perform works of power, as when R. Hanina and R. Oshaia "spent every Sabbath eve in studying the Laws of Creation, by means of which they created a third-grown calf and ate it." As we saw in Chapter 3, such distinctions regarding personnel are typical of elite discourse on the subject of "magic."

[79] The LXX, which otherwise follows the Hebrew fairly closely in this passage, ends with a highly negative view of medical care that is absent from the Hebrew: "Let the one who sins before the one who made him [i.e., God] fall into the hands of a physician" (v. 15).

physician is dependent on God for success (vv. 2, 6, 14). The idea of a secular medical system in which people were healed with skills learned through assiduous study and practice is foreign to this author. Nothing is said about the propriety of consulting a "pagan" physician, but this might be because the author lived in Judea at a time when such healers were scarce or unknown.[80]

Philo, writing some two centuries later in a Greek city where Judeans were a sizeable minority, refers often to physicians and medical healing. The most common Greek word for "physician" (ἰατρὸς) is used fifty-six times in his writings, together with sixty-five instances of cognates. The word for "drugs" or "medicines" (φάρμακα) appears forty-two times. The presence of so many medical references in the writings of a philosopher is not as anomalous as it might seem since ancient medical theory had its roots in philosophy. But the sheer number of references in a corpus that includes no works devoted specifically to medical topics is surprising, particularly when the author is a Judean.

The amount of knowledge that Philo shows regarding the work of physicians is also impressive, though probably not beyond the ken of other educated Greeks. The following list summarizes what can be gleaned from his writings about the work of physicians.

- They conduct studies of the inner workings of the body (which he rightly calls ἀνατομή) that enable them to understand the central role of the heart and the nature of the fetus in the mother's womb. (*Spec. Leg.* 3.20.117, *Leg. All.* 2.3.6)
- They gain employment based on their experience. (*Spec. Leg.* 4.29.153)
- They treat all patients alike, ignoring differences in wealth, position, family, and power. (*Jos.* 14.160, *Prov.* 2.17)
- They diagnose illness by checking the regularity of the pulse, palpating the abdomen, and feeling the patient's temperature. (*Prov.* 2.17)
- Their treatment methods include diet, medicines, purging, fasting, changes of lifestyle, rest, encouragement, amputation, and cauterization. (*Leg. All.* 3.80.226, *Sacr.* 19.70-71, 37.123, *Praem. Poen.* 5.33, *Quaest. in Gen.* 4.204, *Dec.* 2.12)
- They make their own medicines and ointments out of plant and animal substances. (*Aet. Mund.* 16.79, *Conf. Ling.* 37.187, *Quaest. in Gen.* 4.76, *Ebr.* 45.184, *Prov.* 2.60)
- They understand the progress of different types of fevers and skin diseases. (*Spec. Leg.* 4.14.83, *Conf. Ling.* 19.151)
- They vary their treatments according to changes in the patient's condition. (*Jos.* 7.33, *Omn. Prob. Lit.* 9.58)
- They value moderation and slow progress over urgency so as to allow nature time to work. (*Poster. C.* 42.141, *Deus Imm.* 14.65, *Quaest. in Gen.* 2.41, *Quaest. in Exod.* 2.25)

---

[80] The physicians mentioned in Mk 5:26/Lk. 8:43, Mk 2:13/Mt. 9:12/Lk. 5:31, and Lk. 4:23 were presumably Jewish. All three passages treat the presence of physicians in first-century Palestine as a given. The reference in the latter text to the inefficacy and financial impact of medical treatments has parallels in Greek and Roman sources.

- They sometimes lie or withhold information from patients regarding their diagnoses and treatments in order to avoid creating fear or despair. (*Cher.* 5.15, *Quaest. in Gen.* 4.204, *Deus Imm.* 14.65-6)

Not one item in this list is distinctively "Jewish"; all have parallels in the writings and practices of Greek medical theorists and physicians. The same is true for other passages where Philo speaks about physicians or medicine. His statement in *Spec. Leg.* 4.35.186 that physicians should work to help people and not injure them recalls the Hippocratic Oath, as does his comment in *Post. C.* 42.141 that physicians should not seek to show off their skills but do only what is good for their patients. In *Vit. Cont.* 2.16 he actually quotes the famous opening lines of Hippocrates's *Aphorisms*, "Life is short but art long" (Ὁ βίος βραχύς, ἡ δὲ τέχνη μακρή), though he need not have read Hippocrates to know this proverb. He also mentions "Hippocrates the physician" by name in *Op. Mund.* 36.105 when describing the seven seasons of life through which men (using males as the norm) pass. In *Leg. Gai.* 106 and 109, he goes so far as to speak of the god Apollo as the great physician and "inventor of healing medicines."[81] Numerous other passages in his writings describe the workings of the human body in a way that shows familiarity with medical observations and not just lay observation.

In short, Philo's writings suggest that he knew, conversed with, and consulted Greek physicians either predominately or exclusively. He also presumes that his readers share his medical knowledge, as evidenced by his practice of injecting medical references into his arguments without explanation in order to support an unrelated point. While it is possible that he was simply showing off for his audience, a more natural interpretation is that his writings reflect the common practice of elite Judeans in Alexandria who knew about and engaged with Greek medical practitioners. Surely there were Judeans who practiced medicine in Alexandria, but one would never know it from reading Philo.

Philo's trust in Greek medicine, however, was not unbounded. Where Greek physicians credited their knowledge and skills to the god Asklepios and other healing deities, Philo insists that it is the God and Creator of the universe who performs all acts of healing. Physicians should give thanks to this God for restoring the health of their patients rather than praising their own skills or those of other gods (*Mut. Nom.* 39.221, *Leg. All.* 3.178, *Deus Imm.* 19.87-8). People who become sick should turn first to God rather than running off to physicians and returning to God only when their skills prove ineffective (*Sacr.* 19-70-71). Medicine is an unreliable source of healing: some people grow worse or even die under its influence while others are cured without it. In this way "the reasonings of the physician have been utterly found out to be dreams, full of all indistinctness and of riddles" (*Leg. All.* 3.80.226). Physicians cannot even maintain their own health; they, too, are taken away when pestilence comes (*Spec. Leg.* 1.46.252,

---

[81] The latter reference appears in a speech that he claims to have made to Gaius in Rome, so his language should be taken as a rhetorical adaptation to the beliefs of his audience and not as a reflection of his own beliefs. In the same treatise he speaks of how Augustus "healed the pestilences common to Greeks and barbarians" (21.144-5).

Conf. Ling. 7.22). In short, Greek physicians have many useful skills, but they lack the reverence that is due to the one true God.

In short, this most Hellenized of Judeans offers only a qualified endorsement of medical healing. He does not go as far as Sirach who elevates religious healing above medical healing, but he does situate medical healing squarely within a Judean ideological framework. He both mimics and distances himself from the Greeks, whose view of medical healing was filtered through a polytheistic religious lens.

Among the rabbis, the dominant attitude toward physicians and medical care is positive, though discordant voices can be heard here and there. The clearest negative judgment is found in m. Qidd. 4.11, which says, "The best of the physicians (טוב שברופאין) is destined for Gehenna." The broader context is a discussion about what trades are suitable for the son of a rabbi. The author classes physicians alongside donkey drivers, camel drivers, potters, sailors, shepherds, and shopkeepers as professions to be avoided. No reason is given as to why physicians are lumped together with these other occupations, but it is easy to see how some of their work might violate the sole criterion that the passage offers for a suitable trade, that it be "clean and easy." In other words, the text probably reflects the rabbis' class prejudice against certain forms of menial work rather than a comment on the validity of consulting medical healers.

Less easily explained is the inclusion of "the best of the physicians" (טוב שברופאין) in a separate list of occupations whose practitioners "have no share in the World to Come" ('Abot R. Nat. 36:5). The others are the clerk (לבלר), the scribe (or possibly, "schoolteacher") (סופר), the civic judge, the sorcerer (or "magician") (קוסם), the *ḥazzan* (cantor), and the butcher. Given the high regard in which the rabbis held scribes, judges, and *ḥazzans*, it is difficult to guess what the motivation might be for such a statement.[82] The statement is doubly odd in view of a verse in b. Sanh. 17b that lists a court, a physician, and a clerk (using the same Hebrew words as above) among ten things that must be present in a city before a Torah scholar can live there. The discrepancy might signify a disagreement among the rabbis over the propriety of the medical profession or some sort of difference in social context between the two passages, but both presume that people will be using the services of physicians just as they do those of judges and clerks.

Yet another potentially negative statement about physicians appears in b. Pesaḥ. 113a, which reads, "Do not dwell in a town where the leader of the community is a physician." Here, too, the meaning is unclear, though interpreters have suggested that it might reflect the fear that a physician will be so busy caring for patients that civic affairs will be neglected. However it is interpreted, the text says nothing that would dissuade people from seeking medical cures from a physician, though it might point to a degree of discomfort among certain rabbis (and other elites?) regarding the practitioners of medicine.

---

[82] Catherine Hezser notes that all of the positions listed were paid professionals and suggests that the condemnation might have been related to the high fees that they charged or the plebeian nature of their activities as compared with those of the rabbis. See "Jewish Scribes in the Late Second Temple Period: Differences Between the Composition, Writing, and Interpretation of Texts," in *Scriptures in the Making: Texts and Their Transmission in Late Second Temple Judaism*, ed. Raimo Hakola, Jessi Orpana, and Paavo Hakola (Leuven: Peters 2021), 167.

Over against this handful of critical statements stand a host of positive comments in the rabbinic literature about physicians.[83] The previously noted statement in b. Sanh. 17b regarding the necessity of having a physician to serve the needs of Torah scholars certainly fits in this category, as does R. Ashi's passing observation that it is common sense for a person who is sick to visit a doctor (b. B. Qam. 46b). An equally casual acceptance of medical healing can be seen in b. Ber. 60a, which contains prayers that a person should recite before and after going to a physician to have blood let by cupping, and b. B. Qam. 85a, where the rabbis debate at length whether an injured person should receive compensation for medical costs incurred under various conditions. In both of these texts the rulings are justified by reference to an opinion of R. Ishmael's school that inferred from Exod. 21:19 (a text that speaks of an injured man being "completely healed") the conclusion that "permission has been given [by God] to the physician to heal." This is similar to what we saw in Sirach and Philo.

For the most part the Mishnah and Talmud say nothing about the ethnicity or religion of the physicians whose services are under discussion. Given the rabbis' narrow focus on the behavior of Jews, it seems natural to infer that they had Judean physicians in mind.[84] This reading of the evidence is borne out by a handful of passages in which the propriety of visiting gentile physicians is explicitly discussed as a matter of uncertainty. The most extensive treatment is in b. 'Abod. Zar. 26a-29a, which reports a series of opinions by various rabbis concerning the implications of the rather cryptic statement in the Mishnaic *lemma* (m. 'Abod. Zar. 2.1) that Jews may be treated by gentiles where it involves "healing for money" (רִפּוּי מָמוֹן) but not רִפּוּי נְפָשׁוֹת ("healing of persons"?). The rabbis debated the meaning of both phrases, as the distinction is by no means clear. The details of the debate need not concern us here; what matters for our purposes is that the passage provides clear evidence that some Judeans in the rabbinic era were going to gentile physicians for treatment and the rabbis were divided over the propriety of these actions.

The same pattern can be seen in two other passages that discuss the question of whether gentiles can deliver or circumcise the babies of Judean mothers (b. Menaḥ. 42a and 'Abod. Zar. 26b-27a). As in the more general passage, the rabbis offer conflicting opinions on both practices, with those who oppose them expressing concern that the gentile might harm or kill the Judean baby. Whether such fears were warranted is unclear, but the discussion certainly gives the impression that the rabbis were grappling with a real-world situation in which Judeans were using gentile physicians to deliver and circumcise their babies and not merely speculating about a hypothetical question.

---

[83] A good overview of rabbinic references to physicians can be found in Catherine Hezser, "Representations of the Physician in Jewish Literature from Hellenistic and Roman Times," in *Popular Medicine in Graeco-Roman Antiquity: Explorations*, ed. William V. Harris (Leiden and Boston: Brill, 2016), 180-92.

[84] Catherine Hezser discusses several passages in which the Judean identity of a physician is explicitly mentioned or strongly implied in "Representations of the Physician in Jewish Literature from Hellenistic and Roman Times," 181-7.

Conclusion

A careful review of the evidence for Judean healing practices in Greco-Roman antiquity shows clearly that Judeans in both Palestine and the Diaspora made regular use of all three of the overlapping health care systems that were available for treating illness and injury.

Their use of religious healing practices comes as no surprise, since this is the system that is most often recommended and exemplified in the Jewish Scriptures. But whether Judeans limited themselves to Jewish religious practitioners and settings is not entirely clear. Contrary to common presumptions, there is evidence that at least some Judeans visited "pagan" religious sanctuaries and participated actively or passively in cultic rituals honoring deities other than the God of Israel. We cannot therefore rule out the possibility that some Judeans may have consulted Greek religious specialists (e.g., exorcists and purifiers) or traveled to Asklepian sanctuaries in search of healing. The likelihood that they did so increases when we recall that many of the healing techniques employed in these settings did not require direct personal appeals to Greek or Roman deities. But the silence of Judean sources on this topic renders all answers speculative.

The situation is different with regard to "magical" healing, where source material is ample. The openness of Judeans in both the Second Temple and rabbinic eras to practices that most observers would regard as "magical" is remarkable in light of the many biblical texts that condemn "sorcery" and related practices. Closer inspection, however, shows that healing is never mentioned in connection with any of the prohibited acts and that the Bible in fact contains several passages that describe and even commend modes of healing that in other ancient contexts would be labeled as "magical." Whether these texts were ever cited to justify the use of magical healing practices is unclear, but their presence undermines any attempt to assert that there was a clear and consistent biblical prohibition of magical healing that would have been recognized by all ancient Judeans apart from deeply Hellenized renegades and apostates. In fact, both literary and archaeological data show that magical healing was as normal among Judeans as it was among Greeks and Romans.

Equally surprising is the ambivalent attitude toward medical healing in our sources. Most seem to view the practice as uncontroversial, but some authors regard it as secondary to religious healing and criticize those who turn too quickly to physicians. This is true even for Judean physicians, so we cannot attribute their reservations to discomfort with "pagan" practices. In fact, there is ample evidence in our sources that at least some Judeans made regular use of Greek and Roman physicians to treat their health problems. Whether they willingly submitted to whatever treatments these practitioners recommended or resisted some on religious grounds cannot be determined.

In short, there was no unified "Jewish" perspective on sickness and healing in the Second Temple era to which Paul could have turned for guidance as he sought to determine what kinds of treatment were and were not acceptable for himself and his congregations. This distinguishes it from issues like sexuality or sacrificing to pagan deities where Scripture and tradition were clear. We should therefore avoid saying that because Paul was a Jew, he could not possibly have used or condoned this or that healing practice. Other than valuing religious approaches, the attitude of most Judeans to health care seems to have been pragmatic: if a treatment works, it can be used. The importance of this observation for assessing Paul's practices will become clear in Chapter 9.

8

Christian Approaches to Health Care

Introduction

The apostle Paul was not the only Christ-follower who faced questions relating to health care as the Jewish movement that came to be known as Christianity took root and flourished in gentile soil. Others, too, struggled to figure out what elements of Greek and Roman culture were consistent with devotion to the God of Israel and his son Jesus Christ, whom they had come to know through missionary preachers like Paul. The letters that Paul wrote to his churches were copied and used by other Christ-followers as a source of guidance on questions of belief and practice, but they said almost nothing about sickness or healing. Writings by later church leaders filled the gap to some extent, but those writings were not readily accessible to the illiterate masses. As late as the fourth century, leaders were exhorting their congregants against visiting Asklepian temples and engaging in "magical" practices, so it appears that Christ-followers continued to visit Greek and Roman healers long after the time of Paul. Unlike Paul, however, this later generation of leaders felt compelled to confront Christians who behaved in this manner.

This chapter explores what Christian authors in the first few centuries said about health care in order to highlight some of the intellectual and practical resources that might have been available to Paul if he had chosen to speak more directly about matters of sickness and health care in his letters. The question is not whether any of these other authors influenced Paul, since most of them lived long after his era. The aim is rather to hear what these later authors were saying in order to assess whether their approaches are consistent with Paul's theology and praxis and, if they are, to ask why Paul did not use similar arguments in advising his congregations on matters of health care.

Our review will begin with the documents that make up the Christian New Testament, since they show us both what other Christian leaders were thinking and saying about sickness and health around the time of Paul and what resources were available for succeeding generations in the Christian Scriptures as they grappled with such questions. From there the focus will shift to later Christian writings following the same pattern that was used in Chapter 7, with religious healing being treated first, followed by "magical" and medical healing. A concluding section will raise questions about how the chapter's findings might be applied to the writings of the apostle Paul.

Health Care in the Early Christian Era

Virtually all scholars agree that the early Christ-movement used the Scriptures of Judaism as a touchstone for belief and practice in the years prior to the composition of the books that we call the New Testament. Like many commonplaces, however, this one gets as much wrong as it does right. It might have been true in the early days when the movement was essentially a form of Judaism, but the situation quickly changed as the number of Judean members was overwhelmed by gentiles who had little or no prior exposure to the Jewish Scriptures. Few gentile Christ-followers would have been capable of reading and studying the text of Scripture on their own in an era when books were expensive and literacy levels hovered around 5 to 10 percent.[1] If we add to this what we learned in Chapter 7 about the infrequency of comments about health care and healing in the Jewish Scriptures, the possibility that the early Christ-followers used the texts of Judaism to guide their thinking about sickness and healing diminishes to the vanishing point.

How, then, did they know what was and was not acceptable? Unless they were challenged by their leaders to think and act otherwise, there is no reason to think that they would have changed what they were doing before becoming Christ-followers—using some combination of traditional, religious, magical, and medical health care.[2] The earliest Christian writings offer few signs that such challenges were common.

The most obvious place to look for evidence of early Christian beliefs regarding health care is the Gospels, since healing is central to their depictions of Jesus. Their accounts of Jesus's healing activity are not directly pertinent to this study, since our concern is with the movement that developed after Jesus and not with Jesus himself. But the Gospels are a product of that movement and its interests, so it is relevant to observe how much space their authors devoted to stories of healing when shaping their source material into continuous narratives. Miraculous healings occur frequently, instantaneously, and effortlessly in all four Gospels. Both the number of healing narratives and their miraculous nature imply that the authors were writing for an audience that valued physical healing and would be impressed by someone who could restore health so easily. In the Greek view, only gods and heroes could perform such mighty deeds, so the Jesus of the Gospels would have appeared to Greek readers as some type of divine being. At a time when divine healers like Asklepios and Hygieia were attracting large and devoted followings, portraying Jesus as a divine healer was a sure way to gain adherents once the Christ-movement moved to Greek soil.[3]

At the same time, the Gospels offer little guidance for the early Christian community regarding what they themselves should do to address their health needs. All of the

---

[1] This is the conclusion of William V. Harris's monumental study that has gained broad acceptance among classical scholars—see *Ancient Literacy* (Cambridge, MA: Harvard University Press, 1989).
[2] Medical historian Gary Ferngren agrees that this was the norm: "The evidence, scattered and circumstantial as it is, suggests that first-century Christians relied on ordinary means of healing, such as conventional medicine or folk or traditional remedies" (*Medicine and Religion*, 78).
[3] Judean readers, by contrast, would have been more likely to take these stories as evidence that Jesus was a prophet, since, as we saw in Chapter 8, prophets are the only humans who perform miraculous healings in the Jewish tradition.

healings that Jesus performs are miraculous; only three stories include any form of treatment. Two involve relatively simple procedures: in Mk 8:22-26 Jesus applies saliva to a man's eyes and lays his hands on him, while in Jn 9:6-11 he does a similar act using mud made from saliva and dirt, then commands the man to wash in the pool of Siloam. The third story, Mk 7:31-35, relates a more complex series of actions: he inserts his fingers into the ears of a deaf man, spits (on the ground?), touches the man's tongue, looks up toward the sky, and pronounces the Aramaic word "Ephphatha," meaning "be opened!" Saliva is used in many Greek medical remedies,[4] but the other acts have more in common with the magical healing arts that we studied in Chapter 3. None of the stories makes any claim that others could achieve similar results by following Jesus's example, but it is easy to see how they might have been used by later generations to justify "magical" forms of healing.

The same is true for Jesus's exorcistic healings. In theory they could be imitated by others, but the stories offer little guidance about how this should be done other than perhaps repeating the words that Jesus used when commanding demons to leave a sick person and announcing that they are speaking "in the name of Jesus" (Mt. 7:22, Mk 9:38-39/Lk. 9:49, Lk. 10:17). The Synoptics include a story in which Jesus imbues his disciples with power to heal and expel demons (Mt. 10:1-8, Mk 6:7-12, Lk. 9:1-6), but only Luke gives any indication that similar power might be available to Christ-followers after the death of Jesus (Lk. 24:49). Even here the reference is vague; nothing is said about whether this "power from on high" will include the ability to heal and cast out demons as Jesus and his disciples did. Later Christians who looked to the Gospels for instruction about dealing with sickness would have found little guidance other than to expel a demon or pray for a miracle.

The same is true for the book of Acts. Numerous healings are either narrated or referenced under summary statements like the one in Acts 5:16, which reads, "A great number of people would also gather from the towns around Jerusalem, bringing the sick and those tormented by unclean spirits, and they were all cured" (cf. Acts 8:6-7, 28:9). The healings are invariably instantaneous and miraculous. Little is said about how these healings were effected; the only techniques mentioned are verbal command (3:6, 9:34, 9:40, 14:10), touch (3:7, 8:18, 9:41, 28:8), prayer (9:40, 28:8), and exorcising demons (5:16, 8:7, 19:12). The author makes a point of ascribing the healings to the risen Jesus rather than to some innate divinity in the apostles (3:6, 3:16, 4:10, 4:30, 9:34),[5] though this emphasis is undermined somewhat by two stories in which healing power is directly associated with the healer's body (Peter's shadow in 5:15 and cloths that had touched Paul's skin in 19:12). Whether and how ordinary Christ-followers might be able to tap into that healing power is never addressed. As in the Gospels, there is little here to guide later Christians in the treatment of specific cases of illness or injury.

The rest of the New Testament (excluding the genuine letters of Paul, which will be treated in Chapter 9) contains only a handful of references to healing, only three

---

[4] Pliny lists a host of uses for saliva in *HN* 28.7, including both medical and magical functions. Most relevant here is his remark about how people commonly spit three times onto the ground to improve the efficacy of a remedy.

[5] Surprisingly, the healing ministry of the earthly Jesus is mentioned only once in the book (10:38).

of which relate to the treatment of sickness.[6] In the first, 1 Tim. 5:23, the author recommends that Timothy "take a little wine for the sake of your stomach and your frequent ailments." Wine was a common remedy in both traditional and medical forms of healing, so its appearance here is unremarkable except as an implicit endorsement of its use. No mention is made of prayer or other forms of religious healing. The same is true for Rev. 3:18, where the risen Jesus refers metaphorically to the application of a healing salve to cure the (spiritual) eyes of the Laodiceans. Salves and ointments for eye problems are one of the most common remedies described in ancient pharmacological texts.

The situation is different in the third text, Jas 5:13-16, where the author prescribes a ritual that combines techniques seen in other New Testament texts: prayer, physical touch (the laying on of hands), and anointing with oil (cf. Mk 6:13, Lk. 10:34). Oil was used in healing throughout the ancient world, so there is nothing odd in its appearance here. The association of sickness with sin and forgiveness (vv. 15-16) has deep roots in the biblical tradition, as does the idea that healing comes from "the Lord" (v. 15). The only unusual element in the passage is the role of the elders, which probably derives from synagogal practice. The corporate nature of the ritual sets it apart from the individualism of most Greek and Roman healing rituals.[7]

Notably absent from all of these texts is any criticism of the various modes of healing practiced by non-Judeans at the time. We might suppose from their condemnations of idolatry that early Christian authors would have looked askance at practices that involved direct or indirect contact with non-Judean deities, but nothing is said on the subject. In the only text where the healing practices of outsiders come up for discussion, Jesus rallies to the defense of a man who is successfully expelling demons in his name despite not being one of his followers (Mk 9:38-41). The story is set in a Judean (and thus presumably monotheistic) context, so it would be perilous to generalize from it to a gentile setting.

Taking all of the evidence together, it seems that Christians who were seeking guidance from their founding texts about the propriety of various types of healing would have found little to aid them. Whether the omission was accidental or reveals a lack of interest in the topic is hard to judge. But the result was the same: either they had to give up the effort (and presumably continue in their previous practices) or else generalize from texts dealing with similar or related subjects to figure out what their founders might have said if they had chosen to address the topic. The remainder of this chapter will investigate what they actually did.

---

[6] Metaphorical references can be found in Heb. 12:12-13, 1 Pet. 2:24, Rev. 13:3, 13:12, and 22:2. All are quite general; none cite any real-world healing techniques. Some Christians have argued for a literal interpretation of 1 Pet. 2:24 ("by his wounds you have been healed"), but nothing in the context supports such a reading, and the text says nothing about how healing is to be performed even if a literal reading is granted.

[7] For an analysis of this passage through the lens of medical anthropology, see Martin C. Albl, "'Are Any among You Sick?' The Health Care System in the Letter of James," *JBL* 121 (2002): 123-43.

Christians and Religious Healing

References to religious healing are fairly common in patristic texts. This is true even if we exclude the many instances in which authors use healing language metaphorically to describe the spiritual benefits that the church affords to believers (i.e., the "cure of souls") rather than relief from physical sickness. Several patterns can be discerned in the more literal references.

Regarding the causes of sickness, patristic authors generally echo what we saw in our study of Jewish thought: sickness can be an expression of divine displeasure, a test of human faith, the work of demons, or a product of living in a fallen world. Here and there someone notes that sickness can result from a poor lifestyle, whether chosen or circumstantial, but religious explanations dominate. Christians are repeatedly exhorted to despise bodily sufferings while seeking to discern what lessons God might be trying to teach them through their sickness. Sickness, in short, is a school of faith; it should draw people closer to God regardless of whether they are healed.[8] The health of the soul is more important than that of the body. Darrel Amundsen summarizes their opinion well: "An undue concern for the body to the point where one's mind revolves around its needs and a desperate clinging to life are a tragic contradiction of Christian values."[9]

The primary channel for religious healing is prayer. Christians serve a loving God who desires good for them but wants them to pray for healing. Prayer is important not as a way of informing a remote god about one's sufferings or motivating a reluctant deity to act but as a means of submitting oneself to the will of a God who knows what is best. Christians should petition God to deliver them from sickness while at the same time praying for strength to bear it and learn from it if that should be God's will. It is not wrong to seek healing through human channels such as physicians and medicines, but one should not rely on them to the exclusion of prayer and submission.[10] God is the giver of health, regardless of the channels through which it comes.

While miraculous healings are not necessarily to be expected, most Christians believed that they were possible and some actively sought them. In fact, Christian belief in miracles was so well known by the second century CE that it attracted the notice of the Roman physician Galen, who criticized it on the grounds that it "entailed a capricious deity who could overthrow at will the whole 'scientific' basis of the universe, including medicine."[11] Many church fathers assert that miraculous healings were common in Christian circles, and Gary Ferngren has shown that the number of these references actually increased between the second and fourth centuries CE.[12] Stories of healing miracles are especially common in the early monastic era. Popular healing

---

[8] For a review of what individual authors say on the subject, see the excellent survey by Darrell W. Amundsen, "Medicine and Faith in Early Christianity," *Bulletin of the History of Medicine* 56 (1982): 326–50.
[9] Ibid., 342.
[10] As we will see later, there are dissenters on this point: a few authors reject the use of medicine entirely while others recommend avoidance for people like monks who seek to live closer to God.
[11] Nutton, "Medicine in the Greek World, 800-50 BC," 16.
[12] Evelyn Frost, *Christian Healing*, 2nd ed. (London: A. R. Mowbray, 1949); Ferngren, "Early Christianity as a Religion of Healing," 8–15.

practices included invoking the name of Christ, applying the sign of the cross, laying on of hands, prayer and fasting, anointing with oil, wearing amulets, and exorcism.[13] Some even practiced incubation (seeking healing dreams) at Christian shrines.[14]

For those who were not immediately healed by God, divine healing could also come through the tender care of fellow believers. While in practice this approach overlaps with medical healing, the motive for providing such care is religious, and God is credited as the healer when health is restored.[15] Nursing of the sick initially took place in the home, often through the hands of church ministers like widows and deacons, but by the fourth century CE this desire to express God's love for the sick led to the erection of the first Christian hospitals as centers for the delivery of religio-medical health care. Harnack views this concern for the sick as one of the primary channels for attracting new converts to the Christian movement, while Ferngren goes so far as to say that "it was not curing but caring that constituted the chief ministry of the early Christian community to the sick."[16] How far this was the case is disputed, but outsiders were clearly impressed with how much time and effort Christians devoted to tending the sick, including people who were not part of their community.

What about non-Christian modes of religious healing? Did Christians in the first few centuries restrict themselves to Christian healers, or did they continue to visit Asklepian temples and consult with Greek or Roman religious healers? While it is often difficult to speculate on the behavior of the illiterate masses, in this case the sources are clear: gentile Christians continued to use all of the healing techniques that they practiced before joining the movement, including Asklepian temple healing. Numerous church fathers, including Tertullian, Origen, Arnobius, and Athanasius, attacked Asklepios as a demonic being who is in every way inferior to Christ as a healer.[17] The forcefulness and often strained nature of their arguments make little sense unless they were seeking to counter the god's appeal to their followers. The difficulty was compounded by the many similarities that existed in the stories and beliefs surrounding Jesus and Asklepios, similarities that made it harder to draw a sharp distinction between the two or to argue that one was good and the other bad.[18]

---

[13] Ferngren, "Early Christianity as a Religion of Healing," 12. For references, see J. D. King, *Regeneration: A Complete History of Healing in the Christian Church*, vol. 1, *Post-Apostolic through Later Holiness* (Lee's Summit, MO: Christos Publishing, 2017), 40–4, 50–8.

[14] Ferngern and Amundsen, "Medicine and Christianity in the Roman Empire," 2970.

[15] For a good historical survey of Christian philanthropy as it relates to health care, see Gary B. Ferngren, *Medicine and Health Care in Early Christianity* (Baltimore: Johns Hopkins University Press, 2009), 113–39.

[16] Harnack, *Mission and Expansion*, 81–9; Ferngren, "Early Christianity as a Religion of Healing," 18.

[17] For an overview of the evidence, see Edelstein and Edelstein, *Asclepius*, 2.132–4, which includes references to the relevant texts of various church fathers that are quoted in volume 1. The arguments of four specific patristic authors (Justin, Athenagoras, Clement, and Origen) are discussed by Gaetano Spampinato in "The Use of the Figure and the Myth of Asclepius in the Greek Anti-pagan Controversy," *Electra* 5 (2020): 79–101.

[18] The many parallels that existed between the two are highlighted by Edelstein and Edelstein, *Asclepius*, 2.135–7; Hart, *Asclepius, the God of Medicine*, 183–6; and especially René Josef Rüttimann, "Asclepius and Jesus: The Form, Character and Status of the Asclepius Cult in the Second Century CE and its Influence on Early Christianity" (ThD dissertation, Harvard Divinity School, 1986). Two points of difference were highlighted by multiple authors as signs of the superiority of Jesus over Asklepios: (a) Asklepios was killed by Zeus for meddling with the realm of the gods while Jesus died

Even more challenging was the apparent success of Asklepios as a healer, a fact that few Christian authors attempted to deny.[19]

Origen's handling of the subject is typical. In responding to Celsus's observation that "a great multitude both of Greeks and barbarians acknowledge that they have frequently seen, and still see, no mere phantom, but Asklepios himself, healing and doing good, and foretelling the future," he does not dispute the facticity of Celsus's statement but rather denigrates Asklepios's virtue by pointing out that he healed people without regard to their merits, including some who showed by their conduct that they were "not fit to live" (*Cels.* 3.24-25). The fact that Jesus, too, was renowned for ministering to the undeserving apparently does not occur to him. It does, however, to Arnobius, who fifty years later makes exactly the opposite argument: Jesus healed all who came to him, whereas Asklepios healed only the deserving and left many uncured (*Adv. nat.* 49). The contradiction highlights the difficulty that Christian leaders faced as they sought to persuade their followers to break all ties with one of the primary deities that they were trying to persuade outsiders to abandon in favor of Jesus.

How far Christians actually went in their use of Asklepian healing facilities is unclear. Given their leaders' ongoing polemics against idolatry, it seems unlikely that many would have participated willingly and actively in cultic rituals honoring Asklepios as the divine savior. Avoiding such rituals entirely would have been difficult if they spent any time at an Asklepian temple facility, but they might have justified seeking treatment there by citing Paul to the effect that "no idol in the world really exists, and that there is no God but one" (1 Cor. 8:4).[20] It is equally unclear how often such visits occurred or how many people were involved, since even infrequent visits by a handful of Christians to an Asklepian sanctuary could have evoked a sharp and broadly framed reaction from leaders who were struggling to maintain the boundaries between their own community and followers of "pagan" religions. Even if the details are beyond our ability to recover, the very act of asking such questions can help us to entertain possibilities that might otherwise have escaped our notice.[21]

Christians and "Magical" Healing

Condemnations of "magic" are as common in the writings of church fathers as in the rabbinic literature. If we ask what the authors meant by the term "magic," however, we find that they held the same mental reservation as the rabbis: acts that result in healing are not normally included in their condemnations.

---

willingly for the sins of others, and (b) Asklepios required payment for his healing services while Jesus healed for free. Arnobius adds the criticism that Asklepios used medical techniques to restore health whereas Jesus healed miraculously by word and touch (*Adv. nat.* 48).

[19] Noted by Amundsen, "Medicine and Faith in Early Christianity," 346.

[20] Such a mental reservation appears to be implied in 1 Cor. 8:10, which posits a scenario in which a Christ-follower is "eating in the temple of an idol." More will be said on this point in Chapter 9.

[21] René Rüttimann claims that Christians continued to visit the sanctuaries of Asklepios into the fifth century, when they were finally superseded by Christianity (*Asclepius and Jesus*, 205–12).

What Christians Thought

Like the rabbis, the church fathers looked often to Scripture for guidance on matters of conduct. When they did so, they would have found no clear prohibition of "magical" healing in either the "Old Testament" texts that we examined in Chapter 7 or the documents that were eventually canonized as the New Testament. Words based on the Greek μαγ- root appear only eight times in the New Testament, four in Matthew's description of the coming of the Magi and four in the book of Acts (8:9, 8:11, 13:6, 13:8). None of these texts makes any mention of healing. The same is true for the rather odd use of the phrase τὰ περίεργα in Acts 19:19 to designate "magical books" and the warning in 2 Tim. 3:3 against following γόητες who attempt to deceive Christ-followers. Forms of the Greek word φαρμακία, which can refer to the use of medicines, poisons, or magical substances depending on the context, appear five times in the New Testament, all but once in the book of Revelation (Gal. 5:20, Rev. 9:21, 18:23, 21:8, 22:15). The word carries negative connotations in all five passages, but its precise meaning is nowhere spelled out, leaving readers to infer a meaning based on their own cultural competence.

Standing against these vague prohibitions are a number of biblical texts in which healings that could be described as "magical" are recounted with evident approval. The relevant verses from the "Old Testament" were examined earlier, but there are also New Testament passages that could be interpreted as supporting magical healing. All of the exorcistic cures in the Gospels and Acts could be classified under this heading since belief in demonic causality and expelling demons were common features of "magical" healing in Greek and Roman circles. The paucity of information regarding the techniques that were used (apart from verbal adjurations to leave "in the name of Jesus") made these exorcisms less replicable than those reported by Greek and Roman authors, but it is easy to see how gentile Christians could have found in these stories permission to continue using the kinds of exorcistic practices that we examined in Chapter 3, even if this was not the authors' intention.

Several other New Testament texts could be read by willing interpreters as validating the use of "magic." The most obvious is Matthew's extended (and positive) story of foreign "magicians" (μάγοι ἀπὸ ἀνατολῶν) coming to honor the infant Messiah in a visit that Matthew suggests was both motivated and guided by astrological observations (Mt. 2:1-12). More relevant for our purposes are the three Gospel texts cited earlier where Jesus uses healing techniques that resemble those of the μάγοι: applying saliva to the eyes of two blind men; laying hands on one of them (an act that has to be repeated for the healing to be complete) and telling the other to go and wash in a particular pool; inserting his fingers into the ears of a deaf man; spitting (onto the ground?); touching a mute man's tongue; and looking up to the sky while pronouncing a healing word in a foreign language ("Ephphatha!"). None of these texts definitely requires a magical reading, but little imagination is needed to see how ancient Christians could have found in them divine justification for using healing rituals that involved similar actions. The same is true for two texts from the book of Acts that we noted earlier where healings are effected by the passing of Peter's shadow (5:15) and by cloths that had touched Paul's skin (19:12). No rational mode of healing can be posited in either of these cases.

When we combine these examples with the ones from the "Old Testament," the number of texts that could be read as supporting "magical" healing is roughly doubled. Thus there is no basis for thinking that Christians in the Roman era who engaged in "magical" forms of healing were somehow disregarding the teachings of Scripture. In fact, the number and clarity of biblical verses that could be cited in favor of using magical healing techniques vastly outweighed those on the other side.

We should also be careful about assuming that patristic condemnations of "magic" automatically included healing. A few examples will suffice to make the point. In Did. 2:1, the author includes the phrase οὐ μαγεύσεις ("do not practice magic"?) in a long list of biblical laws that should be obeyed by Christians.[22] The phrase does not appear in the LXX, but it was probably intended as an allusion to the verses that we examined earlier that condemn "sorcery" and the like. There is no reason to suppose that any of these prohibitions included healing. The same can be said for several other texts where μαγεία is mentioned, including Barn. 20, where μαγεία appears in a catalog of illicit practices that "destroy human souls" and lead to "eternal death"; Eph. 19.2, where Ignatius classes μαγεία together with "wickedness" and "ignorance" as conditions from which the coming of Jesus freed humanity; 1Apol. 14, where Justin cites "magical arts" (μαγικαί τέχναι) as one of the demonic practices that Christians abandoned in favor of devotion to "the good and unbegotten God"; and several texts from Irenaeus where he accuses opponents of engaging in magical activities (Haer. 1.13.1-3; 1.23.1-5; 1.24.5; 1.25.3, etc.). Not one of these verses mentions healing, and there is no contextual or cultural reason for thinking that the authors intended to include it.

Only a handful of patristic texts speak specifically about magical healing practices. Some are ambiguous, as in Did. 2:1 where οὐ φαρμακεύσεις could refer to the administration of either healing potions or poisons. The latter is more likely here, both because the fear of poisons was common in the Roman world and because a blanket prohibition of medicinal substances would make the text virtually unique among ancient sources.[23] More relevant is the injunction in Did. 3:3 that Christians should not be augurs (οἰωνοσκόκοι), charm-singers (ἐπαοιδοὶ), astrologers (μαθηματικοὶ), or purifiers (περικαθαίρίαι) because such practices can lead to idolatry. Healing is not explicitly named in this list, but charms and purifications played an important role in "magical" forms of healing, so it seems probable that Christian readers would have taken this text as an injunction against being a regular practitioner of these arts. The text says nothing, however, about the propriety of consulting non-Christians who offered these services, and the door remained open for Christians who wished to perform them to argue that they could do so without falling into idolatry.

A more absolute list of prohibited professions is preserved by Hippolytus in Trad. ap. 16, which says that μάγοι should not even be considered for baptism, while enchanters, astrologers, diviners, dream interpreters, "charlatans," and amulet-makers must cease

---

[22] This and the most of the other references in this section were taken from Joseph E. Sanzo, "Early Christianity," in Frankfurter, Guide to the Study of Ancient Magic, 219–31. Sanzo cites many more texts than those listed here.

[23] The same reasoning applies to the inclusion of φαρμακίαι among the practices associated with "the way of death" in 5:1. Tatian, whose views on the subject will be noted later, is the only author who appears to condemn the use of medicinal substances.

their work or be rejected.[24] Amulet-making is clearly a "magical" healing technique, and the same could be true for "enchanters," "dream interpreters," and "charlatans," though the loss of the original Greek text makes certainty impossible. Here again the author says nothing about the propriety of consulting non-Christians who offered such services, but the absoluteness of the prohibition suggests that this, too, would have been discouraged in the church at Rome in the second century CE.

Tertullian appears to go farther in asserting that Christians should not visit poisoners, magicians, diviners, soothsayers, or astrologers (*Apol.* 35:12, 43:1). But none of these practitioners were consistently associated with healing, so it is not clear whether he meant to include healers in his proscription.[25] Tatian is more explicit, charging demons with promoting the idea that "hanging little amulets of leather" on the body of a mentally ill person will elicit a cure (*Or. Graec.* 17). He does not mention any other "magical" remedies or any other illnesses, but the tenor of his argument suggests that he meant for his comments to apply to them as well.

The ambivalence of early Christians toward magical healing is nowhere more evident than in the writings of Origen, especially his *Contra Celsum*. One of his primary concerns in this work is to counter Celsus's claims that Jesus and his followers used magic to manipulate *daimones* to perform miraculous deeds like exorcisms and healings. Origen insists that Christians would never appeal to *daimones* for aid because *daimones* are evil (5.5, 7.69. 8.39). He condemns people who are "curiously inquisitive about the names of demons, their powers and agency, the incantations, the herbs proper to them, and the stones with the inscriptions graven on them" (8.61). People who do such things are "bad and impious" and will in the end "be given over to be torn and otherwise tormented by demons."

Not all forms of magic, however, fall under this heading. Some work through natural channels and do not require interaction with *daimones*. In 1.24, for example, he asserts that "magic is not, as the followers of Epicurus and Aristotle suppose, an altogether uncertain thing, but is, as those skilled in it prove, a consistent system, having words which are known to exceedingly few." Divine names—even those of pagan deities—carry an inherent power when they are "pronounced with that attendant train of circumstances which is appropriate to their nature" (1.24). The phrase "the God of Abraham, and the God of Isaac, and the God of Jacob" is so efficacious in exorcising demons that it is used by "almost all those who occupy themselves with incantations and magical rites" (4.33).[26] Incantations that do not involve divine names can also be efficacious when recited in the proper form: "Those who are skilled in the use of incantations relate that the utterance of the same incantation in its proper language can accomplish what the spell professes to do; but when translated into any other tongue, it is observed to become inefficacious and feeble" (1.26; cf. 5.45).

Healing rituals that involve explicit appeals to *daimones*, however, are unsuitable for Christians. Origen doubts whether *daimones* are capable of curing the body (8.60),

---

[24] Noted by Nutton, "Healers in the Medical Marketplace," 57.
[25] The word *venenarii* can in some contexts refer to providers of healing medicines, but more often it carries the negative sense of "poisoners," as seems likely here.
[26] According to 4.34, similar power is associated with the phrases "the God of Israel," "the God of the Hebrews," and "the God who drowned the king of Egypt and the Egyptians in the Red Sea."

but even if they were, Christians should avoid healers who consort with them because "those who for the sake of bodily health, bodily enjoyment, and outward prosperity busy themselves about the names of demons and inquire by what incantations they can appease them will be condemned by God" (8.61).[27] Christians who need healing should look to God, who by the Holy Spirit enables believers to "expel evil spirits, and perform many cures, and foresee certain events" (1.46).

Origen does not state explicitly what ritual techniques Christian can use to effect cures, but an indirect answer can be found in 1.6, where he answers Celsus's charge that "it is by the names of certain demons and incantations that Christians appear to have power." Origen admits that Christians do indeed "expel evil spirits by incantations" before going on to explain that Christian incantations involve nothing more than adjuring demons "by the name of Jesus" to leave and telling stories about Jesus to those whom they are afflicting.[28] Healing is not explicitly mentioned in this passage, but it is in 3.24, where he tells of how Christians perform cures by invoking over the sick the name of "the God of all things" and the name of Jesus while repeating stories about Jesus. "By this means," he says, "we have seen many people freed from grievous conditions, mental disturbances, madness, and numerous other problems that neither humans nor *daimones* could cure." Similar language can be seen in 8.58, where he recounts how "the utterance of the words 'in the name of Jesus' by the truly faithful has healed not a few from diseases, demon-possession, and other conditions."[29] These words carry so much power, he says, that they are effective even when pronounced by bad people (1.6).

In short, it is perfectly acceptable for Christians to heal by reciting powerful words (the essence of an incantation or charm) and casting out demons, both of which would have qualified as "magical" acts by Greek standards. It is not the act itself that defines what is acceptable but the power that the act seeks to access. Healing rituals that channel the power of the one true God are permissible for Christians, even those that resemble works of "magic," while rituals that seek to manipulate *daimones* are prohibited.

Not until the Constantinian era do we encounter clear and explicit attacks on magical healing. At a time when people were flocking into the newly favored movement and the boundaries between church and society were becoming blurry,

---

[27] The ambivalence that Origen exhibits here is probably due to his earlier admission that Asklepios does seem able to heal (3.24-5) and his concession that sorcerers and magicians also do miracles with the help of *daimones* (5.9, 6.45, 8.47).

[28] Origen does not explain what kinds of stories were used, but it seems likely that he meant stories about Jesus's exorcisms. A similar statement appears in 7.4, where he says that Christians cast out demons "without strange magical arts or secret charms, but by prayer alone and simple adjurations which the simplest person can apply."

[29] Similar phrasing appears in 3.33, where he speaks about "cures wrought in his name." In 1.60, he admits that *daimones* have power that can be accessed by incantations, but he insists that their power cannot withstand that of God: "Should some greater manifestation of divinity be made, then the powers of the evil spirits are overthrown, being unable to resist the light of divinity." Justin (2 *Apol*. 6.6) says much the same: "For numberless demoniacs throughout the whole world, and in your city, many of our Christian men exorcising them in the name of Jesus Christ, who was crucified under Pontius Pilate, have healed and do heal, rendering helpless and driving the possessing devils out of the men, though they could not be cured by all the other exorcists, and those who used incantations and drugs."

leaders like Eusebius of Caesarea, John Chrysostom, and Augustine sought to clarify those boundaries by offering explicit guidance regarding what kinds of behavior were and were not consistent with the Christian faith. Among the topics that they addressed was the use of "magical" practices.

In *Dem. ev.* 3.6, Eusebius argues against claims by outsiders that Jesus was "a magician, an enchanter, a charlatan and a sorcerer." Along the way he remarks that true disciples of Jesus

> will not allow their sick even to do what is exceedingly common with non-Christians, to make use of charms written on leaves or amulets, or to pay attention to those promising to soothe them with songs of enchantment, or to procure ease for their pains by burning incense made of roots and herbs, or anything else of the kind . . . Neither is it ever possible to see a Christian using an amulet, or incantations, or charms written on curious leaves, or other things which the crowd consider quite permissible.

As H. F. Stander astutely observes, "Eusebius is definitely not very honest or objective here."[30] Eusebius himself seems to have recognized that he had overstated his case, as he adds that "all these things at any rate are forbidden by Christian teaching."

In the introduction to his Second Instruction to Catechumens, Chrysostom asserts that omens, incantations, and amulets are "foreign to Christianity." Later in the same document (2.5) he exhorts his catechumens to renounce these practices along with other works of Satan. Instead of trusting in charms and amulets, he says, they should trust God for the health of their bodies. The "drunken and half-witted old women" who trade in incantations have no place in the home of a Christian. This is true even if the women are Christians and recite only the name of the true God, since their activities subject the name of God to mockery. Faithful believers will cleanse themselves of all such practices. The point is developed further in *Hom. Col.* 8, where it is clear that he is speaking about what people in his church are actually doing and not hypothetical or pre-Christian behaviors.[31]

Writing around the same time, Augustine also links "the magical arts" (*magicarum artium*) with the devil (*Doct. chr.* 2.30). Among the activities that he includes under this heading are "all amulets and cures which the medical art condemns." The meaning of this ambiguous expression is clarified by a list of examples: incantations, "marks which they call characters,"[32] "hanging or tying certain articles" on the body, "dancing (or jumping) in a certain way," wearing "earrings on the top of each ear, or the rings of ostrich bone on the fingers," and even a cure for hiccups in which the sufferer is told to "hold your left thumb in your right hand." Augustine classes these and a list of similar practices with idolatry, astrology, and divination as "superstition." Such acts are rooted

---

[30] "Amulets and the Church Fathers," *Ekklesiastikos Pharos* 75 (1993): 59.
[31] Both passages are discussed in Dickie, *Magic and Magicians in the Greco-Roman World*, 271–4, along with a similar text from Athanasius.
[32] The reference is to various esoteric signs and symbols that appear regularly in the *PGM* and on many amulets that are known from archaeological discoveries.

in "a baleful fellowship between men and devils" and should be "utterly repudiated and avoided by the Christian" (2.36).[33]

While these three authors reject many of the same healing practices, their reasons for doing so are different. For Eusebius, sorcery is at root a "base and evil superstition" and thus contrary to Christianity. For Chrysostom, trusting in charms and amulets reveals a lack of trust in God. For Augustine, magical cures are contrary to medical science. Such thinking represents a new development in Christian ethical reflection as earlier authors hardly ever mention magical healing as a cause for concern. As with many other topics, Christian thinking about "magic" and magical healing changed over time as theologians felt compelled to clarify points of doctrine and practice over which earlier generations disagreed. We should therefore be careful about reading the beliefs and prescriptions of leaders like Eusebius, Chrysostom, and Augustine back into earlier periods.

What Christians Did

The relevance of these observations becomes clear when we turn to examine what Christians were actually doing in the patristic era regarding "magical" forms of healing. Numerous church fathers report that Christians in their day were healing and casting out demons, but they say little about how such acts was done. Origen reports that Christians used formulaic language, prayers, and simple adjurations to expel demons and restore people to health, but he says nothing about other forms of magical healing like amulets and dream interpretation. Tertullian relates how a Christian named Proculus was taken under the wing of the emperor Severus after healing him by anointing him with oil (*Scap.* 4.5), and Ireneaus speaks about people being healed by having hands laid on them (*Haer.* 2.32.4).[34] Finally, the *Martyrdom of St. Eugenia* (third century CE) describes how the title character cures a fever by making the sign of the cross over a sick woman. Whether these examples should be classified as "magical" or "religious" depends on one's point of view, but together they reveal the role that ritualized actions played in early Christian healing.

Still, this list tells us only what practices were approved by church leaders, not what people were actually doing. The harsh rhetoric that many church leaders used against practitioners of μαγεία suggests that ordinary Christians continued to consult such people for help with their problems, including sickness. Mutual accusations of magic are also common in the writings of second- and third-century heresiologists.[35] Origen speaks of Christians using spells, incantations, herbs, and engraved stones to channel the power of *daimones*, while Chysostom and Augustine testify to the continuing

---

[33] For a broader discussion of Augustine's views on magical healing techniques, see Dickie, *Magic and Magicians in the Greco-Roman World*, 296–300.
[34] Noted by Frost, *Christian Healing*, 100.
[35] Noted by Morton Smith, *Jesus the Magician* (New York: Harper & Row, 1978), 94. According to Matthew Dickie, "The most common accusation made against members of heretical Christian groups is that they resort to magic to impress people into casting their lot with them" (*Magic and Magicians in the Greco-Roman World*, 174).

popularity of incantations, divination, and amulets among the Christians of their era.[36] A few decades earlier, Basil of Caesarea and Gregory of Nyssa prescribed penance for Christians who visited sorcerers or diviners or who invited outsiders to their homes to perform purificatory or expiatory rites to protect them from demons.[37] Whether these rites were being performed for healing or for other purposes is not stated.

A more tolerant approach can be seen in a Constantinian edict against illicit magical activities that specifically exempts "remedies sought for human bodies" (*remedia humanis quaesita corporibus*). This edict, which was issued in 317 CE, echoes the opinions of Jewish rabbis from the same period that we examined in Chapter 7. According to Matthew Dickie, "There is little room for doubt . . . that for Constantine the forms of activity that he excludes from criminal prosecution are also magic, but differ from the preceding category in that they are aimed at preserving human beings and their crops from harm."[38]

Material evidence also reveals the popularity of "magical" healing practices among Christians in the patristic era, though most of it comes from the later centuries when Christianity in general becomes more visible in the archaeological record. The name of Jesus can be found on healing gems and magical graffiti as early as 200 CE,[39] and distinctively Christian symbols appear on amulets dating from the late second and early third centuries CE.[40] The number of exemplars increases exponentially in the third and fourth centuries, with hundreds of magical gemstones, amulets, and *lamellae* (folded pieces of metal or papyrus inscribed with magical words) marked with Christian words and symbols surviving from this era.[41] Whether the increase reflects the growing popularity of such objects or (more likely) the difficulty of identifying earlier objects as specifically "Christian" is impossible to say. Most interpreters, however, would agree with the judgment of Rangar Cline that "the large number of amulets that survive in multiple forms, the frequent discussions of such objects in Roman and Christian texts, the descriptions of amulets in books of magic, and the discovery of such objects in

---

[36] H. F. Stander summarizes what Christian authors say about how amulets were deployed by Christians: they were worn around the head and feet, tied to the ear, hung around babies' wrists, worn as rings on fingers, hung behind the door of the house or on household items, suspended from bedposts, and even tied around the necks of farm animals. For references, see "Amulets," 61.

[37] Noted by Dickie, *Magic and Magicians in the Greco-Roman World*, 249–50.

[38] *Magic and Magicians in the Greco-Roman World*, 243. The decree is quoted by Eusebius in *Hist. eccl.* 9.16.3. Dickie suggests that the edict was issued in response to pressure from certain church leaders to outlaw practices such as amulets and incantations.

[39] Discussed in Smith, *Jesus the Magician*, 61–4.

[40] Rangar H. Cline, "Amulets and the Ritual Efficacy of Christian Symbols," in *Oxford Handbook of Early Christian Archaeology* (Oxford: Oxford University Press, 2019), 351, 359. According to Cline, "The appearance of the crucifix, cross, anchor, fish, and other Christian symbols on possibly second- and third-century gems, pendants, rings, and similarly amuletic items suggests that such symbols could have appeared on private and household objects prior to their use in public art" (359).

[41] Theodore S. de Bruyn and Jitse H. F. Dijkstra have catalogued 133 amulets and formularies made in Egypt from the third to sixth centuries CE that are definitely or probably Christian. Of the 85 that are definite, 25 pertain to healing, with the earliest from the third century CE. See "Greek Amulets and Formularies from Egypt Containing Christian Elements: A Checklist of Papyri, Parchments, Ostraka, and Tablets," *The Bulletin of the American Society of Papyrologists* 48 (2011): 163–216. For a thorough discussion of these and other Christian amuletic materials, see Theodore S. de Bruyn, *Making Amulets Christian: Artefacts, Scribes, and Contexts* (Oxford: Oxford University Press, 2017).

household contexts suggest that amulets formed part of the fabric of the daily lives of Christians and other Romans in Late Antiquity."[42]

Did Christians use amulets containing "pagan" religious symbols? Determining who might have worn a particular amulet can be difficult, but the available evidence suggests that they did. As late as the fourth century CE, Chrysostom was decrying the practices of Christians who "encircle their heads and feet with golden coins of Alexander of Macedon" to guard against sickness (*Catech. illum.* 2.5) or hang amulets or bells around the wrist of a newborn child to protect it from harm (*Hom. 1 Cor.* 12.5).[43] Rangar Cline describes how "third- and fourth-century amulets with Christian symbols frequently feature them in combination with Greek, Egyptian, and Jewish sacred names, ritual terms and formulae, symbols, deities, and allegorical representations."[44] In fact, the earliest known depiction of the crucifixion, dated to around 200 CE, appears on one of these gems, accompanied by "magic names of the sort found on amulets and papyri in Egypt."[45] Around the same time that this gem was produced, Clement of Alexandria warns his audience against wearing rings marked with symbols of pagan deities and suggests that they instead use symbols that could bear a Christian interpretation such as a dove, a fish, a ship, a lyre, or an anchor (*Paed.* 3.3). Finally, the Greek magical papyri contain numerous examples of amulets, charms, and incantations that combine Christian and "pagan" words and symbols, though it is notoriously difficult to judge which ones might have been used by Christians.

In short, while Christian leaders were struggling to draw lines between permissible and illicit uses of "magic," the people in their churches continued to consult magical practitioners and to engage in ritual practices that many of their leaders would have condemned, including "magical" forms of healing. The reason is not hard to discern—they simply continued following the time-honored healing practices of their culture. Gary Ferngren frames it well: "Some early Christians resorted to the use of amulets or relied on dreams, predictions, and portents, not because their faith encouraged them to do so (in fact, it explicitly forbade some of them) but because they were commonly appealed to in the larger culture of the Roman Empire."[46] The resultant gap between leaders and members is described well by Joseph Sanzo.[47]

> If we read between the lines of these proscriptive Christian texts (and take into consideration the extant material record), we quickly discover that a sizable number of Christians—if not a majority—found nothing incompatible between following Jesus and visiting local specialists to acquire curative or protective objects or to receive information about the future. To the extent that it was known or understood, the emerging conceptualization of illegitimate ritual for many of

---

[42] "Amulets," 351–5.

[43] H. F. Stander points to a number of texts that show the frequency with which protective amulets were applied to infants and children and traces the practice to the high rates of infant and child mortality in the ancient world. See "Amulets," 55–66.

[44] "Amulets," 353.

[45] Jeffrey Spier, "Engraved Gems and Amulets," in *The Routledge Handbook of Early Christian Art*, ed. Mark D. Ellison and Robin M. Jensen (New York: Abingdon/Oxford: Routledge, 2018), 144–5.

[46] Ferngren, *Medicine and Religion*, 81.

[47] "Early Christianity as a Religion of Healing," 238.

these believers would have probably constituted little more than a "highfalutin" abstraction by out-of-touch priests and bishops.

If this is true for the centuries after Paul, it is even more likely to have been the case in Paul's day when Christian leaders were only beginning to reflect on the implications of their faith for the behavior of their followers. The significance of this observation will become evident in Chapter 9.

Christians and Medical Healing

Christian authors express mostly positive opinions of physicians and medical healing throughout the patristic era, though dissenting views do appear from time to time. Fees and availability continued to limit many people's access to physicians,[48] especially in the countryside, and Christians who could afford their services continued to use other modes of healing as well. But the traditional association of medical healing with pagan deities like Asklepios does not seem to have elicited much anxiety about using the services of physicians, to judge from the Christian writings that have reached us.[49]

The latter point deserves further comment in view of the tendency of some historians to speak as if the use of medical healing posed no problems for early Christians. This tendency is especially evident in the writings of Gary Ferngren and Darrel Amundsen, two historians whose writings are frequently cited in discussions of ancient religion and medicine. The following statements from their *ANRW* entry on medicine and Christianity are typical.[50]

> When Christians suffered from disease they are likely to have consulted physicians routinely, as their non-Christian neighbors did. There was nothing in Hippocratic medicine that was antithetical to Christian theology or practice.
>
> Because Hippocratic medicine was secular, Christian physicians were not compelled to detach it from a pagan religious milieu.

Similar claims can be found in the writings of other scholars who have been influenced by their research. Examples include Owsei Temkin, who asserts that "there is no good evidence that the mass of people, especially educated and well-to-do persons, who had recourse to Hippocratic doctors before their conversion to Christianity shunned

---

[48] Norman Underwood cites a number of patristic authors who complain about how the poor cannot afford the fees of physicians, including Chysostom's observation in *Pecc.* 1 that "the poor man often has to go away deprived of treatment since his income does not even cover the preparation of medicine" ("Medicine, Money, and Christian Rhetoric," 370–4).

[49] The earliest known reference to a Christian physician other than Luke in Col. 4:14 dates from the late second century CE, when Eusebius (*Hist. eccl.* 5.1.49) speaks of a physician named Alexander suffering under persecutions in the Rhone Valley around 179 CE (noted by Owsei Temkin, *Hippocrates in a World of Pagans and Christians* (Baltimore, MD: Johns Hopkins University Press, 1991), 114).

[50] "Medicine and Christianity in the Roman Empire," 2965, 2977.

Hippocratic medicine thereafter," and François Retief and Louise Cilliers, who declare that "there was indeed nothing in Hippocratic medicine which could be seen as seriously antithetical to Christian theology or practice, and it is likely that Christians took to secular medicine very early on."[51]

All of these statements are grounded on two faulty presumptions: (a) that most people in the Roman world relied on physicians as their primary health care providers, and (b) that ancient medicine was inherently secular and thus free from entanglement with religion. Both of these presumptions are anachronistic: they impose a modern Western model of health care onto a society where medicine was one of three overlapping systems of healing (or four, if we count traditional remedies) and no mode of treatment held priority over the others.

On the first point, it is simply untrue that the majority of the population turned first to physicians when dealing with illnesses or injuries. Physicians were not readily available in the heavily populated countryside, and many poor city-dwellers could not afford their services. For these people, traditional and religious modes of healing would have been the norm, not medicine. Even among the elite class, it is not at all clear that everyone preferred physicians over other modes of care, though they certainly made more use of medical services than the rest of the population.

It is equally untrue that ancient medicine was "secular" and thus unproblematic for Christians. As we saw in Chapter 5, physicians were devoted to Asklepios as their patron deity, and even the best of them included in their regimen techniques that would today be considered magical or religious, such as dream interpretation, plants harvested by "magical" means, amulets, astrology, and even prayers. It was certainly possible to engage with a physician in specific cases without encountering such practices, but one could not count on it, and most physicians would have attributed their skills (and their success) to Asklepios even if it was not explicitly mentioned. In short, the decision to visit a physician was by no means free from religious implications.

So what did early Christian authors say about medical healing? Instead of evading or ignoring its religious associations, they negated the danger by setting medicine within a new religious framework that "Christianized" the work of physicians. In so doing, they followed a path charted earlier by Judeans who faced similar challenges. The one true God, they said, created the universe and everything in it, including the materials that were employed to treat sickness. This same deity gave medical knowledge and skills to humans as an act of love and mercy. Thus whenever a person was healed by the medical arts, it was the God of the Christians who cured them, not Asklepios or any other deity. This was true even if that work went unrecognized. In short, Christians claimed that they alone understood how medicine worked. Those who accepted this interpretation could consult even the most benighted physician without fear of idolatry since they knew that it was their God who was working through the mind and hands of the physician.[52]

---

[51] Temkin, *Hippocrates in a World of Pagans and Christians*, 126; Francois Retief and Louise P. Cilliers "The Influence of Christianity on Medicine from Graeco-Roman Times up to the Renaissance," ActT 26 (2006): 265.

[52] For a more detailed discussion, see Amundsen, "Medicine and Faith in Early Christianity," 333–4, 338–41.

Examples of this view can be found throughout the writings of the church fathers. Clement of Alexandria, writing around the end of the second century, asserts that medicine, like many other human achievements, is the product of human reason that has "received the kindling spark from God" (*Strom.* 6.17).[53] His pupil Origen goes even farther, framing medical knowledge as the fruit of divine revelation: "God himself gave medical knowledge to humans, just as he assigned both herbs and other things to grow on the earth." In this knowledge, "those who are adorned with religion [i.e., Christians] use physicians as servants of God" (*Adnot. iii kgs* 15.23). Similar ideas are expressed by John Chrysostom, who insists that "God gave physicians and medicines" to humanity (*Hom. Col.* 8), and Basil of Caesarea, who avers that "the medical art has been entrusted to us by God" (*Rule* 55). Basil specifically underlines the value and God-given nature of healing medicines.

> The herbs which are the specifics for each malady do not grow out of the earth spontaneously; it is evidently the will of the Creator that they should be brought forth out of the soil to serve our need. Therefore, the obtaining of that natural virtue which is in the roots and flowers, leaves, fruits, and juices, or in such metals or products of the sea as are found especially suitable for bodily health, is to be viewed in the same way as the procuring of food and drink. (*Rule* 55)

A number of church fathers show significant familiarity with the practice of medicine. Origen comments several times on the existence of conflicting sects among the physicians (*Cels.* 3.12, 5.61, 5.63, *Hom. in Num.* 3, *Adnot. iii kgs* 15.13) and observes that the best physician is one who studies the various sects and chooses wisely among them (*Cels.* 3.13). He also draws on the popular ideal of the "benevolent physician" as one who searches out the sick and cures them rather than confining his practice to a few rich clients (*Cels.* 3.74, 7.59). Here and there he mentions specific aspects of medical practice, including both physical (regulation of diet and lifestyle, surgery, cauterization, etc.) and psychological (threatening and even lying to patients) modes of treatment (*Cels.* 2.24, 4.18, 4.19, 4.73). For him, there is no doubt that "the science of medicine is useful and necessary to the human race" (*Cels.* 3.12).

References to the medical arts are so common in later writers as to excite little attention. The third-century *Didascalia Apostolorum* uses medical imagery so often that scholars have suspected the author of being a physician. Specific details of medical theory are mentioned by Ambrose, who credits "those skilled in the art of medicine" as the source of his knowledge about the internal workings of the human body (*Hex.* 6.61), and Augustine, who names Hippocrates as his authority for concluding that twins experience different diseases not because of bodily differences but because they have different preferences in food and exercise (*Civ.* 5.2).[54] Basil of Caesarea reveals an awareness of Hippocratic humoral theory when he remarks that "the body suffers affliction from both excess and deficiency" and avers that medicine was given to humans "to guide us in the removal of what is superfluous and in the

---

[53] Some of the references that follow are taken from ibid., 333–4.
[54] Noted by Temkin, *Hippocrates in a World of Pagans and Christians*, 133.

addition of what is lacking." He also encourages his followers to submit to medical treatment and to accept with equanimity such painful medical treatments as cutting, burning, "bitter and disagreeable medicines," abstinence from food, and strict bodily regimens (*Rule* 55).

Yet even those who supported medicine recognized that it has limits: medicine can work only if God so ordains it. Origen insists that "the physician's art has no strength if God is not willing, but it is able to do as much as God wills" (*Adnot. iii kgs* 15.23). While it is perfectly acceptable for Christians to consult physicians, it is even better if they will "rise to the higher and better way of seeking the blessing of Him who is God over all, through piety and prayers" (*Cels.* 8.60). In other words, religious healing is preferable to medical treatment. Similar sentiments are expressed by the fourth-century monk Macarius, who regrets how quickly his fellow monks run to physicians rather than to Christ for healing. Physicians and medicines, he says, were given by God "for the weak and unbelieving . . . who could not yet entrust themselves wholly to God." Monks, on the other hand, should rely on God alone for healing, trusting that the one who cured the disorders of their immortal souls will heal their mortal bodies without the need for "medical attentions and remedies" (*Hom.* 48.4-5).

Augustine, too, voices reservations about giving too much credit to physicians and medicines. "The medicines which people apply to the bodies of their companions," he says, "are of no avail unless God gives them virtue. He can heal without their aid, but they cannot without his" (*Doct. chr.* 4.16.33). Basil of Caesarea labors to strike a balance between medical and religious modes of healing. "To place the hope of one's health in the hands of the doctor is the act of an irrational animal," he warns, yet "to reject entirely the benefits to be derived from this art is the sign of a pettish nature." Christians "should neither repudiate this art altogether, nor does it behoove us to repose all our confidence in it. . . . When reason allows, we call in the doctor, but we do not leave off hoping in God" (*Rule* 55).

Not all Christian leaders were willing to grant even this much credit to medicine. The sharpest criticism comes from the second-century author Tatian, who derided all forms of medicine as elements of a demonic plot to use material things to capture the souls of humans. "By their art," he says, "they turn humans aside from honoring God, contriving to make them trust in herbs and roots" (*Or. Graec.* 17.16). Herbs and roots are not themselves evil since "everything which has good qualities" was made by God, but "the profligacy of the demons has made use of the productions of nature for evil purposes" (17.16). "When they see that humans consent to be served by means of such things," he explains, "they take them and make them their slaves" (17.12).

While most of Tatian's language relates to the use of curative drugs, his criticism extends to all aspects of medicine. "Medicine and everything in it is a form of the same contrivance" (18.1), he says, since it leads people to trust in matter (ὕλη) rather than the power of God (18.2). Those who follow this course will be judged by God, since they are consorting with demons and engaging in idolatry (18:5-6). "Why is he who trusts in the system of matter not willing to trust in God? For what reason do you not approach the more powerful Lord, but rather seek to cure yourself, like the dog with grass, or the stag with a viper, or the hog with river-crabs, or the lion with apes?

Why you deify the objects of nature?" (18:6-8). It is hard to imagine a more complete rejection of the medical arts.[55] For Tatian, only religious healing is valid.

Thus we see that medical healing was by no means uncontroversial in the early church. The use of doctors and medicines was roundly rejected by some church leaders and others accepted the practice only grudgingly for those whose faith in God was lacking. Even those who embraced medical healing worried that Christians might credit a physician or a drug for cures that were in fact performed by God. Religious healing alone could claim acceptance in all circles of Christianity.

One final development that should be included in this section concerns the growing use of the term *Christus medicus* as a title for Jesus. The earliest reference to Jesus as a physician (ἰατρός) occurs in Ignatius *Eph.* 7.2, but nothing is made of it there. It becomes increasingly common in the writings of later authors. Only rarely does it refer to acts of bodily healing performed by Jesus, whether as a man walking around in Palestine or as a spiritual presence within the church. Instead, the title is used metaphorically to describe his power to heal souls from the effects of sin through faith in his death and resurrection.[56] As Isabella Bonati puts it, "Christ is the Divine Healer of the spiritually sick mankind and applies remedies or extirpates sin from the soul exactly like a human practitioner does with cautery and knife."[57] Medical language was also applied quite early to the rites of the church. By the early second century Ignatius was describing the Eucharist as "the medicine (φάρμακον) of immortality, the antidote that preserves us from dying so that we may live forever in Jesus Christ" (*Eph.* 20:6). A few decades later, Tertullian speaks of the waters of baptism as having "medicinal value" for both body and spirit (*Bapt.* 4.5, 5.2).

It would be wrong, however, to conclude from these appropriations of medical language that the authors were seeking to replace physical healing with spiritual healing as if the body was unimportant or the healing ministry of Jesus was a thing of the past. As we saw earlier, several church fathers speak of miraculous healings occurring in their churches, and some even cite them as evidence for the truth of their message about Jesus. Irenaeus is typical in insisting that both physical and spiritual healings are available to those who repent of their sins and turn to Christ in faith, citing Lk. 5:31-32 as evidence (*Haer.* 3.5.2).

> How then shall the sick be strengthened, or how shall sinners come to repentance? Is it by persevering in the very same courses? Or, on the contrary, is it by undergoing a great change and reversal of their former mode of living, by which they have brought upon themselves no slight amount of sickness, and many sins? ... Wherefore the Lord used to impart knowledge to His disciples, by which also it

---

[55] Marcion might be viewed as an even more extreme case if he truly embraced the Gnostic belief that all matter is evil, but doubts have been raised about the evidence on this point. See David E. Wilhite, "Was Marcion a Docetist? The Body of Evidence vs. Tertullian's Argument," *VC* 71 (2016): 1–36.

[56] For a good bibliography on the topic, see Isabella Bonati, "The Un(healthy) Poor: Wealth, Poverty, Medicine and Health-care in the Greco-Roman World," *Akroterion* 49 (2019): 29, n. 48. The earliest use of the term (in Greek) appears in Ignatius, *Eph.* 7:1–2.

[57] Ibid., 30.

was His practice to heal those who were suffering, and to keep back sinners from sin.

Clement of Alexandria uses similar language in describing how "the all-sufficient Physician of humanity, the Savior, heals both body and soul," citing Mk 2:11, Jn 11:43, and Mt. 9:2 in support of his argument.[58] Tertullian adds Isa. 53:4 ("Surely, he has borne our infirmities and carried our diseases") to the collection of prooftexts for viewing Jesus as a healer (*Marc.* 3.17). The Acts of Peter and the Twelve Apostles (second to fourth centuries) depicts Jesus as a physician carrying an unguent box who commands his disciples to "heal the bodies first, therefore, so that through the real powers of healing for their bodies, without medicine of the world, they may believe in you, that you have power to heal the illnesses of the heart also" (8:11–12:19). Cyril of Jerusalem (fourth century) even claims (somewhat spuriously) that the Greek name 'Ιησους means "Healer." He goes on to describe Jesus as a "physician of souls and bodies, curer of spirits, curing the blind in body, and leading minds into light, healing the visibly lame, and guiding sinners' steps to repentance" (*Catech.* 10.13). Lest his hearers should think that he was referring only to Jesus's healing activities in the past, he adds, "If any is encompassed also with bodily ailments, let him not be faithless, but let him draw near; for to such diseases also Jesus ministers, and let him learn that Jesus is the Christ."

Statements such as these show clearly that the church fathers never meant for their references to Jesus as a physician of souls to replace the conviction that he cures bodies. In fact, reports of miraculous bodily healings actually increased in the third and fourth centuries at the same time that *Christus medicus* was growing in popularity as a designation for Jesus.[59] But the practice of depicting Jesus as a physician, whether for bodies or for souls, does represent a new development in Christian thought and rhetoric when compared with the New Testament era.

Conclusion

Exploring what patristic authors said about sickness and healing does not give us any direct information about how Paul viewed these issues, but it does alert us to some of the theological and practical options that would have been available to him if he had wanted to address them. Investigating what ordinary Christians were doing during this era is more helpful as it gives us a set of real-world data to guide our speculations about what Paul's followers might have done to treat their health problems.

All of the authors that we examined held positive views of religious healing as long as it centered on the God of the Bible. Appealing to other gods for aid is useless because all healing comes from God, even when it is credited to other deities. Miraculous

---

[58] This and several other references in this section are taken from Christoffer H. Grundmann, "Christ as Physician: The Ancient *Christus Medicus* Trope and Christian Medical Missions as Imitation of Christ," *Christian Journal for Global Health* 5 (2018): 3–11.

[59] The pattern is documented by Gary Ferngern in "Early Christianity as a Religion of Healing," 10–13, and "Medicine and Christianity in the Roman Empire," 2967–8.

healings are possible if God wills it, but prayer and loving care by fellow believers are the usual channels by which God restores health. Christians who are not immediately healed should be patient and trust in God as they seek to learn what lessons God might want to teach them through the experience.

More disagreement can be observed on the subject of magical healing. Patristic authors warned their followers against practicing *mageia*, but few of them included healing under this heading until late in the patristic era. Exorcistic healing was accepted by virtually all Christian authors, but they disagreed over the use of amulets and incantations. Appeals to the Bible were useless for resolving such questions since texts could be cited on both sides of every question. Almost nothing is said about the propriety of consulting experts who used "magical" healing techniques except that rituals involving direct interaction with other gods are to be avoided.

Finally, the use of physicians and medical healing was approved by virtually all patristic authors with the caveat that Christians must recognize that the physician's power to heal comes from the one true God and not from Asklepios or other deities. Whether this approval extended to seeking medical care at Asklepian sanctuaries is unclear. A handful of authors rejected medical healing entirely as a betrayal of Christians' loyalty to God, while others permitted it for ordinary believers while commending religious healing for those with more faith.

When we turn to examine what Christians were actually doing in this era to maintain or restore their health, we find ourselves in a different world. The persistent efforts by patristic authors to lead their congregations away from "pagan" healing practices suggest that a significant percentage of Christians—perhaps even the majority—continued using the same health care methods that they had employed before turning to Christ. Some visited Asklepian temples and healing centers for treatment, a practice that may have included participation in cultic rituals, while others consulted "magical" healers who plied them with spells, incantations, "magical" substances, purifications, exorcisms, and other curative rituals. Virtually everyone wore amulets to cure or protect them from illness and injury, some of which were marked with symbols and language representing pagan deities. Physicians and medical treatment were less available to the laboring masses, and those who could access their services did not necessarily hold them in higher esteem than other practitioners.

In short, there was a substantial gap between the healing practices recommended by Christian leaders and those practiced by their congregations. The leaders fought long and hard to motivate their followers to change their behaviors, but their efforts were slow to bear fruit. As late as the fifth century Christians were still using healing practices that were condemned by church authorities, and many of them survived into the medieval era.

Whether similar conditions prevailed in Paul's churches is unclear, but it is hard to see any reason for supposing that his followers behaved differently than later generations. The idea that Christians were more serious about their faith in the early days is a romanticization that has no place in historical analysis. Even if it were true, it begs the question of whether Paul or anyone else believed that change was needed in this area. The fact that none of these practices are mentioned in the New Testament suggests that they did not. What we should make of this fact will be examined in the next two chapters.

9

Paul and the Greco-Roman Health Care System

Putting Paul in His Place

In the previous chapters we explored the complex array of health care options that was available in the Greco-Roman world around the time of Paul and the diverse ways in which Judeans and Christian engaged with those options. Now the time has come to shift our focus back to Paul himself. What kinds of health care providers might the apostle Paul have consulted when dealing with an illness and injury and which ones might he have avoided? What kinds of treatments might he have accepted or rejected? What might he have taught his followers about these vital matters, and how do we explain his relative silence on the subject in his letters?

Questions such as these have been largely overlooked by historians of early Christianity, whether because they were unaware of the problems or because there is so little direct evidence on which to base our answers. But we do have mountains of indirect evidence about how people viewed and treated sicknesses and injuries in Paul's era, and we know from Paul's letters (and from the book of Acts, insofar as it contains historical material) that he suffered numerous episodes of illness and injury that would have compelled him to seek some form of care. We can also infer from historical patterns that the same would have been true for the people in his churches.

Based on what we have learned about the entanglement of religion with all forms of healing in Greco-Roman antiquity and the consistency of Paul's polemics against non-Christian religions, we might expect that Paul would oppose the use of any health care provider or treatment that was not associated with a Judean or Christian community. But our investigation of what other Judeans and Christians were saying and doing in the centuries before and after Paul has revealed no such pattern. Here and there an elite author voices concern about practices that they deemed particularly egregious—primarily those that involved direct engagement with "pagan" deities or *daimones*—but for the most part they seem to have viewed Greco-Roman health care practices as non-controversial. Certainly their followers did. Virtually all of the evidence shows that ordinary Judeans and Christians used the same health care practices as their friends and neighbors, regardless of what their leaders said on the subject. Such gaps between the ideas of elite authors and the broader populace are common in virtually every culture, past and present.

So where did Paul fit in? Was he one of those leaders who avoided and sought to divert others from using "pagan" healing practices? Or did he pursue a more pragmatic path, allowing and applying whatever health care practices proved effective? Did he limit himself (and his followers) to the religious modes of treatment that he mentions in his letters (prayer and spiritual healing), or did he accept medical and "magical" techniques as well? Did he consult only Judean and Christian healers, or did he also seek treatment from non-Christian practitioners? Did he do whatever they prescribed, or did he follow some of their prescriptions and not others? Would he have had any reservations about following a special dietary regimen or submitting to blood-letting? What if the healer wanted to perform an exorcistic ritual or told him to wear an amulet or recite an incantation? Would it matter to him if the practitioner worked at an Asklepian temple or healing center? What did he think about the miraculous cures that Asklepios was reputed to perform at such places?

And what are we to make of the fact that he says nothing about these matters in his letters? Did he regard them as unimportant, or did the issue simply not come up at the time he was writing the letters that we now possess? Might his own experiences with sickness and healing have led him to think that he had nothing useful to say on the subject? Or had he given his congregations such clear instructions when he was with them that it never again arose as a source of controversy? If the latter was the case, what did he tell them in the first place? Do his passing references to "gifts of healings" and "signs and wonders" give us any insight into his beliefs on the subject?

As we noted in the Introduction, all attempts to answer such questions are speculative, but that does not mean that all answers are equally probable. A careful review of some of the options for making sense of what we do and do not see in Paul's letters can help us to sort out which possibilities have greater historical plausibility and which ones are improbable, anachronistic, tendentious, or otherwise unhelpful.

Following are eight possible explanations for Paul's relative silence on the subjects of sickness and healing in his letters. Some include speculations about what Paul might have thought and done on the subject while others do not. The first three proposals share a belief that Paul was uninterested in such questions, while the others argue that Paul must have had opinions on the subject but for one reason or another did not mention them in his letters. Some of the proposals are mutually exclusive, while others are not. Some are more credible or complete than others, and all involve a certain amount of guesswork. Even those that are less likely contain ideas that have been put forward by interpreters at one time or another, and all of them raise important issues that must be addressed in any serious attempt to make sense of Paul's views.

1. *Paul wanted his followers to focus on right beliefs and right living rather than pursuing divine favors or mystical experiences.* The view of Paul as a rational theologian who championed a rational faith has a long pedigree in post-Enlightenment scholarship, which has focused on explicating Paul's theology and ethics to the neglect of his religious experience apart from his "conversion."[1] The task of the scholar under this model is to clarify and systematize the theological concepts and moral teachings that are stated or implied in Paul's letters, not to speculate about his spiritual life. Passages where Paul speaks of "signs and wonders" and works of "power" accompanying his ministry or about Spirit-given *charismata* in his churches are either explained away

---

[1] Graham Twelftree discusses this trend in *Paul and the Miraculous*, 5–11.

or ignored, as are many other subjects on which he has little to say, including sickness and healing.

Scholars who defend this reading insist that they are being true to Paul's intentions, which were to teach his followers how to understand and live out their Christian faith in a manner that accorded with the will of God. Mystical experiences play at best a minimal role in this interpretation of Paul and his letters, while irrational and superstitious ideas and practices (including "magic") are excluded entirely, especially those linked to pagan deities. In short, Paul is a heroic forerunner of European Protestantism who championed "faith alone" against the magical thinking and superstitious practices that Protestants associated with medieval Catholicism.

This reading of Paul is undoubtedly correct in giving preeminence to Paul's message about the Christ-event and its implications. But it is also reductionistic insofar as it limits Paul's concern to these issues. Paul clearly valued rational argumentation, but he was also a mystic, a man who not only prayed often but also claimed to receive visions and revelations from God, believed that the Spirit of God (or Christ) lived in and spoke through him, "prayed in tongues" on a regular basis, and experienced "signs and wonders" in connection with his preaching. He also exhorted his followers to seek zealously after "spiritual gifts," including the power to heal, and offered practical guidance about how to manage their use so that the entire congregation could benefit from them (1 Cor. 14). Particularly troubling for this interpretation is Paul's repeated description of his preaching as foolishness to the "wise" (1 Cor. 1:18-31) and his insistence that the Corinthians' faith arose not from trusting in "plausible words of wisdom" but from "a demonstration of the Spirit and of power, so that your faith might rest not on human wisdom but on the power of God" (1 Cor. 2:4-5). Texts such as these pose serious problems for any claim that Paul was not interested in or tried to minimize the importance of religious experience in his churches, including miraculous healing.

This interpretation is correct, however, in insisting that Paul limited religious experiences to the God of Israel and his son Jesus Christ; encounters with other deities are off-limits for Christ-followers. Those who sacrifice at pagan temples are in reality "sacrificing to demons and not to God" (1 Cor. 10:20). "I do not want you to be partners with demons," he says. "You cannot drink the cup of the Lord and the cup of demons. You cannot partake of the table of the Lord and the table of demons" (1 Cor. 10:20-21). Whether he would have viewed non-sacrificial rituals such as spells and incantations in the same light is unclear, but the forcefulness of his injunctions suggests that he would at least have probed them for links with other gods.

2. *Paul was concerned about the spiritual health of his followers, not their physical health.* This interpretation rests on a reading of Paul's letters that sees him devaluing material concerns in favor of the spiritual. One version holds that Paul's theology is fundamentally Platonic and anti-material. The body itself is not evil, but it provides a channel for the expression of "fleshly" desires that can undermine the influence of the spirit (or Spirit) and thus needs to be kept in check and not pampered.[2] Another version highlights the apocalyptic nature of Paul's theology, which discourages entanglements

---

[2] This view was championed by Daniel Boyarin in *A Radical Jew: Paul and the Politics of Identity* (Berkeley: University of California Press, 1994).

with the social and material world in order to be ready when a new spiritual kingdom is revealed with the imminent return of Christ and the corresponding end of the present order (1 Cor. 7:17-24, 7:29-35; 2 Cor. 6.14–7.1; 1 Cor. 15). The mortal and suffering body that believers now inhabit is a temporary vessel that will soon be replaced by a new body that is immune to sickness and injury. In the meantime, Christ-followers must wage unceasing war against the demonic forces that would use their bodily desires to entangle them in earthly affairs and distract their attention from the victory of God and the bodily transformation that will soon take place.

Neither of these readings leaves much room for Paul or his followers to be concerned about bodily illness or injury. In fact, excessive concern for physical health could be taken as a sign that one is lacking in faith. Paul's silence about such matters is thus understandable since the body is unimportant to his way of thinking. What matters is the realm of the spirit, or the reign of God. Bodily suffering is endemic to human existence, but Christ-followers can transcend its effect by looking "not at what can be seen but at what cannot be seen; for what can be seen is temporary, but what cannot be seen is eternal" (2 Cor. 4:18).

This proposal can account for a significant amount of the data in Paul's letters, but it says nothing about what Paul might have taught his followers regarding the treatment of physical ailments (including whether it is acceptable to consult "pagan" health practitioners) nor how he might have handled his own illnesses and injuries. It is certainly possible that Paul's anti-material or apocalyptic theology made him uninterested in such questions, but it is hard to see how he could have avoided the subject entirely as his followers surely would have pressed him for guidance in view of the close association between healing rituals and pagan deities. More significantly, it is hard to see how this interpretation accords with Paul's references to "gifts of healings" in 1 Corinthians 12 or his lengthy discussions of such equally physical questions as whether it is appropriate to eat meat that has been ritually offered to a non-Christian deity (1 Corinthians 8 and 10) or to have sex with a prostitute (1 Cor. 6:15-20) or one's spouse (1 Cor. 7:1-6). If Paul cared enough to offer guidance on these bodily issues, why would he remain silent about sickness and healing, where questions of possible idolatry were even more pressing?

3. *Paul said little about healing because he struggled with it in his own life.* While Paul assures the Corinthians that the Spirit of God bestows "gifts of healings" upon members of the local *ekklesia* for the good of others, he gives no sign that either he or his co-workers benefited from these curative powers. When referring to his initial visit to the Galatians δι' ἀσθένειαν τῆς σαρκὸς, for example, he says nothing about anyone in their community attempting to use charismatic gifts to heal him.[3] His statement that his sickness was a "trial" to the Galatians (4:14) suggests that his recovery was long and slow. He must have received some sort of treatment for his illness during this time, but

---

[3] The reference in Gal. 3:5 to the Spirit continuing to perform miracles in the Galatian churches has suggested to some that they experienced *charismata* like those in 1 Corinthians 12, including "gifts of healings."

he says nothing about what it entailed.⁴ The same is true for the many illnesses and injuries that he narrates in 2 Cor. 11:23-9.

Similar observations can be made about Epaphroditus in Phil. 2:25-30: he eventually recovered from his near-fatal illness, but Paul is silent about how it happened. He gives no sign that Spirit-enabled healers were involved, so the natural inference is that Epaphroditus recovered normally under the care of some type of health care provider. Yet another situation in which divine healing was available but proved ineffectual involves Christ-followers in Corinth who experienced sickness and death following what Paul describes as unworthy participation in the communion meal (1 Cor. 11:29-30). The fact that some of their fellow congregants possessed "gifts of healings" appears to have made no difference in their case. Paul's attribution of their fate to sinful conduct does not mitigate the likelihood that some of the Corinthians had tried without success to use "spiritual gifts" to heal them.

Finally, there is Paul's experience with the ailment that he calls a "thorn in the flesh" in 2 Cor 12:7-9. Whether he pursued any form of treatment other than prayer is unclear, but his failure to receive healing from this annoying condition could have undermined his confidence that he had anything meaningful to say about matters of physical healing.

Taken together, these observations have suggested to some interpreters that Paul said little about physical healing in his letters because his own experience had led him to question his competence on the subject. The fact that he refers to "signs and wonders" and acts of "power" occurring in conjunction with his preaching does not undermine this proposal, since Paul never says that he himself initiated these acts nor that they included healing.

Whether such an interpretation makes sense on psychological and historical grounds, on the other hand, is open to question. If his ideas about healing were so deeply grounded in his own experience, we might expect that his failure to receive divine healing would have caused him to question not just his competence in this area but his very claim of being an apostle of Christ and having Christ working through him since the life-giving power of Christ was not evident in his sickly body. We know that his bodily weakness led others to doubt his credentials (2 Cor. 10:10, 13:3-4), and Paul himself acknowledges the problem in 1 Cor. 2:3-4 when he says that it was an unexplained "demonstration of the Spirit and of power" that overcame the negative impression that his weak (or sick) body had made upon the Corinthians.

Yet he never doubts that Christ has called him to serve as his apostle. Instead, he launches a frontal assault on his critics by claiming that his sufferings are a mark of his apostleship (1 Cor. 4:9-13; 2 Cor. 4:7-12; 11:22-28). In this way he rhetorically severs the universally accepted link between physical suffering and divine displeasure. Even when he is not cured, he says, God assists him in his weakness (2 Cor. 12:9-10). Such a claim makes sense when applied to injuries that he received while pursuing his missionary calling, such as when he was stoned and left for dead, but it sounds like special pleading when applied to ordinary bouts of sickness, including the "the previously mentioned 'thorn in the flesh'".⁵ Whether anyone took him seriously is impossible to say.

---

⁴ Some have suggested that Luke "the beloved physician" (Col. 4:14) served Paul in this capacity, but this theory depends (among other things) on what one believes about the authorship of Colossians.
⁵ More will be said later about the lessons that he learned from this particular experience of sickness.

The other problem with this interpretation is that it cannot explain why Paul says nothing in his letters about what healing methods he used. If his theology was rooted in his experience and he had to make decisions about what modes of treatment to accept for his own body, why does he not draw on that experience to offer guidance to his churches regarding which forms of healing are permissible and effective and which are not? Given the deep cultural ties between healing and religion, he would have had to wrestle with these questions himself, and we can be equally sure that people in his churches would have pressed him on this point. The fact that he does offer guidance on other issues with which he had no personal experience (idolatry, adultery, suing fellow believers, etc.) suggests that experience was not vital to Paul's theological reflection. In short, while this interpretation contains useful observations, it leaves unanswered a number of important questions pertaining to Paul's beliefs and practices on matters of sickness and healing.

4. *Paul followed other Jews in rejecting miraculous and magical modes of healing in favor of religious and medical cures.* This explanation, like the previous one, takes Paul's historical setting and experience more seriously than the first two, but its value is undermined by a faulty view of first-century CE Judaism. While it is true that we see a reaction against the miraculous in some rabbinic texts, several lines of evidence show that this was not the case in Paul's day. Josephus reports a number of miraculous events in the course of his narratives, including a series of omens that portended the fall of Jerusalem and his own prophecy of Vespasian's accession to the imperial throne, and not once does he evince the least embarrassment about their supernatural qualities. Several of the Qumran texts show an interest in healing and exorcisms, and even the rabbinic literature tells of men like Honi the Circle-Drawer and Hanina ben Dosa who are reputed to have performed miraculous cures and exorcisms around the time of Jesus.

A similar picture emerges from the Christian Gospels, where not one Judean character argues that the healing miracles of Jesus (or anyone else, for that matter) are inherently impossible. Their complaints pertain rather to the location or timing of his healings, or the source of his power. In fact, Judeans and Christians were so famous for believing in miraculous cures that the second-century Roman physician Galen voiced amazement at their credulity. And of course, we cannot overlook Paul's own language about "gifts of healings" and his references to "signs and wonders" and acts of "power" that occurred alongside his missionary preaching. Paul was, after all, a Judean.

Regarding "magical" healing, we saw in Chapter 7 how many texts from Greek, Roman, and Christian authors testify to the reputation of Judeans as experts in *mageia* who used incantations and spells to heal the sick. The validity of this view is confirmed by Judean texts such as Tobit, Jubilees, Sibylline Oracles, and Josephus that depict Judeans engaging in "magical" healing practices. Two of these texts, Jubilees and Sibylline Oracles, describe the knowledge of magical arts as a divine boon to humanity. Rabbinic texts speak of Torah scholars performing magical rituals, including healings, while other texts indicate that even rabbis who rejected such practices carved out an exception for actions that improved the health of humans or animals. Material evidence confirms what the literary texts tell us about the popularity of protective and curative amulets throughout the Second Temple and rabbinic periods.

Of course, texts can be cited on the other side as well, but the evidence presented here and in Chapter 7 suggests that it would be wrong to presume that Paul's identity as a zealous Jew would have compelled him to avoid (or teach others to avoid) any of the four health care systems described in this study—traditional, magical, religious, and medical. In fact, we cannot say with certainty that he would have discouraged his gentile Christ-followers from seeking treatment at an Asklepian healing center or wearing an amulet marked with "pagan" religious symbols as long as they did not participate in cultic veneration of a non-Christian deity or credit such a god with curing their illness. Both Jewish rabbis and patristic authors acknowledged that people were healed at Asklepian shrines, with some attributing the cures to the God of Israel and others to *daimones*. We also have evidence that at least some Judeans and Christians visited the temples of Greek or Roman deities from time to time, a practice that Paul seems to tolerate in 1 Cor. 8:10 when he mentions without criticism the possibility that a gentile Christ-follower might be "eating in the temple of an idol." It is hard to imagine Paul himself engaging in such activities in view of his polemics against "worthless idols," but we should at least allow for the possibility that he, like the later rabbis, did not include practices that produced healing under the heading of "idolatry."

5. *Paul approved only treatments performed by Christ-followers.* This solution is based on the premise that Paul was a radical sectarian who sought to maintain sharp boundaries between his followers and people outside the Christ-movement. A parallel can be found in his handling of lawsuits between believers (1 Cor. 6:1-8): just as he insisted that disputes should be handled within the church and not by outsiders, so also he would have recommended that illness be treated by fellow Christ-followers and not by people outside the community. What matters, according to this view, is not what healing techniques are used but who performs them. A Hippocratic physician who joined the Christ-movement would gain the right to treat people within the *ekklesia* whereas practitioners who used similar methods but were not part of the community would be excluded. A similar standard would apply to "magical" healers, with the caveat that practices involving direct appeals to non-Christian deities would be prohibited in any event since radical monotheism was a core element of Paul's theology.

Practices that were less overtly religious in nature, such as root-cutting rituals or wearing amulets, would be permissible under this proposal as long as they were performed by Christ-followers, and it is not impossible that religious rituals commonly associated with outsiders might be rendered acceptable if they could be adapted to a Christian theological framework, such as exorcism or incantations. Divine healing by people empowered by God's Spirit (the "gifts of healings" that Paul mentions in 1 Cor. 12:9) would also play a significant role in the community's health care system under this proposal, though whether such methods would be applied first, last, or coincident with other practices is impossible to say.

Implicit in this model is the presumption that outsiders are either incompetent or dangerous due to their association with non-Christian deities, whom Paul derides as harmful "demons" in 1 Cor. 10:20-21, or with Satan himself, whom Paul describes as "the god of this αἰών" (2 Cor. 4:4). What should be done when Christian healers with the requisite skills were unavailable or when their efforts proved unavailing is not addressed by this proposal. A strict interpretation would suggest that he would have counseled his followers to limit treatments to unoffensive methods of self-care coupled with prayers and nursing by family or friends. A more liberal reading might leave room for treatment by Judean physicians on the grounds they, too, are servants of the one true God. Whether other outsiders might have been permitted to treat extreme cases depends on how radically we envision Paul's monotheistic sectarianism.

This reconstruction of Paul's thinking is consistent with his apocalyptic tendency to draw sharp lines between insiders and outsiders (Rom. 9:22-33; 1 Cor. 2:12-16; 5:9-13; 10:14-21; 2 Cor. 4:3-4; 6:14-7:1, etc.), and it also takes seriously the likelihood that he would have felt obligated to offer some sort of guidance to his followers regarding what they could and could not do to treat illness. But the fact that Paul never actually says any of these things leaves the proposal squarely in the realm of speculation.

6. *Paul approved only the modes of health care that he mentions in his letters.* This explanation takes Paul's silence about non-religious modes of treatment as intentional: he expected his followers to use only those remedies that he mentions in his letters and to patiently endure suffering if a cure is not forthcoming. This solution is essentially a more radical version of the previous one, since the range of treatments that Paul explicitly approves is very narrow and (mostly) "Christian."

At the head of this list stands prayer. Paul tells the Corinthians that he prayed repeatedly for God to intervene when he was afflicted by his "thorn in the flesh" (2 Cor. 12:8), and he often asks his hearers to pray that God will protect him from various forms of danger (Rom. 15:30-31, 2 Cor. 1:10-11, Phil. 1:19-20; cf. Eph. 6:19-20). In cases where believers feel unable to pray, he promises them support from the divine Spirit that dwells within them: "The Spirit helps us in our weakness [ἀσθένεια]; for we do not know how to pray as we ought, but that very Spirit intercedes with sighs too deep for words" (Rom. 8:26). The Greek word ἀσθένεια can also be rendered as "sickness," a meaning that would not have escaped Paul's audience.

The second mode of treatment that Paul explicitly approves is the "gifts of healings" that he cites in 1 Cor. 12:9. Paul does not explain what he means by this phrase, and interpreters have understood it differently. Paul includes it in a list of "manifestations of the Spirit" that God distributes to believers for the common good, but it is not clear whether he is referring to the Spirit-guided application of ordinary healing skills or the performance of miraculous cures. The list includes both types of activities, with "gifts of healings" standing at the rhetorical fulcrum between three ordinary human abilities (wisdom, knowledge, faith) and five that require divine action ("works of power," prophecy, discerning spirits, praying in tongues, interpreting tongues). The fact that "works of power" is listed separately has led some to suppose that "gifts of healings" refers to non-miraculous acts, but it is just as possible that Paul coined the phrase as a designation for other types of miracles. However we interpret it, it is clear that Paul is pointing with approval to a distinctly "Christian" mode of healing in which the Spirit of God ministers to the needs of Christ-followers through the hands (and prayers?) of their fellow believers.

Whether the same phenomenon lies behind Paul's references to "signs and wonders" (Rom. 15:18-19, 2 Cor. 12:12) and works of "power" (Gal. 3:5, 1 Cor. 2:4-5, 1 Thess. 1:5; cf. 1 Cor, 4:20, 2 Cor. 6:7) is less clear.[6] Many have taken the duality of the phrase

---

[6] Several of the works cited in this study include extended commentaries on these verses—see Twelftree, *Paul and the Miraculous*, 180–225; Schreiber, *Paulus also Wundertäter*, 181–270; Nielsen, *Heilung und Verkündigung*, 188–206; Gatzweiler, "La Conception Paulinienne du Miracle," 813–46.

"signs and wonders" as a reference to two distinct manifestations of divine activity, generally thought to be healing and exorcism. But the phrase comes directly from the LXX where it never refers to either of these activities,[7] and Paul says nothing about exorcism in any of his letters. The latter observation is inexplicable if demon expulsion played such a vital role in validating his message. In the end, what Paul meant by this term is unknowable.

The same is true for his references to works of "power." Paul uses the word δύναμις in a variety of senses in his letters, most often in relation to God or the Spirit, but the referents are too diverse to shed any meaningful light on what Paul meant in these passages. It is certainly possible that Paul was referring to miraculous healings and that "gifts of healings" was his shorthand designation for the Spirit's ongoing performance of similar miracles in his absence, but there is no evidence to support this reading. In short, none of these cryptic texts add any new information to our understanding of Paul's view of healing.

The only other healing practice that might perhaps be inferred from Paul's language is nursing care. Paul alludes to something like this in Gal. 4:13-15, where he recalls how the Galatians welcomed him in his infirmity and "had it been possible, would have torn out your eyes and given them to me." Nursing the sick would also seem to be implied in his repeated injunctions to believers to care for one another in times of suffering (Rom. 12:13-15, 1 Cor. 12:26, 2 Cor. 1:3-7, Gal. 6:2, Phil. 2:4, 1 Thess. 5:14), while his rhetorical question in 2 Cor. 11:29 ("Who is weak, and I am not weak?") points in the same direction. It is also hard to imagine him sitting back and doing nothing during the lengthy illness of his companion Epaphroditus that he mentions in Phil. 2:25-29. The fact that he never speaks explicitly about caring for the sick and debilitated is curious, but such practices are so crucial to all forms of health care that he might have taken it for granted that his followers would do so.

The most common prescription for suffering in Paul's letters is patient endurance. He does not apply this specifically to health problems, but his own struggles with illness and injury make it highly likely that he would have included them under this heading. If this is correct, we might say that Paul is more concerned with treating the psychological than the bodily aspects of illness. He does not dissuade his followers from attempting to eliminate the cause of their suffering, as he did when he asked God three times to remove his "thorn in the flesh" (2 Cor. 12:8), but he does insist that they learn to accept whatever occurs in the knowledge that God is with them in their suffering and will strengthen them to endure it (2 Cor. 4:17-18, 12:9-10, Phil. 4:12-13). He also assures them that patient endurance will produce positive results for the sufferers even if they are not healed (Rom. 5:3-4, 8:18, 8:28, etc.). He repeatedly cites his own experience as proof of his words, though only once (2 Corinthians 12) does he mention how his own failure to obtain physical healing contributed to his adoption of a more psychological approach to dealing with sickness.

The importance of this latter observation has often been noted by interpreters, many of whom have found in it the key to Paul's view of sickness. It certainly exercised

---

[7] For a brief, but helpful, survey of the evidence, see S. Vernon McCasland, "Signs and Wonders," *JBL* 76 (1957): 149–52. A fuller treatment appears in Eyl, *Signs, Wonders, and Gifts*, 88–122.

a profound influence on the church fathers, as Darrel Amundsen has shown.[8] But it is not clear under this model how Paul would have advised his gentile followers regarding other healing practices that they had used for their entire lives. Is it really possible that he meant for them to avoid all such practices in favor of prayer, nursing, and miraculous cures and to suffer patiently with God's help if those methods did not produce a cure? Such a radical proposal would surely have required a fuller explanation and a more forceful rhetorical effort than we see in Paul's letters, unless we presume that he had already persuaded all of his followers to adopt this view when he was with them. Even then, one would think that periodic reminders would be required to maintain such a sharp rupture with both past experience and present culture, something like Paul's handling of sexual practices. But nothing like this appears in Paul's letters. In short, while it is useful to sift Paul's writings carefully for insights regarding his views on sickness and healing, there is no reason to limit ourselves to that information.

7. *Paul practiced and approved a variety of healing methods but had no reason to discuss them in his letters.* This solution differs from the others that we have examined in two respects: it takes Paul's relative silence on the issue of healing as incidental rather than as evidence that it was unimportant in his ministry, and it reads his lack of commentary on healing techniques through a permissive rather than a restrictive lens.

On the first point, scholars have long debated how much of the ambiguity in Paul's letters is due to their occasional nature. For example, we would have known nothing about what Paul's followers did in their congregational meetings, including the role of "charismatic gifts" in their gatherings, if the latter had not become a source of controversy within their community. The fact that Paul had spent time with most of his addressees also allowed him to allude to prior teachings and events in a way that would have made sense to his audiences but is too vague or ambiguous for modern interpreters to be certain what he meant. Virtually all of Paul's references to sickness and healing fall under this heading, including the apparently miraculous "signs and wonders" that accompanied his preaching and the "gifts of healings" that he mentions in 1 Corinthians 12. The same is true for several texts in which he refers to his own illnesses and bodily weakness and those of his companions, especially Epaphroditus in Philippians 2. Interpreters who wish to paint Paul as a rational theologian have tended to minimize or provide naturalistic explanations for such passages, but it is also possible to read them together with other texts as signs that "miraculous" and even "magical" practices played a greater role in Paul's ministry than many scholars have thought.[9]

Similar observations lie behind the second part of this proposed solution, the idea that Paul used and approved more healing practices than he mentions in his letters. As has been pointed out repeatedly in this study, the question of whether it was appropriate for Christ-followers to continue using traditional modes of healing in view of their association with "pagan" deities must have come up, and the fact that Paul says

---

[8] "Medicine and Christianity in the Roman Empire," 334–7.
[9] This is the argument of Graham Twelftree, whose careful survey of the evidence led him to conclude that "the miraculous was central and profoundly important in his life, theology, and work" (*Paul and the Miraculous*, 314).

nothing about such matters in his letters could be taken as a sign that he saw no reason for them to change what they were doing, apart from avoiding rituals that involved explicit worship of other gods. The same logic would suggest that Paul himself sought healing from a panoply of providers and methods, perhaps even a broader range than he would have used before becoming a Christ-follower.

In short, this model suggests that the distinctly "Christian" modes of healing that Paul mentions in his letters were offered as additions to and not as replacements for traditional methods of health care. Whether he expected his followers to apply these church-based methods as a first or last resort or along with other forms of treatment cannot be determined from the evidence.

While arguments from silence are always precarious, support for this reading might be found in Paul's handling of the "idol meat" question, where he states that eating meat from animals sacrificed to other gods is permissible since the so-called gods of the nations have no real existence (1 Cor. 8:4). The only exception is when eating might lead a fellow believer to act contrary to conscience with regard to the worship of such gods (1 Cor. 8:7-13). Elsewhere he says that they should eat whatever is put before them and not ask questions about its origins (1 Cor. 10:25-27). If we apply this same rationale to the question of healing practices, we might infer that Paul would have counseled his followers to use whatever means of treatment lay at hand without inquiring into the practitioner's religious proclivities or methods. This is precisely the opinion that we find in the later rabbinic corpus, as described in Chapter 7.

If this was his position, however, why does he not mention it in his letters? Again we are left to draw inferences from silence. The most credible explanation is that he had already explained his position to his followers in person and it never again arose as a point of controversy because he was not advising them to change their behaviors. If there was no call for change, there was no reason to discuss the matter further. This answer has the dual benefit of taking seriously the likelihood that healing practices would have arisen early as a cause of concern among Paul's followers and providing a credible explanation for his silence on the subject in his letters. It also accords well with what we saw in Chapters 7 and 8 about how ordinary Judeans and Christians continued to use the same healing methods as their peers in the centuries following Paul.

It is not clear, however, whether this solution takes seriously enough the entanglement of religion in all forms of Greco-Roman health care, and it might also conflict with Paul's reference to φαρμακεία (a word that can refer to the use of medicinal drugs or sorcery) in a list of "works of the flesh" that Christ-followers should avoid (Gal. 5:20). It also leaves open the question of whether there were any limits on what Paul would have accepted as legitimate remedies. There is little doubt that he would have rejected practices that involved direct appeals to other gods, such as presenting offerings to a statue of Asklepios or reciting an incantation that called on a Greek or Roman god to procure healing. But what would he have thought about his followers visiting an Asklepian sanctuary to consult with a physician, or wearing an amulet marked with "pagan" symbols, or consuming a medicine made from a plant that was harvested using "magical" rituals? What about seeking treatment from a doctor who was also a priest of Asklepios, or a Judean who rejected the Christian gospel? Such questions are impossible to answer with confidence, but they are useful as thought-experiments to help us work through the possible implications of this and other interpretations of what Paul does and does not say about sickness and healing.

8. *Paul's opinions about proper and improper modes of healing are beyond recovery since he says virtually nothing about them in his letters.* This last option might sound like a counsel of despair, but it is important to be honest about what we can and cannot achieve when speculating about subjects that Paul addresses only briefly or not at all in his letters. All of our efforts to reconstruct what Paul thought about matters of health care are based on very slender evidence, and good arguments can be made for a variety of different interpretations.

Still, not all of these interpretations are equal; some have more support than others. For example, it is highly improbable that Paul never reflected on the propriety of using "pagan" modes of health care in view of his own experiences with illness and injury, the practical importance of the issue to his followers, and the theological questions that it raised. It is also hard to believe that he gave such clear instruction on the subject when visiting his churches that it never again arose as a point of controversy, with the possible exception of the permissive option that was discussed under the previous heading. Paul himself admits that he was not an especially good orator (1 Cor. 2:1-5, 2 Cor. 10:1, 10:10-11, 11:6), and the disputes that arose after his departure on such topics as circumcision and sexual conduct show that his instruction on these topics was insufficient to forestall further debate. But such observations cannot tell us what he thought and said on the subject, and the paucity of evidence in his letters renders all solutions suspect.

In the end, all that we have is a range of possibilities for which solid evidence is lacking. The options are so diverse and their implications for Paul's theology and practice so significant that even the most creative interpreter might be tempted to declare the situation hopeless. But similar barriers have not prevented historians and theologians from making informed judgments about other thorny issues in Paul's letters and arguing for their interpretations against the differing judgments of other scholars. Speculation is inherent in the historical enterprise, and there is no reason for us to avoid it as long as we recognize the limits of our reasoning. Responsible historiography demands no less.

Weighing the Options

What then can we responsibly say about Paul's views on sickness and healing? A careful sifting of the interpretive options discussed earlier reveals three broad themes that must be included in any valid reconstruction of Paul's thought and several points of difference where judgments must be made among competing viewpoints. A brief review of these themes will give us a set of parameters for assessing the relative validity of the various proposals that we have considered thus far.

The Experience of Suffering

Paul's ideas about sickness and healing were undoubtedly shaped by his bodily experience. He alludes repeatedly to various types of sufferings that he endured while pursuing his evangelistic mission, including sicknesses and injuries. Some of these afflictions were caused by natural forces (heat and cold, storms, shipwreck, etc.), while others were imposed by civic authorities and other opponents. Paul was not the only evangelist who suffered in this way; Epaphroditus was so sick that he nearly died (Phil. 2:25-30), and there is no reason to suppose that his experience was unique.

Several passages in Paul's letters suggest that these sufferings had produced some kind of temporary or permanent bodily disability that caused others to look down on him. The most obvious example is 2 Corinthians 12, where he recalls how God had told him that he would have to live out his life with an unknown bodily ailment that he describes metaphorically as "a thorn in the flesh."[10] This or a similar condition is probably implied in Gal. 6:17, where he speaks of carrying "the marks of Jesus" on his body; 2 Cor. 4:10, where at the end of a list of sufferings he describes himself as "always bearing in the body the death of Jesus"; and 2 Cor. 10:10, where he quotes his opponents as saying that "his bodily presence is weak." His admission in 2 Cor. 13:3-4 that his opponents are demanding proof that "Christ is speaking in me" due to his apparent weakness and his insistence that he, like Christ, lives "by the power of God" also suggest that he had some sort of visible disability that caused others to look down on him as a man who did not fit the dominant social valuation of bodily fitness or appearance.

Whether the physical infirmity from which he was suffering when he arrived in Galatia (Gal. 4:13-15) was temporary or permanent is unclear. Many have argued for the latter, seeing in his statement that the Galatians would have "torn out your eyes and given them to me" a reference to eye problems and taking Gal. 6:11 ("See what large letters I make when I am writing in my own hand") as further evidence that Paul suffered from chronically weak vision. Such a reading is possible but by no means assured.[11] A similar ambiguity is evident in 1 Cor. 2:3, where Paul recalls how he initially came to the Corinthians "in weakness and in fear and in much trembling." The comparison with Gal. 4:13-15 is obvious, but whether Paul was in fact referring to a similar experience of sickness cannot be determined.

Two important conclusions can be drawn from these observations. In the first place, they give us ample reason to wonder whether Paul would have placed much confidence in any mode of healing, whether ordinary or "miraculous." It is certainly possible that his sufferings had led him to trust some types of treatment more than

---

[10] For a helpful discussion of this passage from the perspective of medical anthropology, see Justin M. Glessner, "Ethnomedical Anthropology and Paul's 'Thorn' (2 Corinthians 12:7)," *BTB* 47 (2017): 15–46. A good overview of the history of interpretation can be found in Adela Yarbro Collins, "Paul's Disability: The Thorn in His Flesh," in *Disability Studies and Biblical Literature*, ed. Candida R. Moss and Jeremy Schipper (New York: Palgrave Macmillan, 2011), 165–83. According to Audrey Dawson, the most common contemporary suggestions regarding Paul's ailment are eye disease, chronic malaria, migraines, and epilepsy (*Healing*, 194). J. Keir Howard presents a strong argument for the latter option in *Disease and Healing in the New Testament*, 241–57.

[11] Some interpreters find additional support for this view in Acts 9, where Paul experiences temporary blindness after encountering the risen Jesus, and Acts 23:4-5, where he fails to recognize the high priest. Even if the stories are not historical, they could reflect a genuine historical memory that Paul struggled with eye problems. This would not be at all surprising, since eye ailments are one of the most common health complaints in ancient epigraphic and literary sources. See Chaniotis, "Illness and Cures in the Greek Propitiatory Inscriptions," 327–9.

others, especially when the problem involved common ailments like the bleeding and contusions that resulted from being beaten, but if he did, he never says so. Nothing in his letters suggests that he received more relief from religious remedies than from other modes of care. In fact, the opposite is the case: the one instance where he explicitly mentions using religious methods (the prayers of 2 Cor. 12:8) ended in failure. These observations present serious problems for any suggestion that Paul would have approved only religious treatments to the exclusion of others.

The second notable point about Paul's bodily experience is one that he draws himself. In several places he relates how his experience with suffering has produced in him a reversal of the ordinary societal valuation of bodily debility. The most common explanation for serious illness and disability in antiquity was to regard it as a divine punishment for some sort of religious violation. The presence of such bodily infirmities cast a pall of suspicion over the sufferer, especially if the suffering was extended or chronic. The elite valorization of healthy male bodies that dominated Greco-Roman social discourse also devalued individuals who did not possess these attributes. The devaluation was especially heavy for people whose disabilities were believed to be permanent, while the harshest judgment was reserved for those who suffered the additional social defect of being a woman, a slave, or a foreigner.[12]

If Paul indeed suffered from some sort of visible illness or disability, he would have experienced this devaluation whenever he arrived in a city or met new people who held such views. Societal rejection would not have been entirely new to him since he grew up as a practicing Jew in a Greek city, but to be devalued on the basis of a physical ailment was probably a novel experience.[13] Since his sufferings arose while pursuing his missionary calling, it is understandable that he would explain any resulting infirmities as an outworking of the divine will. This is exactly what we see in his letters. Not only does he valorize his bodily sufferings as a mark of his devotion to God, but he also makes the astounding claim that God is especially present with and for those who suffer similar debilities, whether physical or social (1 Cor. 1:26-31, 12:22-26, 2 Cor. 1:3-11, 4:7-18, 11:23–12:10, Phil. 2:1-13, 4:12-13). This message has deep roots in the Hebrew Bible, where God stands consistently on the side of the weak and powerless, and the story of Jesus, whose Judean lower-class body, physical sufferings, and crucifixion marked him as uniquely disvalued.[14] The result was a "theology of weakness" that offered comfort to those who, like Paul, did not experience full bodily restoration after an illness or injury or who suffered from congenital debilities.

This theology was an integral part of Paul's thinking about sickness and injury and must therefore be included in any reconstruction of what Paul might have thought, said, and done on the topic of healing. It may also have played a role in the success

---

[12] For more on these points, see Arthur J. Dewey and Anna C. Miller, "Paul," in *The Bible and Disability: A Commentary*, ed. Sarah J. Melcher, Mikeal C. Parsons, and Amos Yong (Waco: Baylor University Press, 2017), 379–425, and Nicholas Vlahogiannis, "'Curing' Disability," in *Health in Antiquity*, ed. Helen King (London and New York: Routledge, 2005), 180–91.

[13] He might have faced something analogous when he visited the public baths and exposed his circumcised penis, but this devalued bodily condition was not continually visible as a physical disability would be.

[14] The latter point is emphasized throughout the article by Dewey and Miller cited in note 12.

of his mission, since it offered a sort of psychological cure for disability that would have been attractive to the many people in Greco-Roman antiquity whose bodily conditions subjected them to constant devaluation.[15] But it should not be taken as the quintessence of Paul's thinking on the subject, since it says nothing about the many practical questions that Paul would have been compelled to address regarding the propriety of various types of practitioners and treatments.

The Power of Israel's God

As a Judean whose thinking was shaped by the stories and teachings of his ancestral Scriptures, Paul was deeply imbued with a monotheistic ethos that forbade the worship of other deities besides the God of Israel. He was also aware of the judgments that God had inflicted upon his ancestors when they violated this standard. The frequent denunciations of "idolatry" in his letters show clearly that he carried this worldview with him into the Christ-movement and that he expected his polytheistic gentile converts to adopt similar views.

Included in this worldview was the conviction that God was deeply and lovingly involved in the material world, unlike the sometimes distant and unpredictable gods of other nations. Two implications of this theology are relevant to our investigation. The first is the belief, attested in the writings of both Judean and Christian authors, that the material world and everything in it is essentially good. Thus any material substance that serves to promote health and alleviate sickness can be viewed as a gift from God, even when it comes through "pagan" channels. The second is the conviction that everything that is good and true in the world of humans, including the wisdom of other nations, has its origins with the God of Israel. This view is evident in the writings of several Judean and Christian authors who crafted elaborate histories or philosophical arguments to show how the best ideas and practices of Greece and Rome were taken from Judean heroes like Moses and Abraham, who received them from God.[16]

These beliefs supplied the theological justification for elite Judeans and Christians in the early centuries CE to adopt the best elements of Greek and Roman culture while maintaining their devotion to biblical monotheism. In most cases this included Greek and Roman approaches to healing, as we saw in Chapters 7 and 8. Objections were raised to certain practices on the grounds that they looked too much like (or crossed the border into) idolatry, especially those that involved cultic veneration of other gods or direct appeals to their power. But almost no one argued that Judeans or Christians should avoid such practices entirely.

While it is always possible to argue that Paul was an exception to this trend, there is little in his letters to support such a view and much that tells against it. In 1 Corinthians 8, for example, Paul's monotheistic affirmation in verses 4-8 is followed immediately by

---

[15] From a medical anthropological standpoint, such a social reinstatement of the disabled person could be considered a "cure" even if the person's bodily condition remained unchanged.

[16] Several good examples of Judean texts that do this can be found in the latter pages of volume 2 of Charlesworth's *Old Testament Pseudepigrapha*. Most of the early Christian apologists engage in similar arguments.

a passing reference in verse 10 to the possibility that one of his followers might be seen "eating in the temple of an idol." He goes on to describe a problem that might result from this behavior, but he does not actually prohibit such visits. He also approves the eating of sacrificial meat in general on the grounds that the gods to whom the meat was offered have no real existence (8:4). The only exception is when it might cause a believer to think that worshipping other gods is acceptable for a Christ-follower.[17] A similar openness can be seen in Romans, where the scathing denunciation of idolatry in Rom. 1:18-32 is followed by a recognition that some non-Judeans might have the law of God "written in their heart" and live up to it more faithfully than Judeans who were nurtured in the Torah (2:14-16). In short, Paul's condemnations of gentile religion do not automatically imply a total avoidance of their practices.[18]

A similar attitude can be seen toward "magic." Though Paul lists φαρμακεία (a word that can refer to the use of either medicinal drugs or sorcery) as one of the "works of the flesh" in Gal. 5:20, he periodically uses language, ideas, and practices that are virtually identical to those that elite Greek and Roman authors rejected as μαγεία. The most obvious example is 1 Cor. 5:3-5, where he speaks about projecting his spirit from a distance and pronouncing curses that will elicit divine judgment. Curses also appear in 1 Cor. 16:22 and Gal. 1:8-9. Even his injunction against cursing one's enemies in Rom. 12:12 presumes a belief that such curses could be effective. Magical language is also used in Gal. 3:1, where Paul voices the fear that someone might have "cast an evil eye" upon the Galatians and so clouded their senses,[19] and Gal. 4:14, where the verb ἐκπτύω ("to spit at") likely alludes to the practice of spitting to counteract the effects of a spell cast by an "evil eye." Other possible references to magical practices include 1 Cor. 15:29, where his obscure statement about Christ-followers being "baptized for the dead" carries a strong hint of necromancy, and Rom. 6:2-7, where his claim that baptism eradicates the power of sin in the believer's body echoes stories of magical rituals being used to effect bodily transformation.[20]

A common magical practice that is not mentioned in Paul's letters is exorcism. Only twice does Paul refer to "demons" (1 Cor. 10:20-21), and it is not at all clear whether he has in mind the evil beings of Jewish mythology or the more neutral suprahuman beings (*daimones*) of Greek thought. Patristic authors use it often in the latter sense when referring to cultic worship, but Paul's language could be read either way. He does speak here and there about Christ-followers being engaged in a spiritual war against invisible

---

[17] The tension between these verses and the language of 1 Cor. 10:14-22 about not sharing the "cup" and "table" of demons (or better, *daimones*) has long been noted, and interpreters disagree about how they should be correlated. Guy Williams's observation is better than most: "Idols may be nothing, but that does not demand that the same is true of the demons which lurk behind them. If one behaves inappropriately toward that dead object then they will take advantage" (*The Spirit World in the Letters of Paul the Apostle* [Göttingen: Vandehoeck & Ruprecht, 2009], 147).

[18] Whether there is any truth behind the story in Acts 17 of Paul walking around Athens and scrutinizing the city's "objects of worship" is unclear, but the text shows that at least one early Christian author could imagine Paul touring Greek cultic sites.

[19] The verb that Paul uses here (βασκαίνω), commonly translated as "bewitched," is used in Greek circles to refer to someone "casting the evil eye" toward another person in order to harm them.

[20] A good recent exposition of this view can be found in Eyl, *Signs, Wonders, and Gifts*, 130–43. The most famous stories of magical bodily transformation appear in Apuleius's *Golden Ass* (second century CE).

evil beings ("Satan," "the god of this world," "powers," "authorities," etc.) who hold a certain amount of authority in the world of humans, but he says nothing about them infusing or "possessing" the body of a believer. They can tempt (1 Cor. 7:5), mislead (2 Cor. 11:13-15), hinder (1 Thess. 2:18), and torment (1 Cor. 12:7) Christ-followers, and Satan can even "destroy the flesh" of a person who is ritually cast out of the community (1 Cor. 5:5). But they can be resisted by those who attend to their tricks and persevere in faith and good behavior with God's help (1 Cor. 7:5, 10:13, 2 Cor. 2:11) until the day when God brings the present eon to a close and destroys them forever (Rom. 16:20, 1 Cor. 15:24). Such ideas are thoroughly Jewish and apocalyptic, not "magical." As in other apocalyptic texts, the power of these beings is only temporary, and those who remain faithful to Christ are free from their dominion.[21] Thus we should not expect Paul to approve the use of exorcism rituals to treat the illness of a Christ-follower.

Whether the same is true for other magical healing rituals is less obvious. "Magic" is in the eye of the beholder and can therefore be applied to any type of forbidden ritual. But it is not at all clear that the category of "forbidden ritual" even existed in Paul's thought-world. The only rituals that he expressly forbids are the circumcision of gentiles and the veneration of deities other than the God of Israel, both of which are clearly religious and not "magical" acts.[22] There is also no sign in Paul's letters of any anxiety that people might manipulate evil powers to do harm to others unless we include his passing reference to the "evil eye," nor is there any suggestion that rituals might be used to keep them at bay. When we add to this what we observed in Chapter 7 regarding the openness of Judeans in Paul's day and beyond to healing rituals that Greek or Roman intellectuals might have disparaged as μαγεία, it is hard to see what grounds Paul might have had for opposing the use of "magical" healing practices by his followers. It seems more likely he would have agreed with the later rabbinic judgment that if a remedy worked, it came from God and should therefore be accepted with gratitude.

Life in Community

One of the key insights of modern medical anthropology is its recognition of the communal nature of sickness and healing. Where the Western medical model views sickness as the biological dysfunction of an individual body and healing as the restoration of that body to its pre-sickness state through the intervention of an expert practitioner, medical anthropology sees sickness and healing as discursive concepts that are defined and enacted within a particular community. Different societies and societal subgroups can have different ideas about what counts as sickness and how it should be treated.

---

[21] Graham Twelftree sums up Paul's view well: "As Paul sees all people in relation to either Satan or Christ (2 Cor 6:14-15; cf. Gal 5:16-26), and the Christian has passed from Satan to Christ (Col 1:13), it would be inconceivable for exorcism to appear in Paul's list of *charismata*" ("Healing, Illness," in *Dictionary of Paul and His Letters*, ed. Gerald F. Hawthorne, Ralph P. Martin, and Daniel G. Reid [Downers Grove, IL: InterVarsity Press, 1993], 380).

[22] He does, of course, tell gentiles that they do not need to follow the laws of Torah, but he does not single out legal or religious rituals specifically for criticism.

Paul and his followers lived at the nexus between several different communities—Greek, Roman, Judean, and indigenous—that held different ideas about the nature of reality, including such fundamental beliefs as the nature of the human body and the forces to which it was subject. They also differed in the valuations that they placed on human life and health. Exposure of newborns who were deemed physically deficient was common in Greek and Roman cultures, and those who survived were subjected to mockery and abuse.[23] Elite opinion held that the bodies and minds of those on the lower rungs of society were by their very nature (we might say "genetically") inferior to those at the top, and the same was true for women in relation to men. Sickness and debility were thought to be naturally endemic to the lower classes, and no duty of care existed toward such people.[24]

Judeans and Christians, by contrast, were taught that all humans were made in the image of God and thus worthy of love and respect. Their sacred texts claimed that the divine creator of the universe had a special concern for those on the bottom of society—the poor, the lowly, the weak—and mandated that those who possessed resources should care for those who had little. Less was said about care for the sick, but both communities believed that this was included in the obligation to look out for those in need.

Paul took this a step further in 1 Corinthians 12, comparing the local community of Christ-followers to a human body in which the suffering of one member affects the entire body. His language is metaphorical, but his repeated calls for compassion toward those who are weak or suffering (Rom. 12:15, 15:1, 2 Cor. 11:29, 1 Thess. 5:14, etc.) show that it could be applied to literal bodies as well. When one member of the community was sick, the others were obligated to care for them. In short, sickness and healing were communal rather than individual matters.

Little is known about how this communal nursing of the sick was carried out, but it would have required a significant amount of effort and, in many cases, crossing of social boundaries since Christ-followers would have been scattered across a city or region in households of different social standing. Many would have lived with family members who did not share their beliefs, practices, or values. In the absence of instruction to the contrary, it is reasonable to suppose that Christian compassion would have led them to use any form of treatment that they thought might be effective, whether traditional, religious, magical, or medical. If they had understood and accepted Paul's teachings about "idolatry," they would have avoided prayers and rituals that appealed to non-Christian deities, but apart from this they would have drawn on whatever knowledge or experience they possessed to guide them in treating sickness. At some point they might have appealed to a fellow Christ-believer who possessed the "gifts of healings" that Paul mentions in 1 Cor. 12:28-9, but it is hard to know how this would have worked

---

[23] This point is well developed in Garland, *Eye of the Beholder*, and Nicole Kelley, "Deformity and Disability in Greece and Rome," in *This Abled Body: Rethinking Disabilities in Biblical Studies*, ed. Hector Avalos, Sarah J. Melcher, and Jeremy Schipper (Atlanta: Society of Biblical Literature, 2007), 31–45.

[24] For more on the latter point, see Ferngren and Amundsen, "Medicine and Christianity in the Roman Empire," 2971–5.

since Paul does not say whether the exercise of these gifts was limited to their corporate meetings or if there were people who could apply them in private homes.

Christ-followers would also have been taught to view the causes of sickness differently than people outside their community. Paul says little about causality in his letters, and when he does, his answers vary. Sometimes he attributes sickness to sin (1 Cor. 11:29-30), sometimes to God or Satan (2 Cor. 12:7), and sometimes to bodily stress (2 Cor. 11:23-29, Phil. 2:30). Such explanations are not unique to Paul but are broadly consistent with what we see in both Judean and Greco-Roman literature. The only popular explanation that that they would have had to reject was the belief that sickness could result from committing an offense against one or another of the Greek or Roman gods. Here again their communal understanding of sickness would have been reshaped by their acceptance of Paul's message.

Whether Paul offered any new ideas about what constitutes "being healed" is hard to say, since the subject is mentioned only obliquely in his letters. In the case of Epaphroditus, healing is demonstrated by his ability to resume his work as a traveling missionary (Phil. 2:25-30), and something similar is implied in Gal. 4:13-15, where the presence of a community of Christ-followers in Galatia suggests that Paul was restored sufficiently to have a successful ministry there. Whether either man was fully cured of sickness in the modern medical sense is unclear, but the fact Paul was able to resume his ministry despite not being cured of his "thorn in the flesh" in 2 Cor. 12:8-9 suggests that this may not have been the case. His claim that he prayed to have the "thorn" removed suggests that complete physical restoration was his norm, but he was willing to accept a psychological cure when it was proffered by the divine voice. A similar diversity in the definition of being "healed" can be seen in other writers from the era.[25] On the whole, it seems that Paul's ideas about what it means to be healed were broadly consistent with the norms of both Greco-Roman and Judean cultures.

What Would Paul Say?

While there is always room for disagreement regarding the meaning and implications of Paul's rhetoric, the evidence and arguments presented in this study suggest that number 7 in our list of options offers the best path forward for reconstructing what Paul thought, did, and said on the subjects of sickness and healing. Other options contain valid insights, but their truth is at best partial and limited. For example, option 4 observes rightly that Paul's views were deeply shaped by his ancestral Scriptures and traditions, but he also believed that a new day had dawned in which the Spirit of Israel's god was performing miraculous healings within the community of Christ-followers (option 5). His confidence in these "gifts of healings" might have been tempered by the fact that he himself did not benefit from them (option 3), but his ability to endure

---

[25] Similar reasoning was no doubt common at the shrines of Asklepios, though such mundane "cures" were not recorded by the temple officials whose aim was to extol the god's power. It is noteworthy, however, that Aelius Aristides never recounts a particular moment when he was "healed" in his *Sacred Tales*. His healing appears to have been more psychological than physical.

illness and injury was surely aided by his conviction that God would soon bring the present era to an end and give Christ-followers perfected spiritual bodies that would be free from suffering (option 2). In the meantime they were to devote themselves to serving the God of Israel and guard their bodies from evil influences (option 2).

All of these are valid observations, but they cannot do justice to the full range of issues and evidence surrounding Paul's views of sickness and healing, as should be evident from the critiques that accompanied the various options. Only in option 7 do we find a coherent explanation for Paul's relative silence on these matters that is both consistent with his treatment of similar topics and takes seriously the historical and theological necessity for him to have addressed these issues with his congregations.

The analogy with his treatment of the "idol meat" question is especially helpful as it provides a template for how Paul handled a similar case where a practice that was inoffensive in itself (eating meat) elicited concerns from some of his followers because of its cultic connections (having been offered in sacrifice to a local deity). The analogy is not perfect: few Christ-followers would have been anxious about eating the meat of animals that were slaughtered outside of a cultic setting, while some healing techniques that did not involve explicit cultic activity still had indirect associations with non-Christian deities that might have aroused concerns from some Christ-followers about the possibility of "idolatry." Examples include visiting a physician who credited his healing prowess to Asklepios; wearing an amulet marked with "pagan" religious symbols; ingesting a medicine concocted from plants that were harvested by "magical" techniques; or reciting a spell or incantation to procure healing or protection from harm.

Even these practices, however, have possible parallels in Paul's handling of the meat issue in Romans 14, where he addresses the concerns of a group of Christ-followers who were objecting to eating meat under any circumstances because they viewed it as "unclean" (v. 14). Paul does not explain their reasoning, but the parallel with 1 Corinthians 8 suggests that meat was associated in their minds with the cult, even if the link was indirect. As in the latter passage, Paul insists that the act in itself is not wrong before going on to say that eating meat should be avoided if it harms another person or violates the conscience of the eater. Whether he would have applied similar reasoning to the questionable healing practices cited earlier is unclear, but it seems reasonable to suppose that he would.

This supposition finds support from a review of the kinds of issues that Paul does and does not address in his letters. The instruction that Paul offers in his letters relates almost exclusively to conduct that is addressed explicitly in the Jewish Scriptures or the teachings of Jesus: worshipping other gods, illicit sexual activities, dissensions, drunkenness, caring for the lowly, and so on. Where these sources offer no guidance, Paul is generally silent. In fact, it is hard to find a single place in Paul's letters where he calls for gentiles to change an ordinary non-cultic behavior that does not conflict with either Scripture or earlier Christian tradition. He does speak now and then about Christ-followers (including himself) being guided by the Spirit to know what to do (Rom. 8:5-14, 1 Cor. 2:10-16, 7:40, Gal. 5:16-25, Phil. 3:15, etc.), but there are no clear instances where he relies solely on the Spirit for authorizing a change of conduct.

As we saw in Chapter 7, the Jewish Scriptures say nothing explicit about any of the questionable healing practices that were mentioned earlier, and there is no evidence that pre-Pauline Christian leaders had addressed the topic either (Chapter 8). It would, therefore, be highly uncharacteristic for Paul to have condemned them. Had he done so, we would expect to hear something about it in his letters, since it is hard to see how such a radical change of behavior on matters that affected people's health and possibly their lives would have gone unchallenged. At a minimum, we would anticipate questions about how a Pauline prohibition might apply to practices that he had not specifically mentioned when he was with them. Instead, we hear nothing.

Despite the usual caveats regarding arguments from silence, the utter absence of commentary by Paul about the propriety of Greek and Roman healing practices is hard to explain if he believed that his gentile followers should stop using healing practices that they had trusted for their entire lives, especially when illness, injury, and debilitation were matters of constant concern. It makes perfect sense, however, if he either had no strong views on the subject or viewed healing, like "idol meat," as an area where individual conscience should be respected as long as it did not veer into open idolatry.

What Would Paul Do?

Similar uncertainties arise when we turn to the question of what kinds of treatments Paul might have used or avoided for his own illnesses and injuries since he says nothing on the subject. But we know enough about the healing practices of Judeans and Christians in the centuries before and after Paul to speculate intelligently about what he might have done.

We can be reasonably certain, for example, that Paul used and recommended religious treatments that were approved by both Jewish and Christian traditions, including prayers for divine healing, personal nursing of the sick, and patient endurance, the latter of which can be viewed as a type of psychological health care. There is also no reason why he should have objected to traditional home remedies that had no obvious ties to religion, such as ingesting plant-based medicines or applying ointments to wounds. The same is true for many of the treatments associated with ancient physicians, including eating or avoiding certain foods or medicines, heating or cooling the body, physical exercise, and purging.

At the other end of the spectrum, we can be fairly confident that Paul would have avoided (and taught his followers to avoid) methods of healing that involved presenting sacrifices or offerings to non-Israelite gods or praying or confessing one's sins to them. The same can be said for spells, incantations, charms, and exorcistic rituals that named these deities in an effort to draw on their healing power. Given Paul's deep aversion to "idolatry," it is also highly improbable that he would have visited an Asklepian temple or healing center to seek treatment from one of their resident physicians. It is less clear that he would have prohibited his gentile followers from doing the same since he could countenance the possibility that one of them might eat in the temple of a Greek or Roman god (1 Cor. 8:10).

Similar observations can be made regarding healing dreams. We can be sure that Paul would not have sought after a dream in which a Greek god like Asklepios would appear and either heal him or give him instructions for treatment. But he might have done so in relation to either Jesus or his divine father, since he claimed that he had encountered them in visions (1 Cor. 15:6-8, 2 Cor. 12:1-7, Gal. 1:15-16) and experienced other revelations from God (1 Cor. 2:7-14, Gal. 1:11-12, 2:1-2; cf. Eph. 3:2-5).[26] Whether he used rituals (as some magicians did) to procure these visions and revelations or whether they came to him through dreams or mental reflection is impossible to say since Paul does not address the question.[27] In either case, the transmission of these revelations to his audiences would have been viewed as a type of divination.[28] He also speaks about his followers receiving divine revelations (1 Cor. 14:26, 14:30, Phil. 3:15), so it is not out of the question that he might have encouraged them to seek healing dreams as well. Whether Paul followed other Judeans in giving credence to signs and omens is hard to say, though at least two texts (1 Cor. 14:22, 2 Cor. 12:12) suggest that he might have done so. If he did, there is no reason to think that he would have objected to the common practice of healers using them to predict the course and outcome of a disease.

Finally, it is unlikely, though not impossible, that Paul would have worn an amulet or gem marked with images or symbols of non-Israelite gods to obtain healing or protection. The wearing of an amulet or engraved gem would not itself be problematic, since amulets were used in all forms of ancient health care, including medicine (Chapter 5). There is also ample evidence that Judeans and Christians wore them on a regular basis (Chapters 7 and 8). But questions could arise if the amulet contained religious markings that would have been evident to the wearer. Objects marked with images of a god or goddess would probably have been rejected by Paul in view of the well-known Jewish concern to avoid visible representations of the divine. But images that could be interpreted in different ways might have escaped his scrutiny. Rings and amulets marked with divine symbols like the moon, the phoenix, the lizard, and the goat are common in the archaeological record, as are gems engraved with esoteric characters.[29] Whether Paul would have worn such objects himself depends on how strictly he interpreted the biblical ban on carved images, but he might not have objected

---

[26] The book of Acts depicts several people receiving visions from God (Paul, Ananias, Peter, the centurion), but only one of them pertains to curing sickness (9:10-12). The idea that God might speak in dreams is broadly accepted in the Jewish Scriptures, where it occurs often. It is also referenced six times in the Gospel of Matthew. Acts 2:17 quotes the words of Joel 2:28 ("your old men shall dream dreams") as a sign that God's promise to pour out the divine Spirit upon "all flesh" is being fulfilled in the nascent community of Christ-followers.

[27] Rituals for seeking an encounter with a deity or *daimon* are described in several places in the PGM; see the discussion in Dieleman, "The Greco-Egyptian Magical Papyri," 290–9. Justin Glessner suggests that Paul might have received his revelation about the meaning of his suffering during a trance that Paul had elicited through a healing rite—see "Ethnomedical Anthropology and Paul's 'Thorn,'" 33–4. The possibility that Paul is speaking about dream experiences is strengthened by John Hanson's observation that it is nearly impossible to distinguish between reports of dreams and visions in ancient literature ("Dreams and Visions in the Graeco-Roman World and Early Christianity," 1408, 1421).

[28] This point is developed further in Eyl, *Signs, Wonders, and Gifts*, 144–69.

[29] For more, see the three articles by Véronique Dasen in the Bibliography.

to his followers wearing them since their ties to the divine are less obvious.[30] We know that second-century Christians wore such items because Clement of Alexandria had to advise his audience to stop wearing rings marked with pagan symbols and replace them with images that could bear a Christian interpretation such as a dove, a fish, a ship, a lyre, or an anchor (*Paed.* 3.3). The fact that Paul gives no such instruction to his followers could suggest that he did not see the wearing of non-iconic symbols as problematic, whether because they did not explicitly depict pagan deities or because the gods that they represented did not truly exist (1 Cor. 8:4).

Between these poles lay a variety of healing practices that contemporary interpreters might be tempted to dismiss as distasteful or superstitious. But there is little in any of them that would have aroused the suspicions of a Judean Christ-follower like Paul, much less his gentile followers. In their eyes, such practices were mundane components of a variegated health care system that was utilized by Judeans, Christians, and pagans alike. Interpreters ignore them at their peril.

For example, there is no reason to think that Paul would have objected to the recitation of spells, charms, and incantations like the ones cited in Chapter 3 that do not name any particular deity or appeal explicitly to suprahuman powers to bring healing. This is especially true for the ones that consist mainly of nonsense syllables, letters, or symbols. It was certainly possible to interpret such gibberish as prayers to forbidden gods, but such an interpretation was by no means necessary since virtually everyone in the ancient world believed that words carried power in and of themselves, without reference to any deity.

Similar observations can be made about the use of ritual language in the collection, preparation, and application of medicinal substances, including amulets, since most of these rituals would have been invisible to the patient. The vast majority of amulets mentioned in Greek and Roman pharmacological handbooks consisted of unmarked materials that had no evident links to the divine, such as bundles of plants or animal remains that were tied around the neck or the affected body part. There is no reason to suppose that Paul would have found the wearing of such items objectionable. His handling of the "idol meat" question in 1 Corinthians 8 suggests that he would have advised his followers to accept these treatments without asking how they had been prepared or how they worked.

The same reasoning applies to the practice, common in both magical and medical sources, of using ritualized actions and exotic substances to procure healing or protection. Examples of ritualized actions include removing all bands from the body (girdles, shoes, rings, etc.) in order to release the body from sickness; laying a puppy or duck on a sick person's stomach to absorb the illness; causing a green lizard to bite a sleeping child and then burning the lizard to remove a hernia; kissing the muzzle

---

[30] Judeans in the Diaspora tended to be relatively lenient about such matters, but Josephus reports that some of their compatriots in the homeland cut down a golden eagle that Herod had placed over the gate of the Jerusalem temple (*War* 1.33.2–3), while others were willing to sacrifice their lives if Pilate did not remove some Roman standards bearing images of Caesar that he had secretly introduced to the city (*War* 2.9.2–3). If there is any truth to the statement in Acts 22:3 that Paul was educated in Jerusalem, it is possible that he could have adopted the more conservative interpretation while he was there.

of a mule to cure a cold; and spitting to avert the supposed contagion of epilepsy. Neither Paul nor his followers would have had any way of knowing whether these rituals worked, but there was nothing in them that would have evoked immediate condemnation in a world where belief in such practices was virtually universal.

Examples of exotic substances that were used to procure healing include the blood or sweat of a gladiator, the gall or pelt of a hyena, the stinger of a stingray, the tail of a python, and the heart of a lion.[31] Many of the materials sold under these names were likely fraudulent, as there was no system in antiquity for validating the contents of a medication, and most could be afforded only by the wealthy. But nothing about them was self-evidently problematic for a Judean Christ-follower like Paul, nor is there anything in his letters like the rationalistic criticism of "superstition" that we see in certain Greek and Roman authors. In short, there is no evident reason why Paul would have rejected any of these remedies if he thought that they might work.

Perhaps the thorniest question to answer is what Paul would have thought about using exorcistic and purificatory rituals to cure sickness. Such rituals were not problematic in themselves, since exorcism and purification were practiced routinely in Judean circles around the time of Paul. Purification rites also had deep roots in the Jewish Scriptures. But there are two reasons to think that Paul might have taken a different view. In the first place, Paul never refers to demons causing illness (with the possible exception of 2 Cor. 12:7),[32] nor does he mention exorcism. It is possible that the omissions are accidental, but the fact that demons play at best a minimal role in his broader theology suggests that it is not. In the second place, Paul almost never uses purity language in his letters, and when he does, he generally interprets it in a symbolic or moral sense (1 Cor. 5:7, 2 Cor. 6:6, 7:1, Phil. 1:10, 4:8). Not once does he speak of Christ-followers using purification rituals, which would seem to fall under the "works of Torah" that he says are not required for gentiles (cf. Rom. 14:20, "Everything is indeed clean"). It thus seems unlikely that Paul would have accepted or recommended exorcism or purification as a mode of treatment, though he might not have objected to their use by his followers as long as the rituals did not involve explicit appeals to non-Israelite deities.

Conclusion

Reconstructing what Paul thought and did with regard to sickness and healing is a speculative enterprise that is fraught with uncertainty. But that does not mean that we can say nothing on the subject. Ancient sources tell us a fair amount about what ordinary people, including Judeans and Christians, were doing to treat health problems in the centuries before and after Paul and what elite authors thought about these practices. From these sources we can identify a range of health care options that

---

[31] All of these examples are taken from various sections of Pliny's *Natural History*.
[32] The uncertainty arises from the fact that Paul does not actually say who gave him the "thorn"—the implied subject of the passive verb ἐδόθη could be either God or Satan. See the discussion in Glessner, "Ethnomedical Anthropology and Paul's 'Thorn,'" 23–6.

would have been available to Paul and his followers. We can then examine what Paul did and did not say about sickness, healing, and related subjects and make informed judgments about how he might have viewed each form of treatment. Applying such a comparative approach enables us to situate Paul squarely within his own world rather than reading him through the lens of modern Western medicine.

If the arguments and evidence presented in this chapter are correct, it would seem that becoming a Christ-follower had little impact on Paul's thinking or practices regarding sickness and healing. Despite the availability of a new mode of treatment in the form of Spirit-endowed "gifts of healings" that could be accessed through the local house-churches, there is no evidence that their presence changed the way Paul viewed or treated his own health problems. We can therefore presume that he continued to employ the same Judean or Greek health care practices that he had used before joining the Christ-movement.

He also shows little interest in changing what his followers were doing in this area, though his negative opinion of non-Israelite deities suggests that he would have cautioned them to avoid practices that involved explicit veneration of "idols." Whether they would have heeded such warnings is unclear, since both literary and epigraphic sources testify to the presence of Judeans and Christians at Greek, Roman, and native temples when cultic worship was being performed.[33] The fact that both Judean and Christian authors condemned such practices shows only that there was a significant disjuncture between the ideas and practices of the elite class and those of the masses.

One set of data that has not been clearly addressed in this chapter is the "signs and wonders" and works of "power" that Paul says accompanied his missionary preaching. If these events included healing, as many interpreters have suggested, our judgments about the importance of sickness and health care in Paul's life and ministry might have to be revised somewhat, though it is not clear that these cures were qualitatively different from those that he labels "gifts of healings." Similar adjustments might be needed if we take seriously Luke's depiction of Paul as a miracle-worker and healer in the book of Acts. These and related matters will be examined more fully in Chapter 10.

---

[33] See the evidence cited in Chapters 7 and 8.

10

Sickness, Healing, and the Mission of Paul

Paul the Healer?

In this final chapter we return to a question that was posed at the beginning of our study: what role did physical healing (or the promise of it) play in the evangelistic program of Paul and his followers? The book of Acts shows Paul doing various types of miracles, including healings, as part of his missionary outreach, and Paul himself speaks several times about "signs and wonders" and works of "power" that accompanied his preaching and moved people to accept his message. He also claims that God had given some of his followers the power to heal, a skill that might conceivably have played a role in evangelism since Paul refers to unbelievers being present at their meetings when charismatic powers were on display and some of them becoming Christ-followers as a result (1 Cor. 14:16, 23-25).[1] Taken together, these texts suggest that healings and other miraculous acts were important to the success of Paul's mission.

But there is also evidence pointing in the opposite direction. We have seen how Paul gives no sign that he himself was miraculously cured from any of his sicknesses or injuries, and he never suggests that divine healing should replace or take precedence over other forms of health care. In fact, he shows little interest in physical healing anywhere in his letters. He mentions "gifts of healings" in relation to only one church (Corinth), and he says nothing about these abilities being used for evangelistic purposes. He is equally reticent about the nature of the miraculous "signs and wonders" that he claims aided the success of his preaching. It is possible that they included healing, but he never says so. Finally, he says nothing about Jesus being a healer, nor does he mention any of the miraculous cures that are reported in the Gospels. This is strange if healing played such a vital role in his evangelistic ministry.[2]

How are we to resolve this discrepancy? The most common solutions are either to ignore the question or to discount the role of "miraculous" activity in the mission and ministry of Paul. Regarding the material in Acts, interpreters have pointed to the questionable historicity of the book and its tendency to valorize Paul as reasons for

---

[1] Paul speaks only about prophecy causing unbelievers to acknowledge their God, but it is hard to imagine that he would have seen no evangelistic value in any of the other *charismata* if he recognized it for this one.
[2] While there are many questions regarding how much Paul knew about Jesus, it is inconceivable that he learned nothing about his healings from Peter and others who knew Jesus personally (cf. 1 Cor. 9:5, Gal. 1:18-19, 2:1-10).

rejecting the author's portrait of Paul as a miracle-worker. As for Paul's own references to "signs and wonders," they can be read as metaphorical appropriations of scriptural language to describe the life-changing power of the gospel that miraculously turned polytheistic gentiles into Christ-followers and enabled them to live godly lives. Paul's language in 1 Cor. 12:9-10 about the Spirit giving Christ-followers the ability to heal and perform miracles can be explained similarly as the enhancement of natural healing skills and other undefined abilities that ancient people might regard as "miraculous." Thus the miracle-working Paul can be demythologized into an evangelistic preacher who was overawed by the effects of his own ministry.

More recent interpreters have recognized that such rationalistic interpretations do not do justice either to the language of Paul's letters or to his accounts of his experience. Paul consistently takes for granted that the "signs and wonders" and works of "power" that served to legitimate his preaching were visible, memorable events that both he and his audiences regarded as miraculous and not just the inner stirrings of faith in those who responded to his message. This idea is embedded in the very language that he uses to describe them. The phrase "signs and wonders" appears twenty-three times in the LXX, where it almost always refers to miraculous acts performed by God either directly or through a prophet. Most of its occurrences relate to the Exodus story.[3] It carries the same sense in the two places where it appears in the Gospels (Mk 13:22, Jn 14:48) and the nine instances where similar language is used in Acts (2:22, 2:43, 4:30, 5:12-16, 6:8, 7:36, 8:13, 14:3, 15:12). In Acts 5:12-16, the expression is linked specifically with miraculous acts of healing. Greek authors use the phrase in a similar way, so even gentile Christ-followers who were unfamiliar with its biblical roots could have understood it as a reference to visible miracles performed by divine powers. In short, the meaning of "signs and wonders" was so clearly established in Paul's day that he would have had to signal to his audience that he was using it in a different sense if he wanted them to understand it as referring to an invisible inner transformation produced by faith and the working of the Spirit.

What we see in Paul's letters is the reverse: the "miraculous" significance of the phrase is underlined by linking it with the word "power" (δύναμις) in all three places where it appears. In Rom. 15:18-19, Paul speaks of how Christ had worked through him to bring gentiles to obedience "by word and deed," a phrase that would appear to refer to the complementary role of preaching ("word") and miracles ("deed") in his evangelistic mission. This interpretation finds support in the two phrases that immediately follow ("in the power of signs and wonders, in the power of the Spirit"), which together serve as biblical shorthand for the miraculous acts of God.[4] The same language appears in 2 Cor. 12:12, where he recalls the "signs, wonders, and [works of] power" that he had performed in Corinth as part of a rhetorical effort to shore

---

[3] McCasland, "Signs and Wonders," 150. The word "signs" appears on its own an additional 153 times, while "wonders" appears 58 times. McCasland cites as non-miraculous uses only Isa. 8:18, where it refers to the prophet Isaiah and his children in some obscure manner, and Isa. 20:3, where it appears that he mistakenly consulted the Hebrew text and not the LXX (151).

[4] The fact that he can use such language without explanation when writing to a church that he has never visited implies an awareness that his fame as a wonder-worker had spread as far as Rome (Schreiber, *Paulus also Wundertäter*, 270).

up his credibility as an apostle in the eyes of the Corinthians who had apparently been impressed by similar (or possibly greater) displays of divine power by a group of outsiders whom Paul labels "super-apostles." The argument only works if the events that Paul is recalling were both visible and memorable to the Corinthians. This is even more true in 2 Thess. 2:9, where Paul (or a later author) describes how a Satanic eschatological figure called "the lawless one" will perform "every [kind of] power and signs and lying wonders" that will persuade unbelievers to honor him as divine (2:4, 11-12).

Similar observations can be made regarding other texts in which Paul uses the word "power" (δύναμις) on its own to describe events that accompanied and authenticated his missionary preaching. In 1 Cor. 2:4-5, he recalls how he came to the Corinthians "not with plausible words of wisdom" but "with a demonstration of the Spirit and of power" so that their faith "might rest not on human wisdom but on the power of God." Preaching and acts of power are clearly distinguished in this recollection of his initial evangelistic activity in Corinth. Similar language can be seen in 1 Thess. 1:5, where he recounts how he delivered his initial message to the Thessalonians "not in word only, but also in power and in the Holy Spirit." It was this combination of preaching and acts of power that produced "full conviction" in the minds of the Thessalonians regarding the truth of his gospel. Preaching and power are conjoined again in 2 Cor. 6:7, where Paul lists "the word of truth" and "the power of God" as two separate channels by which his ministry is commended, and in Gal. 3:1-5, where he refers to the continuing activity of God's Spirit performing works of power (δυνάμεις) in the Galatian churches as proof that his law-free gospel was approved by God.[5]

All of these references presuppose that both Paul and his followers could recall and appreciate the fact that his evangelistic preaching was accompanied by some sort of miraculous activity that God used to validate the truth of Paul's message. But did these activities include physical healing? Most interpreters have thought so. Some have even suggested that the phrase "signs and wonders" should be taken as an implicit reference to healing ("signs") and exorcism ("wonders"). This reading is unlikely, however, since as we saw in Chapter 9, Paul shows little interest in demons and none in exorcism.[6]

The evidence for interpreting the entire phrase as a reference to miraculous acts of healing is only slightly stronger. Paul does acknowledge that the Spirit can give Christ-followers the power to heal and do miracles (1 Cor. 12:9-10, Gal. 3:1-5), so there is no reason to suppose that he objected to such acts in principle. But he says nothing about being a healer himself, nor does he indicate that he either sought or experienced miraculous healing for any of his own illnesses and injuries. If he suffered from some sort of visible or recurring disability, as was suggested in Chapter 9, this condition would have made it difficult for him to present himself as a healer since it

---

[5] A similar contrast between speech and power appears in 1 Cor. 4:19-21, but the context relates to the actions of believers rather than the evangelizing of unbelievers.

[6] Luke recounts only one story of Paul casting out a demon (16:18), and nothing is said about it producing converts. In fact, it does the opposite, eliciting bodily attacks and arrest (16:19-24). Exorcisms are also mentioned as one of the miraculous effects produced by contact with cloths that had touched Paul's body (Acts 19:11-12), but Paul did not initiate these acts and no conversions are mentioned.

would have subjected him to the criticism embodied in the ancient dictum, "Physician, heal thyself!"[7] We know from his letters that some of Paul's opponents cited his physical weakness as a reason for questioning his status as a special emissary of Christ, but no such criticisms are voiced about him pretending to be a healer.[8] In fact, the only evidence for viewing Paul as a healer comes from three stories in the book of Acts (14:8-10, 19:11-12, 28:7-8) that are irrelevant to the question at hand since none of them are associated with evangelistic preaching and none yield converts.

In short, the available evidence offers little support for the view that the miraculous acts to which Paul refers in his letters included healing. Some interpreters have given up entirely on the effort to judge what Paul meant by these references while others have proposed different possibilities, none with much conviction. Jennifer Eyl has compiled a helpful list of practices that people in Paul's day regarded as acts of "power," including casting spells, causing the dead to rise or speak, expelling *daimones*, facilitating the possession of a body by deity, healing sick bodies, transmuting materials, and projecting the soul from the body.[9] Other potentially "miraculous" acts that Paul mentions in his letters include prophecy, speaking in tongues, pronouncing curses, and experiencing visions of God. As it happens, Luke shows Paul engaging in all of these activities in the book of Acts, including a possibly relevant story in which a group of newly baptized believers spoke in tongues and prophesied after Paul had laid hands on them (Acts 19:6).[10] This explanation of what Paul meant by "signs and wonders" is attractive in view of his extended discussion of prophecy and tongues in 1 Corinthians 12-14, but it is only a possibility.

Graham Twelftree has proposed another solution that would preserve the idea of Paul as a healer while avoiding many of the criticisms that have been raised against other iterations of this explanation. According to Twelftree, miraculous acts like healings and exorcisms occurred spontaneously during the course of Paul's preaching and not as a result of any action on his part. It was quite literally the power of Christ working through him, independent of his own will or action.[11] Twelftree explains it this way.

> The resolution of this puzzle—the scenario that brings the pieces together—is that although miracles took place in association with his ministry, Paul neither set out to perform them nor orchestrated those that took place. Rather, as he preached, the Spirit's powerful presence was spontaneously manifested in the miraculous. This was God's doing, not Paul's. In the simplest terms, if pressed, Paul might say

---

[7] Noted by Remus, *Jesus as Healer*, 98.
[8] Jacob Jervell suggests that Paul's illness lay behind the criticisms of the "super-apostles" that Paul addresses in 2 Corinthians 10-12, but he offers no evidence for the claim (*The Unknown Paul: Essays on Luke-Acts and Early Christian History* [Minneapolis, MN: Augsburg, 1984], 93–4).
[9] *Signs, Wonders, and Gifts*, 121.
[10] Luke also describes Paul restoring a young man to life (Acts 20:10-22) and resisting the effects of snake venom (Acts 28:5), but these acts are so singular (and so incredible) as to exclude them from consideration here.
[11] A similar idea was proposed three years earlier by Stefan Schreiber (*Paulus also Wundertäter*, 205, 207), but he did not develop it as Twelftree has done. Twelftree lists Schreiber's book in his bibliography, but he does not cite it in the pages where he lays out his argument.

that the gospel was proclaimed when he did the preaching and Christ, through the Spirit, performed the miracles.[12]

In support of this interpretation, Twelftree cites several passages from the New Testament where miracles are said to have occurred without instigation from the performer, including the woman who was cured by touching Jesus's cloak (Mk 5:24-34); the sick people of Jerusalem who were healed when Peter's shadow passed over them (Acts 5:15); the members of Cornelius's household who began speaking in tongues while Peter was preaching to them (Acts 10:44-47); and the residents of Corinth who were cured or exorcised by contact with cloths that had touched Paul's skin (Acts 19:11-12).[13] He also points to verses in Paul's letters where he talks about the Spirit of God or Christ speaking and acting powerfully through him (Rom. 15:18-19, 2 Cor. 5:20, Gal. 2:20, 1 Thess. 2:13) despite the weakness of his body (1 Cor. 2:1-5, 2 Cor. 4:7-12, 12:9-10; cf. 2 Cor. 3:4-6).[14] A similar idea appears in 1 Cor. 12:4-11, where Paul speaks of the Spirit working through the Corinthian believers to heal and perform acts of power (cf. Rom. 8:9-11, 8:26-27, 1 Cor. 4:19-20, Gal. 3:2-5).[15]

According to Twelftree, the presence of such miraculous events was vital not only to the success of Paul's mission but also to his self-understanding. They confirmed to Paul and to his hearers that God was present when he preached and that he and his followers were indeed living in the eschatological age of the Spirit that Paul claimed had begun with the resurrection of Jesus. Their spontaneity was equally crucial since it showed that it was God's Spirit and not Paul who was performing them. In fact, Paul's knowledge and experience of Christ were rooted in a miraculous act of God that turned him from a critic to a partisan of the risen Jesus (1 Cor. 15:3-9, Gal. 1:13-24, Phil. 3:4-11). His preaching promised a similar transformation by the power of God's Spirit to all who "turned to God from idols" (1 Thess. 1:9), and he assured them that the Spirit would continue to do miracles in their midst like the ones that accompanied his missionary preaching (1 Cor. 12:4-11, Gal. 3:1-5). In short, the present and active power of God was an essential element of Paul's gospel (Rom. 1:16). As Twelftree puts it, "Without the miraculous, there was no gospel, only preaching."[16]

There is much to be said for Twelftree's reading of Paul, especially its ability to answer most of the criticisms that were raised earlier against viewing Paul as a healer. According to Twelftree, Paul did not claim to be a miracle-worker (or a healer) because he was not. Miracles happened when he preached, but he was as surprised as anyone else when they occurred. He could not promise anyone that God would heal them or perform other mighty acts on their behalf because such events occurred independently of his will or control. He could pray for God to heal (2 Cor. 12:8-10), but he was just as likely as anyone to be disappointed. He was only a weak vessel through which God's Spirit chose to act; he did not have any power within himself, nor could he control it.

---

[12] *Paul and the Miraculous*, 225.
[13] Ibid., 215-16.
[14] Ibid., 135, 138, 142, 145, 195-200, 213-16, 219-21,
[15] Twelftree discusses the miraculous quality of the *charismata* in ibid., 170-6, but he does not cite them as evidence for Paul's thinking about the power of God working in and through believers.
[16] Ibid., 317. This paragraph summarizes what Twelftree says in pp. 313-23.

The same could be said for those through whom the Spirit chose to exhibit the special abilities described in 1 Corinthians 12: they could ask God to grant them particular *charismata* (1 Cor. 14:1, 13), but the Spirit alone decides how, when, and through whom those powers will be expressed (1 Cor. 12:4-11).[17]

Given this view of the Spirit's activity, it was useless for Paul to tell stories about Jesus healing the sick as if he could somehow replicate what Jesus had done; he could not. There was also no reason for him or his followers to refrain from using ordinary modes of treatment for sickness and injury since there was no way of knowing if, when, or how God might heal them. Only treatments that appealed to divine powers other than the God and Father of Jesus Christ were to be avoided, since Christ-followers were now citizens of a new kingdom where a greater power prevailed. Their bodies remained subject to the sickness, decay, and death that characterized the present age, but they lived in hope that they would soon receive immortal spiritual bodies free from every form of sickness and suffering when their divine Lord defeated every rival power and reigned supreme forever. Until then, they could count on the Spirit of God that inhabited their bodies to give them strength to bear up patiently under bodily afflictions.

While we cannot be sure that this was in fact what Paul thought and experienced, it makes better sense of the data than any other proposal put forward to date. The remainder of this chapter will explore other lines of evidence that lend plausibility to Twelftree's thesis while painting a more nuanced portrait of its potential implications (both positive and negative) for the success of Paul's evangelistic mission.

Miracles and Evangelism

Enticing someone to abandon lifelong familial, social, and religious identities and associations and join a new religious movement is difficult under any circumstances. The difficulty is compounded when the beliefs and practices of the new group diverge so sharply from prevailing norms as those of the Christ-movement did from the polytheism of first-century Greco-Roman society. To become a Christ-follower meant not only changing one's religious views but breaking ties with the entire social system that defined one's identity and gave structure and meaning to every aspect of daily life. It could also mean incurring the ire of people who could make one's life difficult by withholding necessary goods or services or even inflicting pain upon the convert's body, especially if the person was a slave or a woman. Something more than a fine speech was needed to make people embark on such a perilous course.

Yet Paul succeeded in enticing at least a few people here and there to make this leap of faith. What did he say or do to make this happen? Here again we run into the same problem that we met when inquiring about his views of sickness and health care: a lack of source material. Paul's letters give us only brief and tantalizing glimpses of

---

[17] Opinion is divided over whether Paul envisions the "gifts" in 1 Corinthians 12 as being granted permanently to particular individuals or as temporary expressions of the Spirit's power through different people at different times. The latter reading is followed here.

his missionary activities, and our only other source, the book of Acts, is notoriously tendentious and unreliable.

According to Acts, Paul usually began his evangelistic outreach in a new city by visiting the local synagogue, where he delivered a long, scripture-based sermon that ended with an account of the death and resurrection of Jesus. This sermon attracted a few converts from both Judeans and gentile "God-fearers." Encouraged by these results, Paul continued to visit and speak in the synagogue until Judean opposition forced him to either leave the city or move to another venue. If he did the latter, he ended up preaching mostly to gentiles, who received his message with joy. Here and there he performed miracles, including healing the sick, but only a handful were done to advance his message (13:8-12, 14:3, 15:12). Only one took place while he was in the act of preaching (14:8-10), and it involved conscious action by Paul. It was not spontaneous, and it produced no converts.

Paul, on the other hand, says nothing about visiting synagogues as part of his missionary strategy. But he does say that he presented his message to both Judeans and gentiles (Rom. 1:16-17, 10:1-4, 1 Cor. 1:21-25, 9:19-23), and he also speaks often about how the death and resurrection of Jesus relate to the core scriptural teaching that Judeans are God's chosen people, especially in Romans 9-11, so Luke's account is at least plausible. It is unlikely, however, that preaching in Jewish synagogues played such a prominent role in Paul's missionary strategy as Luke indicates, and it is equally improbable that he used such closely reasoned biblical argumentation when preaching to gentiles who knew little or nothing about Judaism or its Scriptures. The only thing that Paul says about the content of his evangelistic preaching (his "gospel") is that it centered on the crucifixion and resurrection of Jesus and his present status as Lord (Rom. 10:9-13, 1 Cor. 1:17-18, 1:23-24, 2:2, Gal. 3:1). He admits that this message sounds foolish to both Judeans and gentiles (1 Cor. 1:18-31), so it is unlikely that the content of his preaching alone was sufficient to persuade many people to abandon their former lives and follow him.

If his message was hard for people to believe, was it perhaps his preaching style that won them over? Not if they were assessing him by conventional norms. The one point on which Paul and his critics appear to have agreed is that his speeches did not measure up to the canons of Greek and Roman rhetoric (1 Cor. 1:17-18, 2:1-5, 2 Cor. 10:10, 11:6). But this does not mean that he was an incompetent speaker; the fact that he won converts suggests that some people found him persuasive. More likely his speaking style resembled that of the popular preachers who plied their trade in the civic agora, a type of oratory that would have been attractive to the masses though it was disdained by the elites.[18] His insistence that he preached only "Christ crucified" (1 Cor. 1:23, 2:1-2) suggests that his speeches included a fair amount of storytelling as he recounted to his hearers how the one true God had sent Jesus to die for human sins, then restored him to life and exalted him to heaven. He might even have acted out parts of the story to make it more vivid for his audience, depending on how literally we take his language in Gal. 3:1 about Jesus being "publicly displayed as crucified" during his initial visit to the Galatians. Another possible channel for evangelistic outreach is suggested in

[18] More will be said on this point later.

1 Thess. 2:9-12, where Paul recalls how he worked with his hands while teaching the Thessalonians about the ways of God (cf. 1 Cor. 4:12, 9:6, Acts 18:1-3). If we take his words literally, we might envision him engaging in private religious conversations with people in his shop as opposed to unidirectional public preaching.[19] The fact that he worked at a trade would have enhanced his appeal to the laboring masses even as it lowered him in the eyes of the local elites.

Preaching alone, however, cannot change lives; there must be some sort of response. Here and there in Paul's letters we see glimpses of the type of language that he might have used when challenging his hearers to make the life-changing decision that was required to become a full-throated Christ-follower. In 2 Cor. 5:20, where he claims to speak as an "ambassador for Christ," he boldly exhorts the Corinthians "on behalf of Christ, be reconciled to God!" This sounds more like the closing appeal of an evangelistic sermon than an injunction directed to Christ-followers. The same is true for his forceful (and contextually awkward) injunction in 2 Cor 6:2, "Look, now is the right time! Look, now is the day of salvation!" The repeated use of ἰδού here would be particularly appropriate if the words were spoken immediately after Paul had acted out some aspect of the story of Jesus in a public setting. In Rom. 10:9, Paul explains what is required to become a follower of Christ: "If you confess with your lips that Jesus is Lord and believe in your heart that God raised him from the dead, you will be saved." It is easy to see how statements like the ones in 2 Cor. 5:20 and 6:2 might elicit such a response.

Yet Paul cannot speak about his evangelistic success without also mentioning the "acts of power" that accompanied his preaching. Paul was keenly aware of the obstacles that hindered his success: he was not a great orator (at least not by elite standards), his physical appearance was unsightly (possibly marked by a visible disability), and his message—that the one true God is offering salvation to humanity through a crucified Messiah—sounded nonsensical or even offensive to faithful Jews and polytheistic gentiles alike. Something greater than speech was needed to persuade people to accept this message and make the radical and costly decision to break with everything that they had known and join this strange new religious movement. According to Paul, that "something" was the power of God.

It would be easy to suppose that Paul's language about "the power of God" is simply a reflection of his amazement that anyone would respond with faith to his preaching in view of the many barriers that limited his effectiveness: it couldn't be him, it had to be God. But this reading begs the question of how Paul was so successful at winning converts. At best, it implies that Paul must have been a better preacher than he realized. But that is not what Paul says; he attributes his success to displays of divine power that were so visible and obvious as to convince people that he was speaking for the one true God and that his words were true despite the oddness of both speaker and message.

---

[19] This point was developed at length by Ronald F. Hock in *The Social Context of Paul's Ministry: Tentmaking and Apostleship* (Philadelphia: Fortress, 1980). A more recent study that focuses more on Paul's view of work than on its role in his preaching is Todd D. Still, "Did Paul Loathe Manual Labor? Revisiting the Work of Ronald F. Hock on the Apostle's Tentmaking and Social Class," *JBL* 125 (2006): 781–95.

This is what led Graham Twelftree to assert that "without the miraculous, there was no gospel, only preaching."[20]

Once we recognize this fact, we can see other places in Paul's letters where he could be alluding to the role that such displays of divine power played in persuading people to accept his message. In Rom. 1:16-17, he famously refers to the gospel as the "power of God for salvation" by which "the righteousness of God is revealed" so as to evoke a response of faith. While it is usual to take this language as referring to the revelation of God's saving purposes in the death and resurrection of Jesus, the close conjunction of "power," "revelation," and "faith" in these verses sounds very much like what Paul suggests is happening when he preaches his "gospel": the truth of his message is made evident (i.e., "revealed) to his hearers by the presence of miraculous acts of divine power that overcome their intellectual objections and motivate them to profess faith in the Christ whom Paul preaches. A similar explanation can be posited for Paul's repeated use of the word "power" in 1 Cor. 1:17-25 in conjunction with his message about the crucifixion of Jesus (vv. 17, 18, 24), since he goes on to insist it was not his own "persuasive words of wisdom" but "a demonstration of the Spirit and power" that provided the grounds for their faith when he first came to them (2:4-5).[21]

It is tempting to suppose that Paul viewed these displays of divine power as signs (in the sense of "evidence") that the Spirit of God or Christ had come to dwell in the bodies of new believers and imbued them with power (Rom. 5:5, 8:9-11, 1 Cor. 3:16-17, 6:19-20, 2 Cor. 5:5, 13:3-4, Gal. 2:19-20; cf. Acts 2:1-33, 10:44-48, 19:1-7). But Paul never makes such a connection. In fact, there is no suggestion in his letters that every person who came to faith through his preaching experienced an "act of power" in their own bodies as this theory would require. He could just as well be referring to a small number of odd events that he and his hearers interpreted as miraculous.

But what were those events? When and how did they occur? What led his hearers to take them as proofs of the validity of Paul's message? Paul's silence on these questions is frustrating, though not insurmountable. We will never be able to answer the first question with any certainty despite the many possibilities that have been suggested, but we can form reasonable conjectures for the other two by examining the findings of scholars who have studied "miraculous" cures in modern times and using their observations as a template to guide us in imagining and interpreting the social context and practices of Paul's evangelistic preaching. The resultant framework can then be used to assess the plausibility of the thesis that healing was one of the experiences included in Paul's "signs and wonders."

---

[20] *Paul and the Miraculous*, 317.
[21] This interpretation might appear to be undermined by Paul's rejection in 1:22 of Jewish demands for "signs." But he cannot be saying that miracles are unnecessary for true faith as some have supposed since he himself claims that "signs and wonders" played a vital role in the success of his missionary preaching (Rom. 15:18-19). More likely he is using the words "signs" in the same sense that we see in the Gospels, where Jesus consistently refuses demands from skeptics that he perform some sort of "sign" to prove the truth of his message (Mk 8:11-12, Mt. 12:38-42/Lk. 11:29-32, Mt. 16:1-4, Lk. 11:16-18, Jn 2:18-19, 4:48, 6:29-33). This makes all the more sense if Twelftree is right in suggesting that Paul was incapable of performing "acts of power" on demand.

On the Making of Miracles

While we can never rule out the possibility that reports of miraculous events in various world religions reflect the activity of divine powers, such explanations lie beyond the ability of historical and scientific methods to assess. But there is still much that can be learned from focusing on the human side of the equation. Social-scientific methods in particular have proved useful for isolating some of the social and psychological factors that predispose individuals and groups to experience such events.

Significant attention has been given in recent years to the role of the placebo effect in healing. Researchers have long observed that a certain percentage of people who are treated with inert substances like sugar pills (i.e., placebos) show improvements in physical and mental health that are greater than can be reasonably attributed to study design or chance. Conditions for which placebos have been shown to be effective include muscular and joint pain, allergies, psoriasis, gastrointestinal problems, rheumatoid arthritis, and the common cold.[22] Estimates of the percentage of patients whose complaints are partially or fully alleviated by this placebo effect range from 33 to 60 percent.[23] This observation has elicited many follow-up studies to investigate what is actually happening in these cases to produce such measurable healing effects. The result has been a growing appreciation of the role of social and psychological factors in producing both sickness and healing.

At the most basic level, these studies have led to a greater appreciation of the link between body and mind and the degree to which both are affected by their physical and social environments.[24] Negative mental states can increase the incidence of stress-related physical ailments like irritable bowel syndrome, ulcers, herpes, colds, and other conditions, while chronic or severe illness can lead to marked declines in psychological well-being, including anxiety, depression, and suicidal ideations. Both physical and mental health are in turn affected by the physical environment, including exposure to toxins, harsh weather, poor sanitation, and vermin. Difficult social environments can also produce high levels of stress that lead to a host of negative health effects.

More important for our purpose is the positive side of this web of associations. Numerous studies have shown that positive mental states can contribute to the maintenance or restoration of bodily health and vice versa. The same is true for

---

[22] The list comes from Dave Newell, Lise R. Lothe, and Timothy J. L. Raven, "Contextually Aided Recovery (CARe): A Scientific Theory for Innate Healing," *Chiropractic & Manual Therapies* 25 (2017): 1–10. For a fuller list of conditions with extended discussion of the evidence for each one, see Fabrizio Benedetti, *Placebo Effects: Understanding the Mechanisms in Health and Disease* (Oxford: Oxford University Press, 2009).

[23] The lower figure is found in two studies cited by John S. Welch in "Ritual in Western Medicine and Its Role in Placebo Healing," *Journal of Religion and Health* 42 (2003): 26. The higher number comes from Robert Buckman and Karl Sabbagh, *Magic or Medicine: An Investigation of Healing and Healers* (Amherst, NY: Prometheus Books, 1993), 39, 172–3, 237.

[24] For helpful overviews of this integrative understanding of sickness and health, see David Landy, "Toward a Biocultural Medical Anthropology," *Medical Anthropology Quarterly* 4 (1990): 358–69; Giovanni A. Fava and Nicoletta Sonino, "Psychosomatic Medicine: Emerging Trends and Perspectives," *Psychotherapy and Psychosomatics* 69 (2000): 184–97; and Marc S. Micozzi, "Culture, Anthropology, and the Return of 'Complementary Medicine,'" *Medical Anthropology Quarterly* 16 (2002): 398–403.

improvements in the physical environment, as factors ranging from changes of season to better sewage systems to moving to a more salubrious climate can produce better health outcomes. Changes in the social environment can also improve physical and mental well-being, including such influences as new relationships, new jobs, and access to better health care.

Social and psychological factors appear to be the dominant forces behind the placebo effect. As we saw in Chapter 2, medical anthropologists have recognized that physical healing is a social process in which various types of social networks interpret and give meaning to the experience of sickness, define and prescribe suitable modes of treatment, support the sick person during the time of illness, and validate claims of healing. Trust (or faith) plays a vital role in all phases of the health care process—trust in the efficacy of the system as a whole, the skills of the healer, the prescribed modes of treatment, and similar factors. This is just as true for medical forms of treatment as for traditional health care systems.[25]

Nicholas Humphrey has laid out a framework that many others have adopted to explain how this biopsychosocial view of sickness and healing relates to the placebo effect.[26] According to Humphrey, placebos works because people are conditioned in a particular social context to believe (or have faith) that the treatment will provide relief. This belief can influence the body to activate its natural powers of self-healing so that a cure that is in fact produced by the sick person's body is wrongly credited to an external treatment. In short, the body is tricked by the social context of treatment into healing itself.[27] All bodies possess such self-healing powers, which explains why most forms of sickness go away on their own. As Humphrey puts it, "When people recover from illness as a result of placebo treatments, it is of course their own healing systems that are doing the job. Placebo cure is self-cure."[28]

---

[25] For a helpful analysis of the medical visit as a type of religious ritual, see Welch, "Ritual," 22–6. For a comparison of the two approaches in a particular setting, see Sipco J. Vellenga, "Longing for Health: A Practice of Religious Healing and Biomedicine Compared," *Journal of Religion and Health* 47 (2008): 326–37. Newell et al. divide the contextual components into three categories: physical signals, verbal cues, and environmental cues ("Contextually Aided Recovery (CARe)," 7). A subsequent analysis by Giacomo Rossettini, Eleonora Maria Camerone, Elisa Carlino, Fabrizio Benedetti and Marco Testa expanded this list to five categories: physiotherapist features, patient features, patient–physiotherapist relationship, treatment features, and health care setting features ("Context Matters: The Psychoneurobiological Determinants of Placebo, Nocebo and Context-Related Effects in Physiotherapy," *Archives of Physiotherapy* 10 [2020]: 1–12).

[26] Humphrey's views are laid out in several articles, including "Great Expectations: The Evolutionary Psychology of Faith-Healing and the Placebo Effect," in *Psychology at the Turn of the Millennium, Vol. 2: Social, Developmental, and Clinical Perspectives*, ed. Claes von Hofsten and Lars Bäckman (London: Psychology Press, 2002), 225–46; "The Placebo Effect," in *Oxford Companion to the Mind*, ed. Richard L. Gregory (Oxford: Oxford University Press, 2004), 735–6; and (with John Skoyles) "The Evolutionary Psychology of Healing: A Human Success Story," *Current Biology* 22 (2012): 695–7. He does not use the term "biopsychosocial" to describe his theory, but the label is common in the literature.

[27] The language of trickery comes directly from Humphrey: see "Evolutionary Psychology of Healing," 696. Medical research has moved beyond Humphrey's vague proposal to identify many of the neurobiological processes that are involved in the placebo effect. For a summary, see Rossettini et al., "Context Matters," 5–7. A fuller discussion can be found in Benedetti, *Placebo Effects*.

[28] *Placebo Effect*, 736.

Humphrey lays out four psychosocial conditions that are typically present when the placebo response is activated.[29]

- The patient is *aware* that the treatment is being given;
- The patient has a certain *belief* in the treatment, based, for example, on prior experience, or on the treatment's reputation;
- The patient's belief leads her to *expect* that, following this treatment, she is likely to get better; and
- The *expectation* influences her capacity for self-cure, so as to hasten the very result that she expects.

A similar process occurs when medically active treatments are applied: part of the cure is caused by the external remedy, but the mental state of the patient also plays a role. According to microbiologist Tirumalai Kamala, "The placebo effect and its evil twin, the nocebo effect, are at play in each and every interaction between doctor and patient. In fact, the placebo effect is an integral part of medical practice itself. Thus, even bonafide drugs and other medical interventions such as surgeries depend to varying degrees on the placebo effect for their action."[30] Some go even farther, suggesting that the placebo effect is so strong, varied, and indeterminable that even double-blind drug trials cannot necessarily be trusted.[31] In short, contemporary medical science recognizes that the placebo effect plays a significant role in the success or failure of health care treatments.

Similar forces appear to be at work in other forms of healing, particularly those associated with religious settings. Social scientists have studied a variety of religious healers and movements in different countries with a view to clarifying the influence of social and psychological factors on the experiences of miraculous healing that are reported in these settings. Some of these reports can be dismissed as wishful thinking or fraud, but there are enough cases of verifiable partial or complete recovery to raise

---

[29] "Great Expectations," 226. Rossettini et al., as medical researchers, use more clinical terminology to describe the same psychological mechanisms: "expectation, learning processes such as classical conditioning and observational learning, reinforced expectations, mindset, and personality traits" ("Context Matters," 3). The only real difference is the addition of "personality traits," with suggestibility and optimism as the primary traits that can make people more open to placebo effects (5). While it is common to suppose that ancient people were more gullible (i.e., suggestible) than modern people, we have no way of assessing the validity of such a claim. In any event, the authors of the study indicate that the correlation between personality traits and placebo responsiveness is weak.

[30] Blog post on *TK Talk* website, Dec. 29, 2019; available at https://tirumalaikamala.wordpress.com/2019/12.

[31] For an example of this viewpoint, see Olov Lindahl and Lars Lindwall, "Is All Therapy Just a Placebo Effect?" *Theoretical Medicine and Bioethics* 3 (1982): 255–9. After surveying a series of clinical trials, they conclude that "the body's reaction to different medicines (positive, negative, or none) is dependent on the simultaneous interaction with a placebo situation; i.e., the real effect is dependent on the placebo dose. Without knowledge of this dose, it is impossible to decide on the grounds of a clinical trial whether the effect of a therapy in a different situation will be positive, negative or none" (257).

questions about what is causing the cures.[32] Disregarding claims of divine causality, social scientists have pointed to aspects of the healing environment that might serve to activate the placebo effect in certain individuals and so produce genuine cures in people seeking to be healed.

Prior belief in the efficacy of the healer, group, or movement is an important factor in virtually all accounts of miraculous healing.[33] In most cases the sick person is already involved with a group that practices religious healing and thus has a preexisting expectation that healing might occur on a specific occasion. Stories of healings that have occurred in connection with a particular healer or sacred site often circulate within these communities, where they serve to increase the level of expectation. In cases that do not involve prior association, the sick person has often been disillusioned by other forms of treatment and is searching for more powerful remedies, including miracle-working religious healers, as a last resort. A degree of faith is required to experience healing; skeptics are rarely cured unless something occurs during the healing ceremony to stimulate their faith in the healer, the process, or both. Many successful healers make a conscious effort to convert such doubters by using carefully honed techniques that appeal to the mind and emotions of the sick person. The precise techniques that are used vary with the beliefs and practices of the religion. Since the present study focuses on Christian forms of healing, our inquiry will be limited to two examples from Christian settings.

In Pentecostal healing services, the most common techniques for evoking faith are emotional music, selective quotations of biblical texts, testimonies about healings that occurred in prior sessions (or the present one), and exhortations to reach out to God in faith and accept (or "claim") the healing that God offers.[34] Other popular practices include laying on of hands (personalized prayers performed while touching the sick person) and "words of knowledge" (claims by the healer that God is healing or about to heal someone in the audience with a particular health condition). Behaviors that are thought to signify the mighty presence of God coursing through the room are also encouraged, including falling to the ground, trembling, weeping, and laughing uncontrollably. Together these practices create an environment in which sick people feel confident that God is present and ready to heal them if they will only open their hearts in faith and allow God to work.

---

[32] For a thoughtful review of historical and contemporary tensions between Christian religious healers and medical science over "proofs" of healing, see Candy Gunther Brown, "Healing Prayer in an Age of Evidence-Based Medicine," *Transformations* 32 (2015):1–16.

[33] For more on this point, see (in addition to the studies cited in the following note) Gaius Davies, "The Hands of the Healer: Has Faith a Place?" *Journal of Medical Ethics* 6 (1980): 185–9.

[34] See, for example, James Peacock, "Symbolic and Psychological Anthropology: The Case of Pentecostal Faith Healing," *Ethos* 12 (1984): 37–53; Margaret M. Poloma and Lynette F. Hoelter, "The 'Toronto Blessing': A Holistic Model of Healing," *JSSR* 37 (1998): 257–72; and Jörg Stolz, "All Things Are Possible": Towards a Sociological Explanation of Pentecostal Miracles and Healings," *Sociology of Religion* 72 (2011): 456–82. For a detailed analysis of the health problems from which people claim to have been healed in a particular movement, see Ella Paldam and Uffe Schjoedt, "Miracles and Pain Relief: Experienced Health Effects of Charismatic Prayer Healing in a Large Collection of Christian Testimonies," *Archiv für Religionspsychologie* 38 (2016): 210–31.

Healing practices in Roman Catholic circles differ markedly from those used by Pentecostals.[35] While the power of God is in principle available to all believers, Catholics tend to associate healing with certain people (priests, nuns, saints) or places (churches, shrines, grottoes) that they regard as especially holy. Places where the Virgin Mary is reported to have appeared (Lourdes, Fátima, Medjugorje, etc.) are particularly potent, along with sites where saints are buried and churches where parts of saints' bodies are venerated as relics. Sick people often make pilgrimages to these sites in search of a cure, encouraged by stories of healings that others experienced while making similar journeys.

At the local level, Catholics offer prayers for healing to Mary and to various saints who have gained fame as healers based on stories of their healing prowess.[36] Rituals involving the Eucharist are crucial to virtually all forms of Catholic healing because of their belief that it carries divine power as the body and blood of Jesus Christ. The sacrament of Anointing the Sick, applied by the sacred hands of a priest or bishop, can be added in more serious cases.[37] Religious gatherings where people are promised immediate healing are virtually unknown in the Catholic tradition apart from masses at pilgrimage sites and the informal healing services that charismatic Catholics sometimes hold under the influence of the Pentecostal movement. Physical and emotional displays are permissible in the latter setting, where they are interpreted as signs of the presence of God, but they play little role in traditional Catholic healing, which views rituals as the primary channel for experiencing the healing power of God.

Despite their obvious differences, both Pentecostal and Catholic healing practices fulfill all four conditions that Nicholas Humphrey has specified for the activation of the placebo effect.

- The person who seeks healing is clearly *aware* that some form of religious treatment is being given, whether it is performed at home through prayers or rituals (cf. taking pills prescribed by a physician) or by an authorized healer at a particular site using specialized practices (cf. visiting a doctor's office).
- The sick person has a certain *belief* in the treatment that is rooted in core convictions about the nature of God (cf. trust in science and the medical system) and reinforced by stories and personal experiences of successful healing through the use of particular practices (cf. bedside manner, reports of clinical drug trials)

---

[35] Catholic healing methods vary widely; for a sampling of analytic studies of particular practices, see Thomas J. Csordas, "Elements of Charismatic Persuasion and Healing," *Medical Anthropology Quarterly* 2 (1988); 121–42; Jason Szabo, "Seeing Is Believing? The Form and Substance of French Medical Debates over Lourdes," *Bulletin of the History of Medicine* 76 (2002): 199–230; and Katharina Wilkens, "Mary and the Demons: Marian Devotion and Ritual Healing in Tanzania," *Journal of Religion in Africa* 39 (2009): 295–318.

[36] For a detailed sociological analysis of the many factors that contributed to the rise and popularity of a particular healing saint, see Mary Dunn, "Making Miracles Efficacious: Kateri Tekakwitha, Miraculous Cures, and Relational Networks in Seventeenth-Century France," in *Intimacies: Intersubjectivity in the Modern Christian West*, ed. Mary Dunn and Brenna Moore (Bloomington, IN: University Press, 2020), 65–86.

[37] Other rituals can also play a role in particular settings. For a discussion of the many rituals employed by the sick at a specific healing shrine, see David J. Hufford, "Ste. Anne de Beaupré: Roman Catholic Pilgrimage and Healing," *Western Folklore* 44 (1985): 194–207.

and/or accounts of the effectiveness of a healer or site (cf. a physician's reputation as a "good doctor").
- This belief leads the sick person to *expect* that, following this treatment, she is likely to get better, an expectation that is especially potent (and difficult to falsify) in religious settings where the healer is an all-knowing, all-powerful divine being rather than a human doctor.
- This *expectation* influences the sick person's capacity for self-cure and thus hastens the result that she expects, even as her underlying belief system causes her to attribute the cure to God (cf. medical cures being credited to an inert substance).

In short, there is ample reason to suppose that the placebo effect lies behind many or most of the apparently "miraculous" healings that have been reported by religious healers and institutions, whether they happen through direct treatment by a healer or spontaneously during religious gatherings. But this does not mean that religious healers are frauds; they are no more fraudulent than physicians who credit their treatments with producing the 35 to 60 percent of healing outcomes that researchers attribute to the social and psychological environments in which the treatments are dispensed. Fraud undoubtedly occurs in both settings, but it is relatively uncommon.

The reality is that healing is a complex process involving forces that are not fully understood. Crediting God as the cause of a particular cure appears nonsensical from a scientific viewpoint, but it makes eminent sense to Jews, Christians, and Muslims who view all of reality, including sickness and healing, through a religious lens. Medical science, for all of its hegemonic claims, cannot negate these claims since they lie beyond scientific falsifiability.

Paul among the Freelance Experts

So what does all of this have to do with the apostle Paul? He clearly was not a physician, even by ancient standards, and there is no evidence that he led healing services in which he urged his listeners to receive the curative power of God, whether in the marketplace or within the walls of the local house-church. The idea that certain people or places are more holy or powerful than others (with the possible exception of himself and other apostles) is likewise hard to square with his constant reference to his followers as "the holy ones" (οἱ ἅγιοι) and his consistently metaphorical interpretations of cultic terms and practices (Rom. 12:1-2, 15:16, 1 Cor. 3:16-17, 6:19-20, 2 Cor. 6:16, etc.). He does acknowledge that certain rituals can have powerful effects on the condition of humans (Rom. 6:4-7, 1 Cor. 5:3-5, 10:14-21, 11:23-32), but he never associates any of them with physical healing.[38]

At a higher level, however, there are similarities between Paul and modern religious healers that should not be overlooked. In fact, given what we know or can reasonably infer about Paul's evangelistic activities and the healing practices of his day, it is possible

[38] He does assert in 1 Cor. 11:27-30 that sickness can arise from wrongful partaking of the Lord's Supper, but he never says the reverse, that one can be restored to health by taking the sacred meal.

to imagine a historically plausible scenario in which social and psychological forces like those identified by Humphrey might have combined to create spontaneous events, including healings, that Paul and his audiences could have regarded as "miraculous."

As we observed earlier, Heidi Wendt has made a strong case for viewing Paul as one of many "freelance religious experts" who plied their trade in the towns and cities of the Roman Empire in an effort to gain converts, fame, money, and other social goods. Some of these experts maintained fixed abodes in a particular location while others traveled from place to place promoting their wares. A large percentage were foreigners seeking to capitalize on the public's interest in novel and exotic teachings and practices, particularly those from the eastern provinces. Their numbers included both men and women who claimed to have superior knowledge or skill in a wide variety of areas, including "self-proclaimed priests, prophets, mystery initiators, *magi*, sacrificers," diviners, astrologers, purifiers, dream interpreters, exorcists, and of course, healers.[39] They could be found wherever people gathered in sufficient numbers to form an audience, including the local agora on market days and the temple precincts during festivals, where they "competed intensely and with great creativity for potential followers or students."[40] Many used popular entertainment techniques to gather an audience, including juggling, sleight of hand tricks, storytelling, acrobatics, music, acting, and marionette shows.[41]

Popular response to these freelance religious experts was divided. The elites disdained them as charlatans and frauds (using the same language that we saw in Chapter 3 for "magicians"), while much of the broader populace found them engaging, entertaining, and even convincing. Their growing numbers and popularity in the first and second centuries CE led to scattered efforts to suppress them, including a few reports of confiscations of materials and forcible removals from cities.[42] Some were even accused of treason.[43] Elite ignorance about who was and was not a threat often led to indiscriminate action against anyone who might be perceived as a member of this class, including itinerant preachers like Paul.

Those who stopped to listen to such people in the marketplace would have been a mixed crowd. Some were bored shoppers or loiterers with nothing better to do, while others came seeking entertainment or to heckle those whom they viewed as frauds. But enough people took them seriously to arouse concern among the civic elites. Some were disenchanted seekers attracted to new ideas, but the majority appear to have been people who were experiencing some sort of personal difficulty from which they sought relief. Addressing these problems was a central concern of freelance religious

---

[39] Summarized from Wendt, *At the Temple Gates*, 10–17, 43–4.
[40] Ibid., 29.
[41] Dickie, *Magic and Magicians in the Greco-Roman World*, 74–5, 233–40.
[42] For more on elite responses and efforts at repression, see Wendt, *At the Temple Gates*, 1–5, 44–54. Much of what we read in Acts about Paul being driven out of cities can be traced to local leaders viewing him as a member of this class of "charlatans and deceivers." Timothy Luckritz Marquis describes well how Paul's "foreignness, his transient lifestyle, his voluntary poverty, and his apparent lack of physical or oratorical impressiveness" could have led the civic elites to regard him as "a charlatan purveyor of an Eastern god" (*Transient Apostle: Paul, Travel, and the Rhetoric of Empire* (New Haven and London: Yale University Press, 2013), 71, 84).
[43] Wendt, *At the Temple Gates*, 55–8.

experts, to judge from the types of services that they offered. Most used some sort of ritual practice to channel the power or wisdom of the gods to humans or to remove impediments to divine activity. Some appealed to the traditional Greek or Roman deities for help while others promoted various foreign deities whose teachings and rituals they claimed were more effective than those of the traditional cult.

Given the frequency of sickness and injury in the ancient world, it is not surprising that many of these religious experts offered remedies for health problems, nor that people came to them seeking cures. In fact, healing was one of the chief benefits that people sought from the gods and their representatives. It is not hard to imagine the anticipation that would have greeted the arrival of a new preacher like Paul who promised access to the power and protection of a supreme deity who cared so much about the welfare of humans that he sent his son to die for them, then elevated him to the heavens where he intercedes with the almighty creator to assist those in need. Such a message would have been deeply inspiring to some in his audience who were desperate to be healed, stirring up hope that such a deity might use his power to cure them.[44] This hope could have been fervent enough in a few cases to activate their body's powers of self-healing and produce a cure that appeared miraculous.

Others who had been disappointed with previous healers might have had their hopes renewed upon hearing about such a person, especially if the news was attended by reports of miraculous events occurring among his listeners.[45] People like this would have come to Paul ready to be cured, and their expectations would have been further enhanced if they found Paul's message persuasive.[46] This restored confidence might in some cases have been sufficient to induce a sudden improvement in their condition that they (and Paul) viewed as a miracle. Still others might have experienced a sense of emotional release while listening to Paul that they interpreted as a liberation from demonic power or the breaking of a curse. In short, "miracles" could have occurred during Paul's preaching in exactly the way that researchers say they happen in Pentecostal and Catholic healing services (or masses): audience members feel themselves touched by the power of God and cured without direct personal contact with the healer.

Miracles of this sort would not have required any conscious effort on Paul's part; their occurrence depended entirely on the personal history and mental condition of the listener, even if Paul credited them to the sovereign intervention of God. Nor would many such events have been required to convince some listeners about the truth

---

[44] The presence of hundreds of healing shrines across central and western Turkey from the Roman era suggests that divine healing was a particular concern for people in this era. For the archaeological evidence, see Nissen, *Entre Asclépios et Hippocrate*, 62–180; Edelstein, *Asclepius*, 1.370–42; Hart, *Asclepius, the God of Medicine*, 165–82.

[45] John Ashton describes Paul's miracles as "attention-grabbers" that "will have made people stop and look, and convinced many to listen also" (*The Religion of Paul the Apostle* (New Haven and London: Yale University Press, 2000), 165). Matthew Dickie makes a similar point about those who (like Paul?) were viewed as "magicians," noting that their public displays of divine power "served to persuade spectators of the skill of the magician and encouraged them to approach him for help with their own problems" (*Magic and Magicians in the Greco-Roman World*, 231).

[46] According to Rossettini et al., "Verbal suggestions are the simplest and most direct way to shape expectations" ("Context Matters," 3).

of Paul's message and his close links to divinity. Even a handful of testimonies from people who had experienced healing or other effects of divine power while listening to Paul could have been sufficient to move a few people to make the fateful decision to abandon friends, family, civic loyalty, and even the gods of their ancestors to follow the deity proclaimed by Paul.

This does not mean that the decision was necessarily immediate. Sometimes a single encounter with a sympathetic or persuasive leader is enough to motivate a person to join a group that others regard as a cult, but more often a longer period of exposure is required. In either case, the initial encounter often takes on a larger-than-life quality in future tellings as the moment when the convert first recognized that this group possessed the truth.

Of course, there is no way to know whether this is in fact what happened in Paul's case, but such a scenario does make sense of much of what we see in Paul's letters. In particular, it explains how he can speak about "signs and wonders" and works of "power" accompanying his preaching without presenting himself as the instigator of these acts. He is not a healer or miracle-worker, nor does he have any control over whether or when such events take place. He is merely a slave of Christ, a vessel through whom the Spirit of God can work if God so chooses. The same observation explains why Paul says nothing about receiving any personal benefit from divine healing: God alone decides when miracles will take place, and God had apparently chosen not to intervene in his case (2 Cor. 12:8-9). It might even explain why he does not talk about Jesus as a healer, since his own failure to benefit from the healing power of the risen Christ could potentially undermine both his claims to be an emissary of Christ and his teachings about the Spirit of Christ living and working in the community of believers. He acknowledges that there are people in his churches through whom the Spirit works more consistently to produce healing and other miracles (1 Cor. 12:9-10), but he cannot give any normative guidance about how to access this power since it depends entirely on the inscrutable will of the Spirit (1 Cor. 12:4-7, 11). There are no rituals or other activities that humans can perform to compel the Spirit to act.

If this reconstruction of Paul's experience is correct, it also suggests an answer to the question that was raised in the Introduction to this volume about whether Paul used offers of physical healing as a strategy for recruiting new people to his movement. In short, the answer is no. Paul could look back on his evangelistic ministry and celebrate how the Spirit had done miracles (possibly including healings) to validate the truth of his message in the eyes of those who became Christ-followers, but he never indicates that this was a conscious strategy on his part or that he counted on such events occurring. In fact, he does not even say that miracles occurred in every case.

Yet without them it is hard to explain his success. He admits that his message sounds ridiculous to Judeans and gentiles alike (1 Cor. 1:22-24, 2:14; cf. 4:10), and he insists that his oratorical skills were inadequate to overcome this difficulty (1 Cor. 1:17-18, 2:1-5, 2 Cor. 10:10, 11:6). In short, he has no rational explanation for why anyone would accept his message about a dying and rising Messiah. It is therefore natural that he would credit the power of the Spirit, whether this power was exhibited in the performance of miracles or the inner persuasion of human hearts.

Historians, by contrast, point to more mundane factors that facilitated the success of early Christian missionary efforts. Some relate to the historical circumstances in which the movement arose: the Pax Romana, the universality of Greek language and thought, the availability of good roads, popular interest in new religions, the quest by some for a secure afterlife, and so on. Others were intrinsic to the movement. Heidi Wendt points to a constellation of factors that could have made Paul more attractive to some audience members than other freelance experts in the competition to be heard: his ethnic coding as a Judean (though this would have cut both ways); his ability to read and interpret oracular writings (the Jewish Scriptures) and apply them to his listeners; his ability to deploy popular philosophical tropes, especially those relating to moral and spiritual transformation; his willingness to suffer for what he believed; his disinterest in financial compensation and the benefits of patronage; the particular benefits that he promised to those who embraced his message (suprahuman powers, bodily healing, immortality, etc.); the support of a community of like-minded people; and, of course, the acts of divine power that accompanied his preaching.[47]

Others have identified additional factors that could have contributed to the success of the early Christian movement, but these two studies are notable for their effort to situate Paul in relation to those with whom he would have been competing most directly in both the physical marketplace (the agora and other public spaces in the city) and the ideological marketplace (other religious and philosophical ideas). Both settings must be considered if we wish to understand why Paul was successful with some listeners and not with others.

Beating the Competition

A number of sociological studies have highlighted the importance of taking market competition into account when discussing the rise of early Christianity, beginning in 1973 with Peter Berger's book, *The Social Reality of Religion*.[48] Berger argued that in pluralistic religious contexts, religions that seek to obtain new adherents must be marketed to a clientele that is not necessarily interested in buying what the religion is offering. As a result, "The religious institutions become marketing agencies and the religious traditions become consumer commodities."[49] Religions that wish to grow must learn and respond to the needs and interests of potential members, a process that tends to produce an increased emphasis on what Berger calls the "moral and therapeutic functions of religion," including treatment of the sick. Similar forces can lead to changes in the structures, practices, and teachings of the religion.[50]

Subsequent studies have offered more detailed theorizations of how religions respond to market forces. The work of Rodney Stark has been particularly influential in this area. In a number of books and articles, Stark analyzes the workings of what he

---

[47] *At the Temple Gates*, 146–86. Jennifer Eyl highlights many of the same factors, though she labels them differently (*Signs, Wonders, and Gifts*, 86–169). A helpful summary chart can be found on p. 9.
[48] *The Social Reality of Religion* (Harmondsworth: Penguin, 1973).
[49] Ibid., 142.
[50] Ibid., 148–9.

called "religious economies" through the lens of supply and demand economics. Central to Stark's analysis is his application of rational choice theory, the idea that "within the limits of their information and understanding, restricted by available options, guided by their preferences and tastes, humans attempt to make rational choices."[51] According to Stark, religious actors apply a form of rationality when considering the competing claims of different religions, even if their choices do not seem particularly "rational" to outsiders. Humans have goals and rewards that they seek to attain in life, and religions that offer the most effective path to achieving these goals will gain more followers.[52] Religions that offer potential consumers a coherent and convincing explanation of human existence will likewise succeed at the expense of those that rely on rituals to manipulate hidden powers to do their bidding.[53] The presence of miracles can enhance the credibility and market appeal of a religion, but miracles cannot replace rational choices.[54] Social connections also play a role in people's decisions to keep or change religions, but conversion is ultimately rooted in individual assessments of potential gains and losses.[55]

According to Stark, the growth and success of Christianity in the Roman world can be traced to the popular judgment that it addressed this constellation of needs and interests more effectively than the competition. Stark's analysis has been criticized on a variety of fronts. Most of the criticisms relate to his views of religion, which are based more on modern examples than a deep understanding of the ancient world. Objections have been raised against his individualistic model of religion that emphasizes beliefs and rationality over tradition, rituals, and miracles; his assumption that religious groups are engaged in a constant competition for followers; his contention that more exclusive religious groups (such as the early Christians) will generate higher levels of commitment than less exclusive groups; his underestimation of popular devotion to traditional religious systems in the Greco-Roman world; and his failure to attend to the effects of power differentials between religious groups, particularly the role of the civic cults.[56]

In spite of these criticisms, the core of Stark's model remains relevant for understanding how Paul and other early Christian preachers were able to attract

---

[51] Rodney Stark and Roger Finke, *Acts of Faith: Explaining the Human Side of Religion* (Berkeley: University of California Press, 2000), 38.
[52] Ibid., 37–8, 85–8, 97–9.
[53] Ibid., 91–6, 115.
[54] As Stark puts it, "If people observe desirable effects that seem not to have naturalistic explanations, and if they attribute these effects to a god, confidence is increased in *all* explanations offered by the religion" (ibid., 109).
[55] Ibid., 116–24.
[56] For more on these criticisms, see Wendt, *At the Temple Gates*, 220–3; Roger Beck, "The Religious Market of the Roman Empire: Rodney Stark and Christianity's Pagan Competition," in *Religious Rivalries in the Early Roman Empire and the Rise of Christianity*, ed. Leif E. Vaage (Waterloo, ON: Wilfred Laurier University Press, 2006), 233–52; Steven C. Muir, "'Look How They Love One Another': Early Christian and Pagan Care for the Sick and Other Charity," in Vaage, *Religious Rivalries*, 213–31; Eva M. Hamberg and A. Thorlief Pettersson, "Religious Markets: Supply, Demand, and Rational Choices," in *Sacred Markets, Sacred Canopies: Essays on Religious Markets and Religious Pluralism*, ed. Ted G. Jelen (Lanham, MD: Rowman & Littlefield, 2002), 91–114; Daniel V. A. Olson, "Competing Notions of Religious Competition and Conflict in Theories of Religious Economics," in Jelen, *Sacred Markets*, 133–65.

converts despite the many obstacles that stood in their way. Stark's model suggests that Wendt and Eyl are correct in crediting Paul's success not to his facility in persuading people to accept the truth of his message but to his personal characteristics (including his ability to access and utilize divine knowledge and power) and the benefits that he promised to those who embraced his message, both in this world and beyond. Paul's occasional laments about the refusal of listeners to embrace his message suggest that most of those who heard him concluded that the benefits of joining such a movement did not outweigh the costs. But a few judged otherwise, enough to form a house-church community that could maintain and extend Paul's influence after he left a city. Reports and experiences of "miraculous" events played a notable role in these initial conversions, to judge from Paul's comments about "signs and wonders" that demonstrated the validity of his message. Whether these acts included physical healing is unclear, though it is a reasonable supposition.[57]

By the third and fourth centuries, on the other hand, healing had become such a vital element of Christian evangelistic and apologetic ministries that church leaders were compelled to grapple with issues and questions that had been neglected earlier. One of the most pressing questions concerned the apparent power of the cult of Asklepios to heal the sick. Such beneficent acts of power by a pagan deity undercut the church's claim that Greek and Roman cults were idolatrous and should be avoided. Knowing that it would be fruitless to deny the power of Asklepios, Christian leaders instead credited the cult's success to evil *daimones* who counterfeited the miracles of Christ in order to lead people astray from the truth of the Christian gospel. Only after decades of repetition did these arguments gain broad acceptance within the church, and even then there were Christians who continued to pray to Asklepios and consult Asklepian healers in times of sickness. Asklepios remained a stiff competitor for Christianity until his temples were shut down or razed along with other pagan shrines as the Roman Empire was increasingly Christianized. Even without temples, his influence was slow to die out among those who benefited from his assistance.[58]

Nothing like this can be found in the letters of Paul. If he viewed Asklepios as a competitor or a threat, he never says so. Nowhere does he attempt to persuade his followers to avoid "pagan" forms of healing, nor does he present Jesus as a divine healer who could replace Asklepios in addressing the health needs of Christ-followers. His strident monotheism makes it unlikely that he would have had anything to do with Asklepios himself, but otherwise he appears to have adopted a pragmatic approach to health care, utilizing whatever treatments or remedies were available to bring relief to his body. Such an attitude is thoroughly consistent with the judgment of the later rabbis who concluded that "whatever is used as a remedy is not forbidden" (b. Šhab. 67a).

---

[57] The reasonability of this supposition, if not its factuality, finds support in a survey cited by Candy Gunther Brown that shows "as many as 80% to 90% of first-generation Chinese Christians today convert to Christianity because either they or members of their families believe themselves to have been divinely healed" ("Healing Prayer in an Age of Evidence-Based Medicine," 1).

[58] While many Asklepian temples were torn down or turned into churches in the post-Constantinian era, the ancient sanctuary at Kos (western Turkey) continued operating until 554 CE, when it was destroyed by an earthquake (Hart, *Asclepius, the God of Medicine*, 196). René Rüttimann claims that Christians continued to visit the sanctuaries of Asklepios into the fifth century ("Asclepius and Jesus," 205–12).

The idea that Christ-followers should avoid "pagan" modes of healing was a later development that probably never occurred to Paul.

Conclusion

This study has sought to make sense of the apostle Paul's silence regarding a vitally important and potentially problematic element of social and religious life in antiquity, the treatment of sickness and injury. This silence is remarkable in view of the pervasiveness of bodily suffering at all levels of Greco-Roman society (including Paul), the prominence of the topic in ancient discourse (including the writings of Judeans and later Christians), the broad range of methods that was available for treating illness and injury, the reputation of Jesus as a healing deity, and the entanglement of "pagan" religion in all aspects of ancient health care. The latter point in particular would have elicited questions from Paul's followers in view of his repeated calls to avoid idolatry, and it seems equally certain that Paul would have had to grapple with such questions himself when deciding what types of treatment to accept for the many illnesses and injuries that he references in his letters. If he had concerns about any of the usual forms of care, one would think that he would have mentioned them somewhere. But he does not.

The most natural inference from this silence is that Paul did not see any serious danger of idolatry in any of the health care practices that were common in his day, with the exception of those that involved direct appeals to pagan deities. His silence on the latter point is surprising, but he might have thought that the point was so obvious that he had no reason to mention it. It seems unlikely, however, that he would have made the same presumption regarding more subtle questions such as whether it was acceptable for Christ-followers to take medicines or wear amulets that had been prepared using pagan rituals or to recite healing incantations to channel unnamed powers to drive away an illness or restore the sufferer to health. It is equally improbable that neither Paul nor his followers ever thought about such matters or that Paul had given such clear instructions on the subject when he was with them that it never again arose as a matter of concern.

The only explanation that makes sense is that Paul saw no problem with such practices. This interpretation is consistent with what we saw in Chapter 7 regarding how other Judeans in Paul's day (and subsequent centuries) approached the subject of health care, and it also agrees with what we observed in Chapter 8 regarding the views and practices of many Christians in the first few centuries CE. Christian leaders began to raise questions about the propriety of certain healing practices as the movement grew in both numbers and theological sophistication, but there is no evidence that such concerns were raised in Paul's day. The very fact that later leaders found it so hard to stamp out practices that they considered "idolatrous" suggests that earlier leaders (including Paul) had given little instruction on the subject. It certainly does not appear in any of the documents that were included in the Christian New Testament.

Whether Paul's references to "signs and wonders" and works of "power" that accompanied his preaching included healing cannot ultimately be answered, but the available evidence suggests that he did not promote himself as someone imbued by God with the power to heal.[59] It is nevertheless possible that healings occurred in his presence without his direct intervention as sick people came to believe that they were being touched by the power of the god that he proclaimed and this belief initiated a placebo response in their bodies. It is also possible that genuine miracles occurred in these settings, though such claims are beyond historical investigation. Under either explanation the events occurred outside of Paul's control, so they could not have played any conscious role in his evangelistic strategy. But this did not stop him from citing them after the fact as evidence for the truth of his message.[60]

Further reflection on these experiences led Paul to regard preaching and miracles as two prongs of a divine strategy for leading people to faith in Christ. This view is expressed clearly in Rom. 15:18-19, where he assures the Christ-followers in Rome that he does "not venture to speak of anything except what Christ has accomplished through me to win obedience from the Gentiles, by word and deed, by the power of signs and wonders, by the power of the Spirit of God." In a later era, similar acts of power would be cited to counter the appeal of Asklepios and other wonder-working deities to gentile Christ-followers who were accustomed to seeking divine aid when they were sick or facing other insurmountable difficulties.[61]

For Paul, however, they served as evidence that Christ was working through his weak and sickly body in the brief time that remained before God brought the present era to a close and gave Paul and other Christ-followers immortal bodies that would never again suffer sickness or death. Until then, they were free to use every resource that God had placed in the world, including the wisdom of human healers, to keep their bodies healthy so that they could use them in serving God (Rom. 12:1-2). When they were sick, they could rest secure in the knowledge that their bodily suffering "is preparing us for an eternal weight of glory beyond all measure, because we look not at what can be seen but at what cannot be seen" (2 Cor. 4:18-19). Viewed in this light, the health of mortal bodies fades into insignificance.

---

[59] Apart from Acts, later Christian texts show little memory of Paul as a wonder-worker. For the evidence, see Twelftree, *Paul and the Miraculous*, 298–303.

[60] Comparative evidence suggests that offers of physical healing can be a potent tool for recruiting new converts to a religion, especially if it is cheaper and more readily available than other options—see Avalos, *Health Care and the Rise of Christianity*, 1–3, 68–70, 93–5, 103–6.

[61] René Rüttimann puts it well: "When the followers of Jesus entered this religious setting [the Greek world], they were confronted with the people's attitude and the religious expectations to provide healing, and were forced to prove that their god was also a healer" ("Asclepius and Jesus," 6).

Bibliography

Ager, Britta. "Roman Agricultural Magic." PhD diss., University of Michigan, 2010. https://deepblue.lib.umich.edu/bitstream/handle/2027.42/75896/bager_1.pdf
Ahmadi, Amir. "The 'Magoi' and 'Daimones' in Column VI of the Derveni Papyrus." *Numen* 61 (2014): 484–508.
Albl, Martin C. "'Are Any among You Sick?' The Health Care System in the Letter of James." *JBL* 121 (2002): 123–43.
Allan, Nigel. "The Physician in Ancient Israel: His Status and Function." *Medical History* 45 (2002): 377–94.
Alonso, María Ángeles. "Greek Physicians in the Eyes of Roman Elite (from the Republic to the 1st Century AD)." *Annales Universitatis Mariae Curie-Skłodowska* 73 (2018): 119–37.
Amundsen, Darrel W. "Medicine and Faith in Early Christianity." *Bulletin of the History of Medicine* 56 (1982): 326–50.
Angel, Joseph. "The Use of the Hebrew Bible in Early Jewish Magic." *Religion Compass* 3/5 (2009): 785–98.
Ashton, John. *The Religion of Paul the Apostle*. New Haven, CT, and London: Yale University Press, 2000.
Aune, David E. "The Apocalypse of John and Revelatory Magic." In *Apocalypticism, Prophecy, and Magic in Early Christianity: Collected Essays*, 347–67. Grand Rapids, MI: Baker, 2006.
Aune, David E. "Magic in Early Christianity." In *Apocalypticism, Prophecy, and Magic in Early Christianity: Collected Essays*, 368–420. Grand Rapids, MI: Baker, 2006.
Aune, David E. "'Magic' in Early Christianity and Its Ancient Mediterranean Context: A Survey of Some Recent Scholarship." *Annali di storia dell'esegesi* 24 (2007): 229–94.
Avalos, Hector. *Health Care and the Rise of Christianity*. Peabody, MA: Hendrickson, 1999.
Avalos, Hector. *Illness and Health Care in the Ancient Near East: The Role of the Temple in Greece, Mesopotamia, and Israel*. Atlanta: Scholars Press, 1995.
Bailey, Aleshia Jayne. "*Medicina Domestica*: Medicine and Power in the Urban and Non-urban Roman Household." MA thesis, Australian National University, 2012.
Bailliot, Magali. "Rome and the Roman Empire." In *Guide to the Study of Ancient Magic*, edited by David Frankfurter, 175–97. Leiden and Boston: Brill, 2019.
Baker, Patricia A. *The Archaeology of Medicine in the Greco-Roman World*. Cambridge: Cambridge University Press, 2013.
Beck, Roger. "The Religious Market of the Roman Empire: Rodney Stark and Christianity's Pagan Competition." In *Religious Rivalries in the Early Roman Empire and the Rise of Christianity*, edited by Leif E. Vaage, 233–52. Waterloo, ON: Wilfred Laurier University Press, 2006.
Belfiore, Elizabeth. "Epode, Elenchus, and Magic: Socrates as Silenus." *Phoenix* 34 (1980): 128–37.
Berger, Peter L. *The Social Reality of Religion*. Hammondsworth: Penguin, 1973.
Betz, Hans Dieter, ed. *The Greek Magical Papyri in Translation, Including the Demotic Spells*. Chicago and London: University of Chicago Press, 1986.

Betz, Hans Dieter. "Magic and Mystery in the Greek Magical Papyri." In *Magika Hiera: Ancient Greek Religion and Magic*, edited by Christopher A. Faraone and Dirk Obbink, 244–59. New York and Oxford: Oxford University Press, 1991.

Boeft, Jan den. "Asclepius' Healings Made Known." In *Wonders Never Cease: The Purpose of Narrating Miracle Stories in the New Testament and its Religious Environment*, edited by Michael Labahn and Bert Jan Lietaert Peerbolte, 20–31. London and New York: T. & T. Clark, 2006.

Bohak, Gideon. *Ancient Jewish Magic: A History*. Cambridge: Cambridge University Press, 2008.

Bohak, Gideon. "Jewish Exorcism Before and After the Destruction of the Second Temple." In *Was 70 CE a Watershed in Jewish History?: On Jews and Judaism before and after the Destruction of the Second Temple*, edited by Daniel R. Schwartz and Zeev Weiss, 277–300. Leiden: Brill, 2012.

Bohak, Gideon. "Jewish Magic in the First and Second Temple Periods." In *Angels and Demons: Jewish Magic through the Ages*, edited by Filip Vukosavović, 12–15. Jerusalem: Bible Lands Museum, 2010.

Bohak, Gideon. "Prolegomena to the Study of the Jewish Magical Tradition." *Currents in Biblical Research* 9 (2009): 107–50.

Bohak, Gideon. "The Use of Engraved Gems and Rings in Ancient Jewish Magic." In *Magical Gems in their Contexts*, edited by Kata Endreffy, Árpád M. Nagy, and Jeffrey Spier, 37–45. Budapest: L'Erma di Bretschneider, 2019.

Bonner, Campbell. *Studies in Magical Amulets*. Ann Arbor, MI: University of Michigan Press, 1950.

Brockmann, Christian. "A God and Two Humans on Matters of Medicine: Asclepius, Galen and Aelius Aristides." In *In Praise of Asclepius: Aelius Aristides*, Selected Prose Hymns, edited by Donald A. Russell, Michael Trapp, and Heinz-Günther Nesselrath, 116–27. Tübingen: Morh Siebeck, 2016.

Brown, Candy Gunther. "Healing Prayer in an Age of Evidence-Based Medicine." *Transformations* 32 (2015): 1–16.

Burford, Freya. "Greco-Roman Healing Miracles." MA thesis, University of Kent, 2017. https://www.scribd.com/document/461814258/Greco-Roman-Healing-Miracles.

Caldwell, Lauren. "Roman Medical Sects: The Asclepiadeans, the Methodists, and the Pneumatists." In *The Oxford Handbook of Science and Medicine in the Classical World*, edited by Paul Keyser and John Scarborough, 637–54. Oxford: Oxford University Press, 2018.

Calvo Martínez, José L. "The 'Philinna Papyrus': A New Interpretation." Unpublished paper, accessed at https://www.academia.edu/42592163/The_Philinna_Papyrus.

Case, Shirley Jackson. "The Art of Healing in Early Christian Times." *JR* 3, no. 3 (1923): 238–55.

Chaniotis, Angelos. "Illness and Cures in the Greek Propitiatory Inscriptions and Dedications of Lydia and Phrygia." In *Ancient Medicine in its Socio-Cultural Context*, edited by Philip J. van der Eijk, H. F. J. Horstmanshoff, and P. U. Schrijvers, 323–44. Amsterdam and Atlanta: Editions Rodopi, 1995.

Chase, John Michael. "Notes on Squill in Antiquity." In *Miroirs de la mélancholie*, edited by H. Cazes and A.-F. Morand, 29–48. Paris: Hermann, 2015.

Collins, Derek. *Magic in the Greek World*. Malden, MA: Blackwell, 2008.

Compton, Michael T. "The Association of Hygieia with Asklepios in Graeco-Roman Asklepieion Medicine." *Journal of the History of Medicine and Allied Sciences* 57 (2002): 312–29.

Compton, Michael T. "The Union of Religion and Health in Ancient Asklepieia." *Journal of Religion and Health* 37 (1998): 301–12.
Cotter, Wendy. *Miracles in Greco-Roman Antiquity: A Sourcebook for the Study of New Testament Miracle Stories*. London and New York: Routledge, 1999.
Craffert, Pieter F. *Illness and Healing in the Biblical World: Perspectives on Health Care*. Pretoria: Biblia Publishers, 1999.
Craffert, Pieter F. *The Life of a Galilean Shaman: Jesus of Nazareth in Anthropological-Historical Perspective*. Eugene, OR: Cascade, 2008.
Croon, J. H. "Hot Springs and Healing Gods." *Mnemosyne*, 4th ser., 20 (1967): 225–46.
Dasen, Véronique. "Healing Images. Gems and Medicine." *Oxford Journal of Archaeology* 33 (2014): 177–91.
Dasen, Véronique. "Magic and Medicine: Gems and the Power of Seals." In *"Gems of Heaven": Recent Research on Engraved Gemstones in Late Antiquity, AD 200–600*, edited by Chris Entwistle and Noel Adams, 69–74. London: British Museum Press, 2011.
Dasen, Véronique, and Árpád Nagy. "Gems." In *Guide to the Study of Ancient Magic*, edited by David Frankfurter, 416–55. Leiden and Boston: Brill, 2019.
Davies, Gaius. "The Hands of the Healer: Has Faith a Place?" *Journal of Medical Ethics* 6 (1980): 185–9.
Davies, Owen. *Magic: A Very Short Introduction*. Oxford: Oxford University Press, 2012.
Dawson, Audrey. *Healing, Weakness and Power: Perspectives on Healing in the Writings of Mark, Luke and Paul*. Milton Keynes: Paternoster 2008.
Delatte, Armand. *Herbarius: Recherches sur le Cérémonial Usité chez les Anciens pour la Cueilette des Simples et des Plantes Magique*. 3rd edn. Brussels: Palais des Académies, 1961.
Dewey, Arthur J., and Anna C. Miller. "Paul." In *The Bible and Disability: A Commentary*, edited by Sarah J. Melcher, Mikael C. Parsons, and Amos Yong, 379–425. Waco, TX: Baylor University Press, 2017.
Dickie, Matthew W. *Magic and Magicians in the Greco-Roman World*. London and New York: Routledge, 2001.
Dieleman, Jacco. "The Greco-Egyptian Magical Papyri." In *Guide to the Study of Ancient Magic*, edited by David Frankfurter, 283–321. Leiden and Boston: Brill, 2019.
Dillon, Matthew. *Omens and Oracles: Divination in Ancient Greece*. London and New York: Routledge, 2017.
Draycott, J. "Literary and Documentary Evidence for Lay Medical Practice in the Roman Republic and Empire." In *Homo Patiens: Approaches to the Patient in the Ancient World*, edited by Georgia Petridou and Chiara Thumiger, 432–450. Brill: Leiden, 2016.
Dvorjetski, Estee. "Medicinal Hot Springs and Healing Spas in the Graeco-Roman World." In *Leisure, Pleasure and Healing: Spa Culture and Medicine in Ancient Eastern Mediterranean*, 83–123. Leiden: Brill, 2007.
Eckert, Jost. "Zeichen und Wunder in der Sicht des Paulus und der Apostelgeschichte." *TThSt* 88 (1979): 19–33.
Edelstein, Emma J., and Ludwig Edelstein. *Asclepius: Collection and Interpretation of the Testimonies*. With a new introduction by Gary B. Ferngren. 2 vols. Baltimore and London: Johns Hopkins University Press, 1998.
Edelstein, Ludwig. "Greek Medicine in its Relation to Religion and Magic." In *Ancient Medicine: Selected Papers of Ludwig Edelstein*, edited by Owsei Temkin and C. Lilian Temkin, translated by C. Lilian Temkin, 205–46. Baltimore and London: Johns Hopkins University Press, 1967.

Edelstein, Ludwig. "The Methodists." In *Ancient Medicine: Selected Papers of Ludwig Edelstein*, edited by Owsei Temkin and C. Lilian Temkin, translated by C. Lilian Temkin, 173–91. Baltimore and London: Johns Hopkins University Press, 1967.

Eijk, Philip van de. "Cure and (In)curability of Mental Disorders in Ancient Medical and Philosophical Thought." In *Mental Disorders in the Classical World*, edited by W. V. Harris, 307–38. Leiden and Boston: Brill, 2013.

Eshel, Hanan, and Rivka Leiman. "Jewish Amulets Written on Metal Scrolls." *Journal of Ancient Judaism* 1 (2010): 189–99.

Evans, Craig A. "Paul the Exorcist and Healer." In *Paul and His Theology*, edited by Stanley E. Porter, 363–79. Leiden and Boston: Brill, 2006.

Eyl, Jennifer. *Signs, Wonders, and Gifts: Divination in the Letters of Paul*. Oxford: Oxford University Press, 2019.

Faraone, Christopher A. "Magic and Medicine in the Roman Imperial Period: Two Case Studies." In *Continuity and Innovation in the Magical Tradition*, edited by Gideon Bohak, Yuval Harari, and Shaul Shaked, 135–58. Leiden: Brill, 2011.

Fee, Gordon D. *God's Empowering Presence: The Holy Spirit in the Letters of Paul*. Peabody, MA: Hendrickson, 1994.

Ferngren, Gary B. "Early Christianity as a Religion of Healing." *Bulletin of the History of Medicine* 66 (1992): 1–15.

Ferngren, Gary B. *Medicine & Health Care in Early Christianity*. Baltimore, MD: Johns Hopkins University Press, 2009.

Ferngren, Gary B. *Medicine and Religion: A Historical Introduction*. Baltimore, MD: Johns Hopkins University Press, 2014.

Ferngren, Gary B., and Darrel W. Amundsen. "Medicine and Christianity in the Roman Empire: Compatibilities and Tensions." *ANRW* 37.3.2957-80. Part 2, *Principat*, 37.3. Edited by Wolfgang Haase. Berlin: Walter de Gruyter, 1996.

Flemming, Rebecca. *Medicine and the Making of Roman Women*. Oxford: Oxford University Press, 2000.

Fox, Sherry C. "Health in Hellenistic and Roman Times: The Case Studies of Paphos, Cyprus, and Corinth, Greece." In *Health in Antiquity*, edited by Helen King, 59–82. London and New York: Routledge, 2005.

Frankfurter, David. "Ancient Magic in a New Key: Refining an Exotic Discipline in the History of Religions." In *Guide to the Study of Ancient Magic*, edited by David Frankfurter, 3–20. Leiden and Boston: Brill, 2019.

Frankfurter, David. "Introduction." In *Guide to the Study of Ancient Magic*, edited by David Frankfurter, 29–35. Leiden and Boston: Brill, 2019.

Frankfurter, David. "Magic as the Local Application of Authoritative Tradition." In *Guide to the Study of Ancient Magic*, edited by David Frankfurter, 720–45. Leiden and Boston: Brill, 2019.

Frankfurter, David. "The Magic of Writing in Mediterranean Antiquity." In *Guide to the Study of Ancient Magic*, edited by David Frankfurter, 626–58. Leiden and Boston: Brill, 2019.

Frankfurter, David. "Spell and Speech Act: The Magic of the Spoken Word." In *Guide to the Study of Ancient Magic*, edited by David Frankfurter, 608–25. Leiden and Boston: Brill, 2019.

Frede, Michael. "The Method of the So-Called Methodical School of Medicine." In *Science and Speculation: Studies in Hellenistic Theory and Practice*, edited by Jonathan Barnes, Jacques Brunschwig, Myles Burnyeat, and Malcolm Schofield, 1–23. Cambridge:

Cambridge University Press, 1982; Paris: Editions de la Maison des Sciences de l'Homme, 1982.
Frost, Evelyn. *Christian Healing*. 2nd edn. London: A. R. Mowbray, 1949.
Gaillard-Seux, Patricia. "Magical Formulas in Pliny's Natural History: Origins, Sources, Parallels." In *'Greek' and 'Roman' in Latin Medical Texts*, edited by Brigitte Maire, 201–23. Leiden: Brill, 2014.
Garland, Robert. *The Eye of the Beholder: Deformity and Disability in the Graeco-Roman World*. London: Bristol Classical Press, 2010.
Gatzweiler, Karl. "La conception paulinienne du miracle." *ETL* 37 (1961): 813–46.
Glessner, Justin M. "Ethnomedical Anthropology and Paul's 'Thorn' (2 Corinthians 12:7)." *BTB* 47 (2017): 15–46.
Gordon, Richard L. "Archaeologies of Magical Gems." In *'And These the Gems of Heaven': Proceedings of the British Museum Byzantine Seminar*, edited by Chris Entwistle and Noel Adams, 39–49. London: British Museum Press, 2011.
Gordon, Richard L. "From Substances to Texts: Three Materialities of Magic in the Roman Period." In *The Materiality of Magic*, edited by Jan N. Bremmer, 133–76. Munich: Paderborn Fink, 2015.
Gordon, Richard L. "The Healing Event in Graeco-Roman Medicine." In *Ancient Medicine in its Socio-Cultural Context*, edited by Philip J. van der Eijk, H. F. J. Horstmanshoff, and P. U. Schrijvers, 363–76. Amsterdam and Atlanta: Editions Rodopi, 1995.
Gorrini, Maria Elena, and Milena Melfi. "L'archéologie des cultes guérisseurs." *Kernos* 15 (2002): 247–65.
Gourevitch, Danielle. "Popular Medicines and Practices in Galen." In *Popular Medicine in Graeco-Roman Antiquity: Explorations*, edited by William V. Harris, 251–71. Leiden and Boston: Brill, 2016.
Graf, Fritz. "Excluding the Charming: The Development of the Greek Concept of Magic." In *Ancient Magic and Ritual Power*, edited by Marvin Meyer and Paul Mirecki, 30–42. Leiden and New York: Brill, 1995.
Graf, Fritz. "Greece." In *Guide to the Study of Ancient Magic*, edited by David Frankfurter, 115–38. Leiden and Boston: Brill, 2019.
Graf, Fritz. *Magic in the Ancient World*. Translated by Franklin Philip. Cambridge and London: Harvard University Press, 1997.
Graf, Fritz. "Prayer in Magic and Religious Ritual." In *Magika Hiera: Ancient Greek Religion and Magic*, edited by Christopher A. Faraone and Dirk Obbink, 188–213. New York and Oxford: Oxford University Press, 1991.
Graf, Fritz. "Theories of Magic in Antiquity." In *Ancient Magic and Ritual Power*, edited by Marvin Meyer and Paul Mirecki, 93–104. Leiden and New York: Brill, 1995.
Gregory, Andrew. "Magic, Curses, and Healing." In *A Companion to Science, Technology, and Medicine in Ancient Greece and Rome*, edited by George L. Irby, 418–33. New York: Wiley-Blackwell, 2016.
Grmek, Mirko. *Diseases in the Ancient Greek World*. Translated by Mireille Muellner and Leonard Muellner. Baltimore and London: Johns Hopkins University Press, 1989.
Hahn, Frances Hickson. "Performing the Sacred: Prayers and Hymns." In *A Companion to Roman Religion*, edited by Jörg Rüpke, 235–48. Malden, MA: Wiley-Blackwell, 2011.
Hamberg, Eva M., and A. Thorlief Pettersson. "Religious Markets: Supply, Demand, and Rational Choices." In *Sacred Markets, Sacred Canopies: Essays on Religious Markets and Religious Pluralism*, edited by Ted G. Jelen, 91–114. Lanham, MD: Rowman & Littlefield, 2002.

Hanson, John S. "Dreams and Visions in the Graeco-Roman World and Early Christianity." *ANRW* 23.2.1395-1427. Part 2, *Principat*, 23.2. Edited by Wolfgang Haase. Berlin: Walter de Gruyter, 1980.

Harari, Yuval. "Ancient Israel and Early Judaism." In *Guide to the Study of Ancient Magic*, edited by David Frankfurter, 139–74. Leiden and Boston: Brill, 2019.

Harari, Yuval. *Jewish Magic before the Rise of Kabbalah*. Translated by Batya Stein. Detroit: Wayne State University Press, 2017.

Harms, Paul Jonathan. "The Logic of Irrational Pharmacological Therapies in Aretaeus of Cappadocia, Scribonius Largus and Dioscorides of Anazarbus." PhD diss., University of Calgary, 2010. https://prism.ucalgary.ca/handle/1880/104384.

Harris, William V. *Dreams and Experience in Classical Antiquity*. Cambridge, MA, and London: Harvard University Press, 2009.

Harris, William V. "*Manteis* and Medicine." *Menemosyne* 73 (2020): 21–35.

Harris, William V. "Popular Medicine in the Classical World." In *Popular Medicine in Graeco-Roman Antiquity: Explorations*, edited by William V. Harris, 1–64. Leiden and Boston: Brill, 2016.

Hart, Gerald D. *Asclepius, the God of Medicine*. London: Royal Society of Medicine Press, 2000.

Hezser, Catherine. "Representations of the Physician in Jewish Literature from Hellenistic and Roman Times." In *Popular Medicine in Graeco-Roman Antiquity: Explorations*, edited by William V. Harris, 173–97. Leiden and Boston: Brill, 2016.

Horsley, Richard A. *Jesus and Magic: Freeing the Gospel Stories from Modern Misconceptions*. Eugene, OR: Cascade Books, 2014.

Howard, J. Keir. *Disease and Healing in the New Testament: An Analysis and Interpretation*. Lanham, MD: University Press of America, 2001.

Humphrey, Nicholas K. "Great Expectations: The Evolutionary Psychology of Faith-Healing and the Placebo Effect." In *Social, Developmental, and Clinical Perspectives*. Vol. 2 of *Psychology at the Turn of the Millennium*, edited by Claes von Hofsten and Lars Bäckman, 225–46. London: Psychology Press, 2002.

Humphrey, Nicholas K. "The Placebo Effect." In *Oxford Companion to the Mind*, edited by Richard L. Gregory, 735–6. Oxford: Oxford University Press, 2004.

Humphrey, Nicholas K., and John Skoyles. "The Evolutionary Psychology of Healing: A Human Success Story." *Current Biology* 22 (2012): 695–7.

Israelowich, Ido. *Patients and Healers in the High Roman Empire*. Baltimore: Johns Hopkins Press, 2015.

Israelowich, Ido. *Society, Medicine and Religion in the Sacred Tales of Aelius Aristides*. Leiden and Boston: Brill, 2012.

Jackson, Ralph. *Doctors and Diseases in the Roman Empire*. Norman and London: University of Oklahoma Press, 1988.

Janowitz, Naomi. *Magic in the Roman World: Pagans, Jews and Christians*. London and New York: Routledge, 2001.

Jervell, Jacob. *The Unknown Paul: Essays on Luke-Acts and Early Christian History*. Minneapolis, MN: Augsburg, 1984.

Jocks, Ianto. "The *Compositiones Medicamentorum* of Scribonius Largus." MRes thesis, University of Glasgow, 2013. http://theses.gla.ac.uk/4892.

Jones-Lewis, Molly. "Pharmacy." In *A Companion to Science, Technology, and Medicine in Ancient Greece and Rome*, edited by George L. Irby, 402–17. New York: Wiley-Blackwell, 2016.

Jones-Lewis, Molly. "Physicians and 'Schools.'" In *A Companion to Science, Technology, and Medicine in Ancient Greece and Rome*, edited by George L. Irby, 386–401. New York: Wiley-Blackwell, 2016.

Jouanna, Jacques. "The Typology and Aetiology of Madness in Ancient Greek Medical and Philosophical Writing." In *Mental Disorders in the Classical World*, edited by William V. Harris, 98–118. Leiden and Boston: Brill, 2013.

Kee, Howard Clark. *Medicine, Miracle and Magic in New Testament Times*. Cambridge: Cambridge University Press, 1986.

Kelley, Nicole. "Deformity and Disability in Greece and Rome." In *This Abled Body: Rethinking Disabilities in Biblical Studies*, edited by Hector Avalos, Sarah J. Melcher, and Jeremy Schipper, 31–45. Atlanta: Society of Biblical Literature, 2007.

Keyser, Paul T. "Science and Magic in Galen's Recipes (Sympathy and Efficacy)." In *Galen on Pharmacology: Philosophy, History and Medicine*, edited by Armelle Debru, 175–98. Leiden: Brill, 1997.

King, Helen. "Comparative Perspectives on Medicine and Healing in the Ancient World." In *Religion, Health and Suffering*, edited by John R. Hinnells and Roy Porter, 276–94. London and New York: Kegan Paul, 1999.

King, J.D. *Post-Apostolic through Later Holiness. Vol. 1 in Regeneration: A Complete History of Healing in the Christian Church*. Lee's Summit, MO: Christos Publishing, 2017.

Kleinman, Arthur. *Patients and Healers in the Context of Culture: An Exploration of the Borderland between Anthropology, Medicine, and Psychiatry*. Berkeley: University of California Press, 1980.

Kollman, Bernd. *Jesus und die Christen als Wundertätter: Studien zu Magie, Medizin und Schamanismus in Antike und Christentum*. Göttingen: Vandenhoeck & Ruprecht, 1996.

Koloski-Ostrow, Ann Olga. *The Archaeology of Sanitation in Roman Italy: Toilets, Sewers, and Water Systems*. Chapel Hill, NC: University of North Carolina Press, 2015.

Kotansky, Roy. "Greek Exorcistic Amulets." In *Ancient Magic and Ritual Power*, edited by Marvin Meyer and Paul Mirecki, 243–77. Leiden and New York: Brill, 1995.

Kotansky, Roy. "Incantations and Prayers for Salvation on Inscribed Greek Amulets." In *Magika Hiera: Ancient Greek Religion and Magic*, edited by Christopher A. Faraone and Dirk Obbink, 107–37. New York and Oxford: Oxford University Press, 1991.

Kotansky, Roy. "Textual Amulets and Writing Traditions in the Ancient World." In *Guide to the Study of Ancient Magic*, edited by David Frankfurter, 507–54. Leiden and Boston: Brill, 2019.

Lehrich, Christopher I. "Magic in Theoretical Practice." In *Defining Magic: A Reader*, edited by Bernd-Christian Otto and Michael Stausberg, 211–28. Sheffield: Equinox, 2013.

Leith, David. "How Popular Were the Medical Sects?" In *Popular Medicine in Graeco-Roman Antiquity: Explorations*, edited by William V. Harris, 231–50. Leiden and Boston: Brill, 2016.

Lennon, Jack J. *Pollution and Religion in Ancient Rome*. Cambridge: Cambridge University Press, 2014.

LiDonnici, Lynn R. "Beans, Fleawort, and the Blood of a Hamadras Babboon: Recipe Ingredients in Greco-Roman Magical Materials." In *Ancient Magic and Ritual Power*, edited by Marvin Meyer and Paul Mirecki, 359–77. Leiden and New York: Brill, 1995.

LiDonnici, Lynn R. *The Epidaurian Miracle Inscriptions: Text, Translation and Commentary*. Atlanta: Scholars Press, 1995.

Lincicum, David. "Scripture and Apotropaism in the Second Temple Period." *BN* 138 (2008): 63–88.

Lindahl, Olov, and Lars Lindwall. "Is All Therapy Just a Placebo Effect?" *Theoretical Medicine and Bioethics* 3(1982): 255–9.

Lloyd, G. E. R. *In the Grip of Disease: Studies in the Greek Imagination*. Oxford: Oxford University Press, 2004.

Longrigg, James. *Greek Medicine from the Heroic to the Hellenistic Age: A Source Book.* New York: Routledge, 1998.

Luck, Georg. *Arcana Mundi: Magic and the Occult in the Greek and Roman Worlds.* Baltimore and London: Johns Hopkins University Press, 1985.

Luke, Trevor S. "A Healing Touch for Empire: Vespasian's Wonders in Domitianic Rome." *Greece & Rome*, 2nd ser., 57 (2010): 77–106.

Marquis, Timothy Luckritz. *Transient Apostle: Paul, Travel, and the Rhetoric of Empire.* New Haven and London: Yale University Press, 2013.

Martin, Dale B. *The Corinthian Body.* New Haven, CT: Yale University Press, 1995.

Martin, Dale B. *Inventing Superstition: From the Hippocratics to the Christians.* Cambridge, MA, and London: Harvard University Press, 2004.

Martínez, Isabel Canzobre. "Magical Amulets User's Guide: Preparation, Utilization, and Knowledge Transmission in the *PGM*." In *Magikè téchne : formación y consideración social del mago en el Mundo Antiguo*, edited by Emilio Suárez de la Torre, Miriam Blanco Cesteros, Eleni Chronopoulou, and Isabel Canzobre, 177–92. Madrid: Editorial Dykinson, S.L., 2017.

McCasland, S. Vernon. "Signs and Wonders." *JBL* 76 (1957): 149–52.

McNamara, Leanne, "'Conjurers, Purifiers, Vagabonds and Quacks'? The Clinical Roles of the Folk and Hippocratic Healers of Classical Greece." *Iris: Journal of the Classical Association of Victoria* 16-17 (2003–2004): 2–25.

Meggitt, Justin J. "Did Magic Matter? The Saliency of Magic in the Early Roman Empire." *JAH* 1 (2013): 170–229.

Meggitt, Justin. "Magic, Healing and Early Christianity: Consumption and Competition." In *The Meanings of Magic: From the Bible to Buffalo Bill*, edited by Amy Wygant, 89–114. New York and Oxford: Berghahn Books, 2006.

Micozzi, Marc S. "Culture, Anthropology, and the Return of 'Complementary Medicine.'" *Medical Anthropology Quarterly* 16 (2002): 398–403.

Mitchell, Piers D. "Human Parasites in the Roman World: Health Consequences of Conquering an Empire." *Parasitology* 144 (2017): 48–58.

Mitchell, Stephen. *Anatolia: Land, Men, and God in Asia Minor.* 2 vols. Oxford: Clarendon, 1995.

Moyer, Ian. "Thessalos of Tralles and Cultural Exchange." In *Prayer, Magic, and the Stars in the Ancient and Late Antique World*, edited by Scott Noegel, Joel Walker, and Brannon Wheeler, 39–56. University Park, PA: Pennsylvania State University Press, 2003.

Muir, Steven C. "'Look How They Love One Another': Early Christian and Pagan Care for the Sick and Other Charity." In *Religious Rivalries in the Early Roman Empire and the Rise of Christianity*, edited by Leif E. Vaage, 213–31. Waterloo, ON: Wilfred Laurier University Press, 2006.

Newsom, S. W. B. "Hygiene and the Ancient Romans." *British Journal of Infection Control* 5 (2004): 25–7.

Nielsen, Helge Kjaer. *Heilun und Verkündigung: Das Verständnis der Heilung und ihres Verhältnesses zur Verkündigung bei Jesus und in der Ältesten Kirche.* Leiden: Brill, 1987.

Nikita, Efthymia, Anna Lagia, and Sevi Triantaphyllou. "Epidemiology and Pathology." In *A Companion to Science, Technology, and Medicine in Ancient Greece and Rome.* Edited by George L. Irby, 465–82. New York: Wiley-Blackwell, 2016.

Nissen, Cécile. *Entre Asclépios et Hippocrate: Études des cultes guérisseurs et des médecins en Carie.* Liège: Centre International d'Étude de la Religion Grecque Antique, 2009.

Nuffelen, Peter van. "Galen, Divination, and the Status of Medicine." *Classical Quarterly* 63 (2014): 337–52.

Nutton, Vivian. *Ancient Medicine*. London and New York: Routledge, 2004.
Nutton, Vivian. "The Drug Trade in Antiquity." *Journal of the Royal Society of Medicine* 78 (1985): 138–45.
Nutton, Vivian. "Folk Medicine in the Galenic Corpus." In *Popular Medicine in Graeco-Roman Antiquity: Explorations*, edited by William V. Harris, 272–9. Leiden and Boston: Brill, 2016.
Nutton, Vivian. "Galenic Madness." In *Mental Disorders in the Classical World*, edited by William V. Harris, 119–27. Leiden and Boston: Brill, 2013.
Nutton, Vivian. "Healers in the Medical Marketplace: Towards a Social History of Graeco-Roman Medicine." In *Medicine in Society: Historical Essays*, edited by Andrew Wear, 15–58. Cambridge: Cambridge University Press, 1992.
Nutton, Vivian. "Medicine in Late Antiquity and the Early Middle Ages." In *The Western Medical Tradition, 800 BC to AD 1800*, edited by Lawrence I. Conrad, Michael Neve, Vivian Nutton, Roy Porter, and Andrew Wear, 71–87. Cambridge: Cambridge University Press, 1995.
Nutton, Vivian. "Medicine in the Greek World, 800–50 BC." In *The Western Medical Tradition, 800 BC to AD 1800*, edited by Lawrence I. Conrad, Michael Neve, Vivian Nutton, Roy Porter, and Andrew Wear, 11–38. Cambridge: Cambridge University Press, 1995.
Nutton, Vivian. "Roman Medicine, 250 BC to AD 200." In *The Western Medical Tradition, 800 BC to AD 1800*, edited by Lawrence I. Conrad, Michael Neve, Vivian Nutton, Roy Porter, and Andrew Wear, 39–70. Cambridge: Cambridge University Press, 1995.
Oberhelman, Steven M. "Anatomical Votive Reliefs as Evidence for Specialization at Healing Sanctuaries in the Ancient Mediterranean World." *Athens Journal of Health* 1 (2014): 47–62.
Oberhelman, Steven M. "The Diagnostic Dream in Ancient Medical Theory and Practice." *Bulletin of the History of Medicine* 61 (1987): 47–60.
Ogden, Daniel. *Magic, Witchcraft, and Ghosts in the Greek and Roman Worlds: A Sourcebook*. Oxford: Oxford University Press, 2002.
Olson, Daniel V. A. "Competing Notions of Religious Competition and Conflict in Theories of Religious Economics." In *Sacred Markets, Sacred Canopies: Essays on Religious Markets and Religious Pluralism*, edited by Ted G. Jelen, 133–65. Lanham, MD: Rowman & Littlefield, 2002.
Otto, Bernd-Christian, and Michael Stausberg, ed. *Defining Magic: A Reader*. Sheffield: Equinox, 2013.
Panagiotidou, Olympia. "Asclepius: A Divine Doctor, A Popular Healer." In *Popular Medicine in Graeco-Roman Antiquity: Explorations*, edited by William V. Harris, 86–104. Leiden and Boston: Brill, 2016.
Panagiotidou, Olympia. "Religious Healing and the Asclepius Cult: A Case of Placebo Effects." *Open Theology* 2 (2016): 79–91.
Parker, Holt. "Women and Medicine." In *A Companion to Women in the Ancient World*, edited by Sharon L. James and Sheila Dillon, 107–24. New York: Blackwell, 2012.
Parker, Robert. *Miasma: Pollution and Purification in Early Greek Religion*. Oxford: Clarendon, 1983.
Parkin, Tim G. *Demography and Roman Society*. Baltimore: Johns Hopkins University Press, 1992.
Parkin, Tim G. "The Demography of Infancy and Early Childhood." In *Oxford Handbook of Childhood and Education in the Classical World*, edited by Judith Evans Grubb, Tim Parkin, and Roslynne Bell, 40–61. New York and Oxford: Oxford University Press, 2013.

Peacock, James. "Symbolic and Psychological Anthropology: The Case of Pentecostal Faith Healing." *Ethos* 12 (1984): 37–53.

Peerbolte, Bert Jan Lietaert. "Paul the Miracle Worker: Development and Background of Pauline Miracle Stories." In *Wonders Never Cease: The Purpose of Narrating Miracle Stories in the New Testament and its Religious Environment*, edited by Michael Labahn and Bert Jan Lietaert Peerbolte, 180–99. London: T. & T. Clark, 2006.

Penso, Giuseppe. *La médecine romaine: L'arte d'Esculape dans la Rome antique.* 2 vols. Paris: Les Éditions Roger Dacosta, 1984.

Petridou, Georgia. "Asclepius the Divine Healer, Asclepius the Divine Physician: Epiphanies as Diagnostic and Therapeutic Tools." In *Medicine and Healing in the Ancient Mediterranean World*, edited by Demetrios Michaelides, 291–301. Oxford: Oxbow Books, 2014.

Petridou, Georgia. "Healing Shrines." In *A Companion to Science, Technology, and Medicine in Ancient Greece and Rome*, edited by George L. Irby, 434–49. New York: Wiley-Blackwell, 2016.

Petsalis-Diomidis, Alexia. "The Body in Space: Visual Dynamics in Graeco-Roman Healing Pilgrimage." In *Pilgrimage in Graeco-Roman & Early Christian Antiquity: Seeing the Gods*, edited by Jas Elsner and Ian Rutherford, 183–218. Oxford: Oxford University Press, 2005.

Pilch, John J. *Healing in the New Testament: Insights from Medical and Mediterranean Anthropology.* Minneapolis: Fortress, 2000.

Pilkington, Nathan. "Growing Up Roman: Infant Mortality and Reproductive Development." *Journal of Interdisciplinary History* 44 (2013): 1–36.

Pollard, Elizabeth Ann. "Charms, Spells, Greece and Rome." In *The Encyclopedia of Ancient History*, edited by Roger S. Bagnall, Kai Brodersen, Craige B. Champion, Andrew Erskine, and Sabine R. Huebner, 1444. Malden, MA: Wiley-Blackwell, 2013.

Prioreschi, Plinio. *Greek Medicine.* Vol. 2 of *A History of Medicine.* Lewiston, NY: Edwin Mellen Press, 1994.

Prioreschi, Plinio. *Roman Medicine.* Vol. 3 in *A History of Medicine.* Omaha: Horatius Press, 1998.

Raphals, Lisa. "Divination and Medicine in China and Greece: A Comparative Perspective on the Baoshan Illness Divinations." *East Asian Science, Technology, and Medicine* 24 (2005): 78–103.

Remus, Harold. *Jesus as Healer.* Cambridge: Cambridge University Press, 1997.

Retief, Francois, and Louise P. Cilliers. "The Influence of Christianity on Medicine from Graeco-Roman Times up to the Renaissance." *ActT* 26 (2006): 259–77.

Retief, Francois P., and Louise Cilliers. "Medical Dreams in Graeco-Roman Times." *South African Medical Journal* 95 (2005): 841–4.

Retief, François P., and Louise Cilliers. "Tumours and Cancers in Graeco-Roman Times." In *Health and Healing: Disease and Death in the Graeco-Roman World*, 200–21. Bloemfontaine: Publications Office of the University of the Free State, 2005.

Ricks, Stephen D. "The Magician as Outsider in the Hebrew Bible and the New Testament." In *Ancient Magic and Ritual Power*, edited by Marvin Meyer and Paul Mirecki, 131–43. Leiden and New York: Brill, 1995.

Riethmüller, Jürgen W. *Asklepios: Heiligtümer und Kulte.* 2 vols. Heidelberg: Verlag Archäologie und Geschichte, 2005.

Risse, Guenter B. "Asclepius at Epidaurus: The Divine Power of Healing Dreams." Unpublished paper, last modified March 10, 2015. https://www.researchgate.net/publication/273440826_Asclepius_at_Epidaurus_The_Divine_Power_of_Healing.

Rives, James B. "*Magus* and its Cognates in Classical Latin." In *Magical Practice in the Latin West*, edited by R. L. Gordon and F. Marco Simón, 53–77. Leiden: Brill, 2010.
Rives, James B. *Religion in the Roman Empire*. Malden, Mass.: Blackwell, 2007.
Rostad, Aslak. "Confession or Reconciliation: The Narrative Structure of the Lydian and Phrygian Confession Inscriptions." *Symbolae Osloenses* 77 (2002): 145–64.
Russell, Donald A., Michael Trapp, and Heinz-Günther Nesselrath, ed. *In Praise of Asclepius: Aelius Aristides, Selected Prose Hymns*. Tübingen: Morh Siebeck, 2016.
Rüttimann, René Josef. "Asclepius and Jesus: The Form, Character and Status of the Asclepius Cult in the Second Century CE and its Influence on Early Christianity". Th.D, diss., Harvard Divinity School, 1986.
Sanchez, Magali de Haro. "Between Magic and Medicine: The Iatromagical Formularies and Medical Receptaries on Papyri Compared." *ZPE* 195 (2015): 179–89.
Sanzo, Joseph E. "Early Christianity." In *Guide to the Study of Ancient Magic*, edited by David Frankfurter, 198–239. Leiden and Boston: Brill, 2019.
Scarborough, John. "Adaptation of Folk Medicines in the Formal 'Materia Medica' of Classical Antiquity." *Pharmacy in History* 55 (2013): 55–63.
Scarborough, John. "Drugs and Drug Lore in the Time of Theophrastus: Magic, Botany, Philosophy and the Rootcutters." *Acta Classica* 49 (2006): 1–29.
Scarborough, John. "The Pharmacology of Sacred Plants, Herbs, and Roots." In *Magika Hiera: Ancient Greek Religion and Magic*, edited by Christopher A. Faraone and Dirk Obbink, 138–74. New York and Oxford: Oxford University Press, 1991.
Scarborough, John. *Roman Medicine*. Ithaca, NY: Cornell University Press, 1969.
Scarborough, John. "Romans and Physicians." *The Classical Journal* 65 (1970): 296–306.
Scarborough, John. "Theophrastus on Herbals and Herbal Remedies." *Journal of the History of Biology* 11 (1978): 353–85.
Schäfer, Peter. "Magic and Religion in Ancient Judaism." In *Envisioning Magic: A Princeton Seminar and Symposium*, edited by Peter Schäfer and Hans J. Kippenberg, 19–43. Leiden: Brill, 1997.
Scheid, John. *An Introduction to Roman Religion*. Translated by Janet Lloyd. Bloomington: University of Indiana Press, 2003.
Scheidel, Walter. "Disease and Death in the Ancient City of Rome." *Princeton/Stanford Working Papers in Classics* (2009): 1–14.
Schreiber, Stefan. *Paulus also Wundertäter: Redakstiongeschichtliche Untersuchungen zur Apostelgeschichte und den authentischen Paulusbriefen*. Berlin and New York: Walter de Gruyter, 1996.
Scobie, Alex. "Slums, Sanitation, and Mortality in the Roman World." *Clio* 68 (1986): 399–43.
Shaily, Shashikant Patel. "Magical Practices and Discourses of Magic in Early Christian Traditions: Jesus, Peter, and Paul." PhD diss., University of North Carolina, 2017. https://cdr.lib.unc.edu/downloads/bc386k15p?locale=en.
Simboli, Cesidio R. "Disease-Spirits and Divine Cures among the Greeks and Romans." PhD diss., Columbia University, 1921. https://archive.org/details/diseasespiritsa00simbgoog.
Skinner, Stephen. "Refining the Definition of Amulet, Phylactery, Charm, Lamen and Talisman as They Appear in the PGM and the Grimoires." Unpublished paper accessed September 29, 2020, https://www.academia.edu/34736473367.
Smith, Jonathan Z. "Trading Places." In *Ancient Magic and Ritual Power*, edited by Marvin Meyer and Paul Mirecki, 13–27. Leiden and New York: Brill, 1995.
Smith, Morton. *Jesus the Magician*. New York: Harper & Row, 1978.
Spampinato, Gaetano. "The Use of the Figure and the Myth of Asclepius in the Greek Anti-pagan Controversy." *Electra* 5 (2020): 79–101.

Stafford, Emma. "Cocks to Asklepios: Sacrificial Practice and Healing Cult." In *Le sacrifice antique: Vestiges, procédures et strategies*, edited by Véronique Mehl and Pierre Brule, 205–21. Rennes: Presses Universitaire de Rennes, 2008.
Stanley, Christopher D. *A Bull for Pluto*. Buffalo, NY: Amelia Books, 2020.
Stanley, Christopher D. *A Rooster for Asklepios*. Buffalo, NY: Amelia Books, 2020.
Stanley, Christopher D. "Paul and Asklepios: The Greco-Roman Quest for Healing and the Mission of Paul." *JSNT* 42 (2019): 1–31.
Stannard, Jerry. "Medicinal Plants and Folk Remedies in Pliny, 'Historia Naturalis.'" *History and Philosophy of the Life Sciences* 4 (1982): 3–23.
Stark, Rodney, and Roger Finke. *Acts of Faith: Explaining the Human Side of Religion*. Berkeley: University of California Press, 2000.
Stern, Karen B. "Harnessing the Sacred: Hidden Writing and 'Private' Spaces in Levantine Synagogues." In *Inscriptions in the Private Sphere in the Greco-Roman World*, edited by Rebecca Benefiel and Peter Keegan, 213–47. Leiden: Brill, 2015.
Stolz, Jörg. "All Things Are Possible": Towards a Sociological Explanation of Pentecostal Miracles and Healings." *Sociology of Religion* 72 (2011): 456–82.
Stratton, Kimberly B. "Magic Discourse in the Ancient World." In *Defining Magic: A Reader*, edited by Bernd-Christian Otto and Michael Stausberg, 243–54. Sheffield: Equinox, 2013.
Styers, Randall. "Magic and the Play of Power." In *Defining Magic: A Reader*, edited by Bernd-Christian Otto and Michael Stausberg, 255–62. Sheffield: Equinox, 2013.
Temkin, Owsei. *Hippocrates in a World of Pagans and Christians*. Baltimore, MD: Johns Hopkins University Press, 1991.
Thomassen, Einar. "Is Magic a Subclass of Ritual?" In *The World of Ancient Magic: Papers from the First International Samson Eitrem Seminar at the Norwegian Institute at Athens 4–8 May 1997*, edited by David R. Jordan, Hugo Montgomery, and Einar Thomassen, 55–66. Bergen: Paul Astroms, 1999.
Thumiger, Chiara. "The Early Greek Vocabulary of Insanity." In *Mental Disorders in the Classical World*, edited by William V. Harris, 62–95. Leiden and Boston: Brill, 2013.
Totelin, Laurence M. V. *Hippocratic Recipes: Oral and Written Transmission of Pharmacological Knowledge in Fifth- and Fourth-Century Greece*. Leiden: Brill, 2008.
Totelin, Laurence M. V. "*Pharmakopōlai*: A Re-Evaluation of the Sources." In *Popular Medicine in Graeco-Roman Antiquity: Explorations*, edited by William V. Harris, 65–85. Leiden and Boston: Brill, 2016.
Trachtenberg, Joshua. *Jewish Magic and Superstition: A Study in Folk Religion*. New York: Behrman's Jewish Book House, 1939. Reprint, New York: Atheneum, 1979.
Twelftree, Graham H. "Healing, Illness." In *Dictionary of Paul and His Letters*, edited by Gerald F. Hawthorne, Ralph P. Martin, and Daniel G. Reid, 378–81. Downers Grove, IL: InterVarsity Press, 1993.
Twelftree, Graham H. *Jesus the Exorcist: A Contribution to the Study of the Historical Jesus*. Peabody, MA: Hendrickson, 1993.
Twelftree, Graham H. *Paul and the Miraculous: A Historical Reconstruction*. Grand Rapids, MI: Baker, 2013.
Twelftree, Graham H. "Signs, Wonders, Miracles." In *Dictionary of Paul and His Letters*, edited by Gerald F. Hawthorne, Ralph P. Martin, and Daniel G. Reid, 875–7. Downers Grove, IL: InterVarsity Press, 1993.
Underwood, Norman. "Medicine, Money, and Christian Rhetoric: The Socio-Economic Dimensions of Healthcare in Late Antiquity." *Studies in Late Antiquity* 2 (2018): 342–84.

Versnel, H. S. "The Poetics of the Magical Charm: An Essay in the Power of Words." In *Ancient Magic and Ritual Power*, edited by Marvin Meyer and Paul Mirecki, 105–58. Leiden and New York: Brill, 1995.
Vlahogiannis, Nicholas. "'Curing' Disability." In *Health in Antiquity*, edited by Helen King, 180–91. London and New York: Routledge, 2005.
Wainwright, Elaine M. *Women Healing/Healing Women: The Genderization of Healing in Early Christianity*. London: Equinox: 2006.
Wallace, Ella Faye. "The Sorcerer's Pharmacy." PhD diss., Rutgers University, 2018. https://rucore.libraries.rutgers.edu/rutgers-lib/59256/PDF/1/play/
Watson, Lindsay C., ed. *Magic in Greece and Rome*. London and New York: Bloomsbury, 2019.
Watson, Patricia. "Animals in Magic." In *Magic in Greece and Rome*, edited by Lindsay C. Watson, 127–65. London and New York: Bloomsbury, 2019.
Wells, Louise. *The Greek Language of Healing from Homer to New Testament Times*. Berlin and New York: Walter de Gruyter, 1998.
Wendt, Heidi. *At the Temple Gates: The Religion of Freelance Experts in the Roman Empire*. Oxford: Oxford University Press, 2016.
Wickkeiser, Bronwen L. "The Appeal of Asklepios and the Politics of Healing in the Greco-Roman World." PhD diss., University of Texas, 2003. https://repositories.lib.utexas.edu/bitstream/handle/2152/12602/wickkhiserbl032.pdf?sequence=2&isAllowed=y
Williams, Guy. *The Spirit World in the Letters of Paul the Apostle*. Göttingen: Vandenhoeck & Ruprecht, 2009.
Yamauchi, Edwin. "Magic in the Biblical World." *Tyndale Bulletin* 34 (1983): 169–200.
Zucconi, Laura M. *Ancient Medicine: From Mesopotamia to Rome*. Grand Rapids, MI: William B. Eerdmans, 2019.

Index of Ancient Authors

Aelian 102
Aelius Aristides 100 n.41, 103, 111 n.15, 122, 128 n.10, 206 n.25
Apuleius 66 n.54
Aretaeus of Cappadocia 48, 118
Aristotle 57, 175
Arnobius 171, 172
Artemidorus 46 n.64, 71, 72, 78, 102
Asklepiades 110 n.12, 111
Athanasius 171, 177 n.31
Augustine 177–9, 183, 184
Aulus Cornelius Celsus 23 n.29, 42, 48–9, 109 n.10, 117, 118

Basil of Caesarea 179, 183, 184

Cato the Elder 31 n.12, 36–7, 49 n.81
Celsus 147, 172, 175, 176
Clement of Alexandria 57 n.20, 180, 183, 186, 210
Columella 39, 42 n.56

Dioscorides 38–40, 42–3, 46 n.69, 48, 74 n.94, 117, 118

Eusebius 177–8, 179 n.38, 181 n.49

Galen 42, 48, 69–70, 102, 107 n.5, 109 n.10, 118–21, 129 n.14, 170, 193
Gregory of Nyssa 179

Herodotus 57, 58, 70 n.72
Herophilos 30 n.10, 110 n.12, 120
Hippocrates 15 n.2, 16, 17 n.10, 18, 21 n.21, 33, 61–3, 69, 106–7, 110, 115, 129, 161, 183
Hippolytus of Rome 174–5

Irenaeus 158, 178

John Chrysostom 177–8, 180, 183
Josephus 143, 149–50, 153–4, 193, 210 n.30

Justin Martyr 158, 174, 176 n.29
Juvenal 69 n.69, 70, 71 n.81

Lucian of Samosata 77 n.106, 92 n.14, 147

Macarius 184
Menander 90–1, 102

Origen 147–8, 158, 171, 172, 175–6, 178, 183–4

Pausanius 101 n.48, 103, 129 n.17
Philo 146, 151, 160–1
Philostratus 47 n.73, 77 n.106, 92 n.14, 102
Plato 22 n.25, 35–6, 58–63, 65–6, 69, 78, 121–2
Plautus 70, 71, 78, 102
Pliny the Elder 30–1, 37–43, 48, 49, 63 n.43, 64–6, 74–5, 77–84, 113 n.19, 117, 147, 156, 168 n.4, 211
Polybius 69
Posidonius 147
Pythagoras 121

Rufus of Ephesus 119, 120 n.46

Scribonius Largus 40, 48, 75, 117, 118
Soranus of Ephesus 37, 48, 106, 114, 120 n.45
Strabo 99 n.37, 147

Tatian 174 n.23, 175, 184–5
Tertullian 171, 175, 178, 185, 186
Theophrastus 38, 73, 90, 120
Thucydides 69

Varro 17 n.7, 37 n.27, 108 n.8

Xenocrates of Aphrodisias 121
Xenophon 57

Subject Index

amulets   24–5, 41–3, 78, 80–3, 93–4
   Christian use   85–6, 147–8, 171, 174–5, 177–80, 187, 194
   Jewish use   153–8, 193
   medical use   117–18, 124, 127
Asklepios   32, 45, 46, 94, 98–103
   Christians and   3 n.13, 50, 105, 166, 167, 171–2, 176 n.27, 187, 207, 233, 235
   healing centers   95, 100–3
   Jews and   144–6, 161, 194
   Paul and   189, 194, 198, 207–9, 233–4
   physicians and   8, 33, 128–30, 182
   temples   8, 77, 95, 98

chants, *see* incantations
charismata   3, 5, 6, 8, 29, 189–90, 197, 205 n.21, 213, 217 n.15, 218, 226
charms, *see* incantations

daimones/demons   91–2, 103, 146, 149, 184, 188, 190, 194, 209 n.27, 233
   causing sickness   44, 47, 61, 88 n.4, 137, 147, 149, 173, 211
   exorcism   47, 68, 93–4, 142, 147, 152–4, 158, 168–9, 173, 175–6, 178, 196, 203–4, 215 n.6, 216, 229
dietary treatments   24, 32, 33, 101, 108–9, 115–16, 123–4, 128, 160, 183, 189
disabilities   3 n.18, 10, 22, 24, 200–2, 205, 215–16, 220
divination   6, 45–6, 58–60, 67–72, 77, 85, 95–6, 119–21, 139, 151, 152, 174–5, 177–9, 209
diviners, *see* divination
dream interpretation   45–6, 70–2, 85, 97, 100–5, 119–20, 127–9, 144–5, 147, 171, 174–5, 178, 180, 209
drug-sellers   60, 67, 72–3, 75–6, 85, 117

evil eye   11, 76 n.103, 203, 204
exorcism, *see daimones*/demons

freelance religious experts   5–6, 59, 69–72, 84–5, 89–94, 104, 139, 228–9, 231

gems and rings   41–2, 57–8, 79, 81–2, 93–4, 179–80, 209
gifts of healing, *see charismata*

healing and health care, definitions of   4 n.23, 19–20, 26–34, 125
Hippocratic Corpus   16–17, 23 n.29, 36, 42, 48 n.78, 61, 69 n.68, 72, 109, 110, 113 n.19, 114, 117, 118 n.38, 119–22, 129–30
home remedies   11, 26–51, 67, 208
humoral theory   88, 107–9, 115–16, 119 n.43, 120, 183
Hygieia   94, 99, 129, 145, 167

incantations   32, 34–8, 40, 41, 46, 56 n.18, 57–60, 64–6, 71, 74–83, 90–4, 121–2, 126
   use by Christians   10, 85–6, 174–80, 187, 189–90, 194, 198, 203, 207–8, 210, 216, 234
   use by Jews   147, 149–51, 153, 157–8, 193

Judean, use of the term   12 n.54, 135 n.1

literacy/illiteracy, effects   33, 37 n.28, 43, 46, 48, 58, 59, 76–8, 81, 85, 104, 109, 111, 114, 125, 126, 136, 166, 171

mageia/magia, *see* magic and magicians
magi, *see* magic and magicians

252 Subject Index

magic and magicians 34–43, 49, 56–86, 91, 126–8
   Christians and 50, 166, 168, 172–81, 187, 205
   definitions 26, 32, 35, 52–6, 59 n.29, 65–7
   Jews and 138–40, 142, 144, 147–59, 162, 164
   Magi 43 n.58, 49, 56–7, 79–81, 147
   Paul and 10–11, 85, 193–4, 203–4, 207, 209–11
   philosophers and 58–64
   physicians and 30, 33, 61–2, 117–22, 124, 127, 128
   training 30, 58, 78
   women and 32, 57, 67, 69 n.70, 71, 78, 84–5, 90–3, 139, 150 n.44, 151, 177
magical papyri 36, 47 n.74, 71, 74–5, 78–83, 92–3, 154 n.59, 158, 177 n.32, 209 n.27
medical anthropology 4, 18–20, 27–9, 67 n.57, 76 n.103, 87, 169 n.7, 200 n.10, 202 n.15, 204, 223
medical tourism 8, 23 n.28, 99–100
medicine
   Christians and 168 n.2, 170, 181–7
   definitions 33, 66–7, 124, 130–1
   Jews and 140–2, 159–64
   Paul and 124, 193–5, 208
   schools 30 n.10, 110–13, 115–23, 125
midwives 10, 30, 36–7, 50, 57, 114–15, 121, 130, 140
miracles
   Asklepios and 8, 22 n.24, 32, 98, 101, 128
   and magic 54, 66, 77
   Christians and 29, 167–8, 170–1, 175, 185–7, 233
   Jews and 137–8, 141–2, 148–9, 155
   modern explanations 8, 12, 222–7
   Paul and 3–6, 9, 190, 193, 195–7, 200–1, 206–7, 213–21, 230
   physicians and 107, 129
   role in Christian evangelism 1–2, 4, 9, 213–21, 228–30, 233

Paul
   Asklepios and 189, 194, 198, 207–9, 233–4
   and magical healing 10–11, 85, 193–4, 203–4, 207, 209–11
   and medical healing 124, 193–5, 208
   and miracles 3–6, 9, 190, 193, 195–7, 200–1, 206–7, 213–21, 230
   possible disability 3 n.18, 10, 200–2, 215–16, 220
   and religious healing 8, 10–11, 85, 189, 193–6, 198, 201, 205, 208
   and suffering 3, 7, 124, 191–2, 195–7, 199–202, 205, 209 n.27, 218
PGM, see magical papyri
pharmacology 22 n.25, 38–9, 42–3, 47–8, 72–6, 85, 116–18, 169, 210
pharmakopolai, see drug-sellers
physicians 18, 22–5, 30–1, 42, 70, 77, 88, 97, 101, 106–31, 140–2, 159–63, 181–5, 187
   and magical healing 30, 33, 61–2, 117–22, 124, 127, 128, 182
   methods 35–6, 42, 46–8, 61, 108–11, 115–23
   and religious healing 106–7, 110, 112, 122, 124, 127–9, 182
   social location 112–15
   training 30, 111–12
   women 114–15
placebo effect 100 n.40, 222–7, 235
prayer and healing 3, 4, 8, 24, 29, 32, 34, 36, 40, 44–5, 47, 72, 74, 93, 95–8, 104, 122, 130, 137–8, 141–3, 153, 159, 163, 168, 170, 184, 186–7, 195, 205, 208, 217, 225–6, 233
purification rituals 46–7, 57–8, 61–2, 64, 67–9, 74, 89–91, 93, 97–8, 138, 151, 164, 174, 179, 211

rabbis
   Asklepios and 144 n.23, 145–7
   and magical healing 148, 155–9, 164, 179, 193, 204
   and medical healing 162–3
   and religious healing 193, 194
religious healing 8, 10–11, 26–7, 32–3, 44–7, 87–105, 126–7, 130–1, 222–7, 229–30
   Christians and 170–2, 182–4, 186–7, 233
   Jews and 137–8, 141–7, 162, 164–5

Paul and   8, 10–11, 85, 189, 193–6, 198, 201, 205, 208, 228–30, 233–4
physicians and   106–7, 110, 112, 122, 124, 127–9
religious markets theory   231–4
rhizotomists, *see* root-cutters
root-cutters   67–8, 72–6, 85, 117, 150, 183–4, 194

sacrifices and offerings   24, 26, 32, 45, 58–9, 65–6, 74, 95–8, 100, 104, 122, 126, 129–30, 139, 142, 208
sickness in Antiquity

causes   15–17, 23–5, 38, 44, 46–7, 68, 88–9, 91–3, 95–7, 107–11, 120–1, 129, 136–7, 147, 170
common forms   18–22
definitions   18–20
signs and wonders   3–6, 9, 12, 189–90, 192, 193, 195–7, 212–18, 221, 230, 233, 235
sorcerers   6, 8, 59 n.28, 60, 76–86, 138–9, 148–50, 152, 155–6, 159, 164, 174, 178, 179, 203
spells, *see* incantations

votive offerings   20, 96–8, 100–1, 103, 129, 145

www.ingramcontent.com/pod-product-compliance
Lightning Source LLC
Chambersburg PA
CBHW062134300426
44115CB00012BA/1924